# INTERNAL MEDICINE

# Mastering The Boards And Clinical Examinations

# HEPATOBILIARY AND PANCREATIC DISEASES

---

## A. B. R. Thomson

www.giandhepatology.com

athoms47@uwo.ca

i

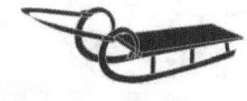

# INTERNAL MEDICINE

# Mastering the Boards and Clinical Examinations

# HEPATOBILIARY AND PANCREATIC DISEASES

## This book compliments

## Mastering the Boards and Clinical Examinations
## GASTROENTEROLOGY

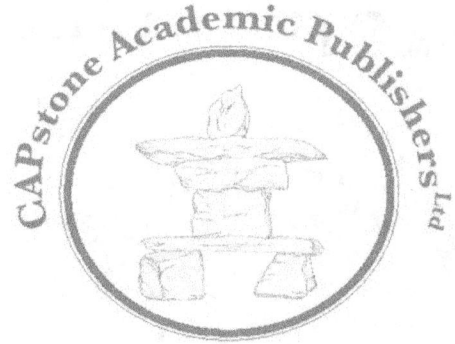

*CAPstone (Canadian Academic Publishers Ltd) is a not-for-profit company dedicated to the use of the power of education for the betterment of all persons everywhere.*

*"For the Democratization of Knowledge"*

© *A.B.R. Thomson*

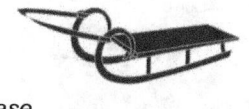

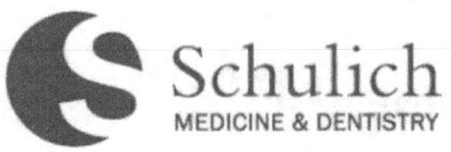
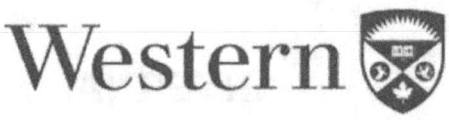

# THE WESTERN WAY

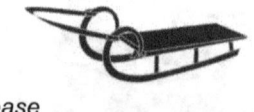

## ARE YOU PREPARING FOR EXAMS IN GENERAL INTERNAL MEDICINE OR IN GASTROENTEROLOGY AND HEPATOLOGY?

See the full range of examination preparation and review publications from CAPstone on Amazon.com

For no cost viewing, please consult: www. giandhepatology.com

### Gastroenterology and Hepatology

Endoscopy and Diagnostic Imaging Part I (ISBN: 978-1477400579)

Endoscopy and Diagnostic Imaging Part II (ISBN: 978-1477400654)

First Principles of Gastroenterology and Hepatology in Adults and Children – Volume I - Gastroenterology, 7th edition (ISBN: 978-1494345624)

First Principles of Gastroenterology and Hepatology in Adults and Children - Volume II - Hepatology and Paediatrics, 7th edition (ISBN: 978-1494345501)

Guideline – Based Therapy in Gastroenterology (ISBN: 978-1515078623)

Guideline – Based Therapy in Hepatology (ISBN: 978-1502928078)

Mastering The Boards and Clinical Examination –Gastroenterology (ISBN: 978-1515386636)

Medical Mini Review Series in Gastroenterology and Hepatology: Efficient Refresher for the Busy Clinical Gastroenterologist (ISBN: 978-1502472199)

Practice Review in Gastroenterology, 3rd edition (ISBN: 978-1500855321)

Scientific Basis for Clinical Practice in Gastroenterology and Hepatology (ISBN: 978-1475226645)

The Physiology and Pathophysiology of Gastrointestinal and Hepatopancreaticobiliary Disorders (ISBN: 978-1500298265)

### General Internal Medicine

Achieving Excellence in the OSCE. Part I. Cardiology to Nephrology (ISBN: 978-1475283037)

Achieving Excellence in the OSCE. Part II. Neurology to Rheumatology (ISBN: 978-1475276978)

Bits and Bytes for Rounds in Internal Medicine (ISBN: 978-1478295365)

Mastering The Boards and Clinical Examinations – Cardiology (ISBN: 978-1516842155)

Mastering The Boards and Clinical Examinations In Internal Medicine - Hematology, Nephrology, Infectious Diseases (ISBN: 978-1516961795)

Mastering The Boards and Clinical Examinations In Internal Medicine - Rheumatology and Endocrinology (ISBN: 978-1516959792)

Mastering the Boards and Clinical Examinations. Neurology (ISBN: 978-1517268411)

v

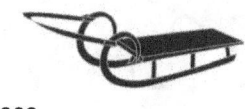

*MASTERING THE BOARDS*
*Hepatology & Pancreaticobiliary Disease*

A.B.R. Thomson

## DISCLAIMER

The primary purpose of this publication is education. The author, editor and publisher acknowledge that the development of new material opens to way for possible errors – what is correct today might not be the standard of care tomorrow. Readers are advised to ensure that the doses of drugs which they use are in compliance with their country's product information, and that the use of any therapeutic agent, be it a pharmaceutical or a technology, should be guided by local guidelines. There is often a wide diversity of professional opinion, and guidelines from one country are not always congruent with another.

The author, editor and publisher do not guarantee the safety, reliability, accuracy, completeness or usefulness of this material.

They disclaim any and all liability for damage and claims that may result from the use of information, publications, technologies, products, and for series provided in this publication.

We have made every attempt to trace the holders of copyright for material reproduced in this book. If by some oversight we have omitted a copyright holder, please contact us.

Thank you

A. B. R. Thomson

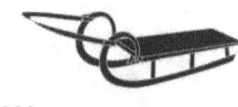

# TABLE OF CONTENTS

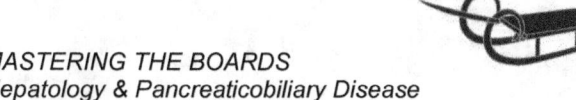

*MASTERING THE BOARDS*
*Hepatology & Pancreaticobiliary Disease*

A.B.R. Thomson

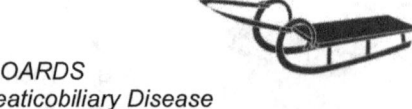

*MASTERING THE BOARDS*
*Hepatology & Pancreaticobiliary Disease*

A.B.R. Thomson

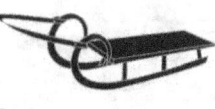

x

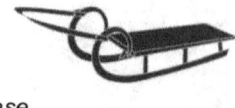

Available online at www.giandhepatology.com

# GI PRACTICE REVIEW AND THE CANMED OBJECTIVES

## Medical Expert
The discussion of complex cases provides the participants with an opportunity to comment on additional focused history and physical examination. They would provide a complete and organized assessment. Participants are encouraged to identify key features, and they develop an approach to problem-solving.

The case discussions, as well as the discussion of cases around a diagnostic imaging, pathological or endoscopic base provides the means for the candidate to establish an appropriate management plan based on the best available evidence to clinical practice. Throughout, an attempt is made to develop strategies for diagnosis and development of clinical reasoning skills.

## Communicator
The participants demonstrate their ability to communicate their knowledge, clinical findings, and management plan in a respectful, concise and interactive manner. When the participants play the role of examiners, they demonstrate their ability to listen actively and effectively, to ask questions in an open-ended manner, and to provide constructive, helpful feedback in a professional and non-intimidating manner.

## Collaborator
The participants use the "you have a green consult card" technique of answering questions as fast as they are able, and then to interact with another health professional participant to move forward the discussion and problem solving. This helps the participants to build upon what they have already learned about the importance of collegial interaction.

## Manager
The participants are provided with assignments in advance of the three day GI Practice Review. There is much work for them to complete before as well as afterwards, so they learn to manage their time effectively, and to complete the assigned tasks proficiently and on time. They learn to work in teams to achieve answers from small group participation, and then to share this with other small group participants through effective delegation of work. Some of the material they must access demands that they use information technology effectively to access information that will help to facilitate the delineation of adequately broad differential diagnoses, as well as rational and cost effective management plans.

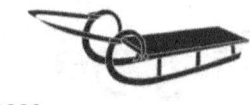

## Health Advocate
In the answering of the questions and case discussions, the participants are required to consider the risks, benefits, and costs and impacts of investigations and therapeutic alliances upon the patient and their loved ones.

## Scholar
By committing to the pre and post-study requirements, plus the intense three day active learning GI Practice Review with colleagues is a demonstration of commitment to personal education. Through the interactive nature of the discussions and the use of the "green consult card", they reinforce their previous learning of the importance of collaborating and helping one another to learn.

## Professional
The participants are coached how to interact verbally in a professional setting, being straightforward, clear and helpful. They learn to be honest when they cannot answer questions, make a diagnosis, or advance a management plan. They learn how to deal with aggressive or demotivated colleagues, how to deal with knowledge deficits, how to speculate on a missing knowledge byte by using first principals and deductive reasoning. In a safe and supportive setting they learn to seek and accept advice, to acknowledge awareness of personal limitations, and to give and take $360^0$ feedback.

## Knowledge
The basic science aspects of gastroenterology are considered in adequate detail to understand the mechanisms of disease, and the basis of investigations and treatment. In this way, the participants respect the importance of an adequate foundation in basic sciences, the basics of the design of clinical research studies to provide an evidence-based approach, the relevance of their management plans being patient-focused, and the need to add "compassionate" to the Three C's of Medical Practice: competent, caring and compassionate.

-----------------------

"They may forget what you said, but they will never forget how you made them feel."

Carl W. Buechner, on teaching.

"With competence, care for the patient. With compassion, care about the person."
Alan B. R. Thomson, on being a physician.

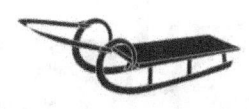

# PROLOGUE

Like any good story, there is no real beginning or ending, just an in-between glimpse of the passing of time, a peek into a reality of people's minds, thoughts, feelings, and beliefs. The truth as I know it has a personal perspective which drifts into the soul of creation. When does life begin, when does an idea become conceived, when do we see love or touch reality? A caring, supportive, safe, and stimulating environment creates the holding blanket, waiting for the energy and passion of those who dream, invent, create – disrupt the accepted, challenge the conventional, ask the questions with forbidden answers. Be a child of the 60's. Just as each of us is a speck of dust in the greater humanity, the metamorphosis of the idea is but a single sparkle in the limitlessness of the Divine Intelligence. We are the ideas, and they are us. No one of us is truly the only parent of the idea, for in each of us is bestowed the intertwined circle of the external beginning and the end....

....during a visit to the Division of Gastroenterology at the University of Ottawa several years ago, the trainees remarked how useful it would be to have more than two hours of learning exchange, a highly interactive tutorial with concepts, problem solving, collegial discussion, the fun and joys of discovery and successes. Ms. Jane Upshall of BYK Canada (Atlanta, Nycomed), who had sponsored two of these visiting Professorships, encouraged the possibility of the development of a longer program. Her successor, Lynne Jamme, supported the initial three day educational event for the trainees enrolled in the GI training program at the University of Ottawa. With her entrepreneurial forsight, wisdom, and enthusiasm, the idea began. Lynne's commitment to an event which benefited many of the future clinicians, who will care for ourselves and our loved ones, took hold. Then, thanks to the GI program directors in Ottawa and the University of Western Ontario, Nav Saloojee and Jamie Gregor, more trainees were exposed, future GI fellows talked with other trainees, and a grassroots initiative began. Had it not been for Nav and Jamie's willingness to take a risk on something new, had they not believed in me, then there would have been no further outreach. Thank you, Lynne, Nav, and Jamie. You were there at the beginning. I needed you.

By 2008, all but one GI program in the country gave their trainees time off work to participate in the three-day event, GI Practice Review (GI-PR). The course is 90% unsponsored, and is gratis to the participants, (except for the cost of their enthusiastic participation!) I am happy to give back to the subspecialty that gave me so much for 33 years. I hope GI-PR is helpful to all trainees. I know that from these future leaders there will arise those who will continue to dedicate and donate their time, energy, and ability to the betterment of those who contribute to the continued improvement of our medical profession. The clinicians, the teachers, the researchers.

In the short span of six years, more than 250 fellows, coming from all the 14 training programs in Canada, have participated in the small group sessions in the GI practice review. I thank the training program directors who have supported GI-PR. Special appreciation as well to their many staff physicians who worked without their trainees for the three days of each program.

The idea for the electronic and hard copy summary of the "list of facts" came from the trainees who wished for an aide memoir. But the GI-PR is about more than lists and facts - it is about problem formulation, case discussions, review of endoscopy, histopathology, motility, diagnostic imaging. It is about having fun working together to learn. The subterfuge to gain interest in the basic sciences is the use of clinical scenarios to show the way to the importance of first principles. While the lists are here, the experience is in the performance.

The child will grow, the images will expand, the learning of all aspects of our craft will develop and flourish amongst persons of good will. Examinations will become second nature, as each clinical encounter, each person, each patient, becomes our test, the determination of clinical competence, of caring, of compassion. May these three C's become part of each of our live's narrative. And from this start comes Capstone Academic Publishing, an innovation for the highest quality and value in educational material, made available at cost, speaking in tongues, in the languages of many cultures, with the dialect of the true North strong and free, so that knowledge will be free at last.

Outstanding medical practice and true dedication to those from whom we receive both a privilege and pleasure of care, comes from much more than the GI-PR can give you, much more than Q & As, descriptions of diagnostic imaging or endoscopy stills or videos, histopathology or motility. True, we need all of these to jump over a very high bar. But to be a truly outstanding physician, you need to care for and care about people, and you must respect the dignity and rights of all others. You must strike a balance between love and justice, and you place your family and friends at the top of your wish-list of lifetime achievements.

For the skeptics who ask "What do you want from me?" I simply say "You are the future; I trust that in time you too will help young people to be the best they can be."

May good luck, good health, modesty, peace, and understanding be with you always. Through medicine, all persons of the world may come to share caring, respect, dignity, and justice.

Sincerely,

Alan Thomson

Emeritus Distinguished University Professor, U of A

Adjunct Professor, Western University

XV

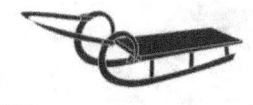

## DEDICATION

Dedicated to Jeannette Rita Cécile Mineault

My life began when I met you:

Your wit, your charm, your laughter,

Your love for children, your caring, your common sense.

As always, all ways, thank you for saying I do.

– – – – – – – – – –

For the parents who gave us life.

For the children and grandchildren who give us hope.

For the teachers who gave us knowledge.

For the partners who give us confidence, encouragement and meaning.

## ACKNOWLEDGEMENTS

Patience and patients go hand in hand. So also does the interlocking of young and old, love and justice, equality and fairness. No author can have thoughts transformed into words, no teacher can make ideas become behavior and wisdom and art, without those special people who turn our minds to the practical – of getting the job done!

Thank you, Naiyana and Duen, for translating those scribbles (called my handwriting), into the still magical legibility of the electronic age. Sarah, thank you for your hard work and creativity.

My most sincere and heartfelt thanks go to the excellent persons at JP Consulting, and CapStone Academic Publishers. Jessica, you are brilliant, efficient, dedicated, and caring. Thank you most sincerely.

When Rebecca, Maxwell, Megan Grace, Henry, Felix, Toby, Grady, and Jasper ask about their Grandad, I will depend on James and Anne, Matthew and Allison, Jessica and Matt, and Benjamin to be understanding, generous, kind and forgiving. For what I was trying to say and to do was to make my professional life focused on the four C's and an "H"; competence, caring, compassion, and composure, as well as humour – and to make my very private personal life dedicated to family – to you all.

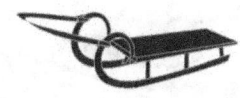

*MASTERING THE BOARDS*
*Hepatology & Pancreaticobiliary Disease*

A.B.R. Thomson

# LIVER

# TABLE OF CONTENTS

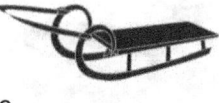

*MASTERING THE BOARDS*
*Hepatology & Pancreaticobiliary Disease*

A.B.R. Thomson

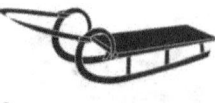

*MASTERING THE BOARDS*                         A.B.R. Thomson
*Hepatology & Pancreaticobiliary Disease*

4

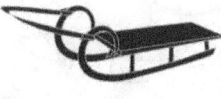

# HISTOLOGY

## Hepatocytes

- Polygonal cells, 20 to 30 μm in diameter
- Organized into "plates" of cells, 1-2 hepatocytes thick
- Sinusoidal membrane
    - Dynamic polarization due to exo-/endocytosis
    - Endocytosis is non-selective, or selective by way of RME (receptor-mediated endocytosis).
    - Molecules, ligands bind to their membrane receptor and are taken up into the membrane.
    - Clathrin coated vesicles enter the cytoplasm, loose the clathrin coat, travel along the microtubular.
- Canalicular membrane of the hepatocytes
    - Secrets products into the bile canaliculus
    - Flow across the canalicular membrane is unidirectional.
    - Bile flows into the terminal canals of Hering which are lined and formed by hepatocytes and cholangiocytes.
    - Both the canalicular and sinusoidal membranes of the hepatocyte have microvilli.
- The nuclei of the hepatocytes have round nuclei
- The nuclei vary in size, and 30% of hepatocytes may have 2 nuclei
- These proteins are coated by COP (coatamers) to form vesicles
- These vesicles move from cis, to medial- and then to trans Golgi stacks (trans- Golgi network), and then to the cell membrane for exocytosis.
- Protein synthesized from the RER traffic to Golgi complex the cis side of outer membrane of nucleus is in continuity with the ER (endoplasmic reticulum).
- The ER contains cisternae
    - Rough ER (RER)
        - Attached ribosomes
        - Protein synthesis
    - Smooth ER (SER)
        - Lipid synthesis
        - Detoxification
        - Calcium regulation

5

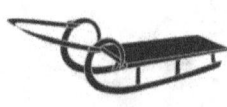

- The endothelial cells of the sinusoids have fenestrae (pores).
- The size of the fenestrae can be changed
- The individual hepatocytes are joined by desmosomes ("..... specialized membrane structures that anchor intermediate filaments to the plasma membrane and link cells in the tight junctions").
- $Ca^{2+}$ and calmodulin act on filaments of actin to change the size of the fenestrae
- CMA (chaperone-mediate autophagy). "...... is a selective mechanism for the degradation of altered cytosolic proteins in lysosomes" (Sleisenger and Fordtran's Gastrointestinal and Liver Disease. 10th Edition. Saunders/Elsevier, Philadelphia, 2016, page 1231).
- The ubiquitin / proteasome pathway
    - Binds to misfolded proteins and directs proteasome-dependent proteolysis.
    - Regulate cytoplasmic protein trafficking

## Kupffer Cells

- Kupffer cells are tissue macrophage
- The Kupffer cells includes
    - Remove old red blood cells
- Function
    - Line the sinusoids along with the sinusoidal membranes of the hepatocytes arise
    - Tissue macrophages arise from monocytes and bone marrow stem cells
    - Secrete lymphokine mediators
    - The Kupffer cell lymphokine mediators influence the hepatocytes to synthesize
        - Proteins
        - Mediators of inflammation
        - Prostaglandins
        - LDL (low-density lipoproteins)

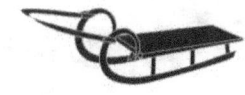

**Stellate Cells** (HSC, Hepatic Stellate Cells; aka Ito Cells)

- Give functions of the hepatic stellate cells.
  - Surround the wall of the sinusoids (perisinusoidal)
  - Control the diameter of the lumen of the sinusoidals
  - May become activated and express desmin and actin
  - HSCs are activated by
    - Sinusoidal endothelial cells
    - ↑ fibronectin
    - Convert latent TGF-B to active fibrogenic active TGF-B
    - Intestinal LPS (lipopolysaccharides → absorbed in portal blood → binds to hepatocyte TLR4 (toll-like receptor 4)
    - LPS bound to TLR4, in the presence of MyD88 (myeloid differentiation response protein) activates NFkB (nuclear factor kappa B)
    - NFkB-downregulates pseudotumour Bambi (bone-morphogenic protein and the actin membrane-bound inhibitor)
    - Kuppfer cells
      - Chemokines expression by HSC attracts kupffer cells
      - Kupffer cells secret TGF-B
    - Hepatocytes
    - Platelets and WBC
  - Downregulation of Bambi-sensitized HSCs to TGF-B
  - HSCs alter cytoskeleton assembly increase extracellular matrix proteins (collagenous and non-collagenous glycoproteins, proteoglycans and glycosaminoglycans).
  - Receptors for vitamin A
  - Store vitamin A

**Sinusoidal cells**
  - Sinusoidal cells (aka HSECs [hepatic sinusoidal epithelial cells])
  - HSECs overlap, and form fenestrae by having
    - No junctions
    - No basement membrane

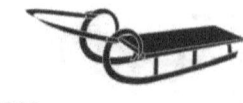

**The Spaces of Disse**

- o Is between the lining of the sinusoidals and the hepatocytes

- o Contains plasma and collagen

- o This collagen in the space of Disse (type I, III and V) forms the scaffolding (skeleton) of the liver.

- o "There is bidirectional exchange of liquids and solutes between the plasma [in the portal vein blood] and hepatocytes at the sinusoidal surface [of the hepatocytes] (Sleisenger and Fordtran's Gastrointestinal and Liver Disease. 10th Edition. Saunders/Elsevier, Philadelphia, 2010, page 1207).

- o The skeleton is comprised of
  - – Microfilaments
    - ▪ Polymers of G-actin
    - ▪ Acts as highways for trafficking of intracellular proteins
    - ▪ α/β polymerized dimers of tubulin
    - ▪ ATP-driven motor proteins
  - – Intermediate filaments
    - ▪ Lamins
    - ▪ Cytokeratins
      - – Hepatocytes: CK8, CK18
      - – Bile duct epithelium: CK8, CK18, CK19
    - ▪ Vimetin
    - ▪ Plectin

**Pit Cells** (aka Liver NK [Natural Killer] Cells)

- • Give functions of the hepatic pit cells.
  - o Express Ox-8 antigen

  - o Kill tumour cells

  - o Remove hepatocytes infected by virus

  - o Intracytoplasmic membrane-bound sacs that contain protein kinase for protein degradation (autophagic lysosomal pathway)

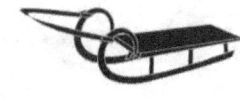

**Central Vein** (aka Terminal Hepatic Venule)

- o At the periphery of the acinus
- o Between the portal tract and the central vein are the 3 zones of hepatocytes
  - – Periportal
  - – Intermediate
  - – Perivenular
- o Riedel lobe
  - – A variant of normal development, leading to a large right lobe of the liver.

- Give the detailed laboratory and diagnostic imaging investigation of the patient with suspected chronic liver disease.

  - o History and physical examination
    - – Fatigue, malaise, anorexia, fever, weight loss/gain, ankle swelling
    - – Following blood donation-positive hepatitis B or C test
    - – Blood transfusions
    - – Drug abuse
    - – MSM (men who have sex with men)
    - – Extrahepatic manifestations
    - – Following acute hepatitis-failure of recovery, whether clinical or biochemical or both

  - o Abnormal liver enzyme or function tests, or positive hepatitis B or C viral markers at routine check-up

  - o Physical findings
    - – Hepatomegaly
    - – Knobby liver with umbilication – pathognomonic of hepatic metastases (2°)
    - – Signs of portal hypertension
      - ▪ Splenomegaly
      - ▪ Jaundice
      - ▪ Peripheral edema
      - ▪ Ascites
      - ▪ Hepatic encephalopathy
      - ▪ Renal dysfunction
      - ▪ Bleeding (varices, coagulopathy)

    - o Umbilicus
      - – Common site of infiltration by cancer metastases

9

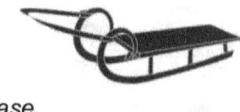

- o Direction of flow of blood in veins of abdominal wall
    - Flow below umbilicus is down into saphenous veins.
    - Above umbilicus flow is upwards into veins of thoracic wall.
    - In portal hypertension, dilated veins show normal direction of flow
    - In IVC obstruction, flow in veins below umbilicus is reversed, i.e., flows upwards
- o Spider nevi
    - Telangiectases
- o Leuconchyia-white nails, beginning at the lunula-may be normal; seen in cirrhosis, leprosy, arsenic poisoning, vasomotor disturbance of fingers
    - Finger clubbing with portal cirrhosis.
    - Dupuytren contracture is suggestive of alcoholic cirrhosis
    - Patients with hemolytic jaundice do not have pruritus or bradycardia
    - Parotid enlargement is common in liver disease, as is fever, even in absence of infection (look for spontaneous bacterial peritonitis)
- o Jaundice with hepatic 2° is usually due to
    - Lesions at hepatic fissure
    - Ascites due to portal vein obstruction by glands
    - Peritoneal deposits
    - Endocrine changes
        - Gynecomastia
        - Testicular atrophy
        - Impotence
        - Amenorrhea
- o Cutaneous signs of chronic liver disease.
    - Clubbing
    - Dupuytren contracture
    - Excoriations
    - Hyperpigmentation
    - Jaundice
    - Loss of lunulae
    - Palmar erythema
    - Parotid enlargement
    - Spider angiomata
    - Telangectasia
    - White nails
    - Xanthelasma
    - Xanthomata

10

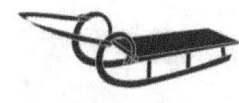

- Give clinically significant extrahepatic manifestations of acute and chronic liver disease.
  - CNS: depression, anxiety, hepatic encephalopathy (HE)
  - Lung: portopulmonary hypertension, hepatopulmonary syndrome, pleural effusion, congestive heart failure, aspiration
  - Heart: prolonged QT (from low Mg 2+); endocarditis; peripheral intravascular vasodilation, ↓ systemic vascular resistance, ↑ HR, ↑ BP, ↑ CO, vitamin K,
  - Blood: Coagulopathy (DIC, fibrinolysis), thrombocytopenia, Hypersplenism, ↓ thrombopoetin, immune mediated destruction, ITP (especially with use of interferon for HCV), direct effect of alcohol, cryoglobulinemia
  - GI
    - Esophageal ulcers from sclerotherapy, GERD, varices
    - Stomach: delayed gastric emptying, PHG, GAVE
    - Small bowel: slow transit, bacterial overgrowth
  - Bone: osteoporosis, osteomalacia: cholestasis, liver Tx, malnutrition, alcohol, tobacco, ↓ motility, hypogonadism, malabsorption
  - Kidney: hyponatremia, ascites, hepatorenal syndrome, glomerulosclerosis (HCV), nephritic syndrome, amyloid
  - Muscle: spastic paraparesis (from demyelination of corticospinal tracts and posterior columns), wasting; arthritis (hemochromotosis)
  - Gonads; hypergonadism, amenorrhea

Abbreviations: GAVE, gastric antral vascular ectasia; PHG, portal hypertensive gastropathy

"When originality may not be genuine, check it on "Turn it in.com". Even Deans deviate.

Grandad

11

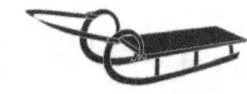

*MASTERING THE BOARDS*
*Hepatology & Pancreaticobiliary Disease*

A.B.R. Thomson

# HEPATIC LABORATORY TESTS

- o Liver function tests
    - Bilirubin
    - Albumin
    - INR
- o Liver enzymes
    - Aspartate transaminase (AST; SGOT)
    - Alanine transaminase (ALT; SGPT)
        - R value
            - ALT/AP
            - >5, hepatocellular disease
            - <2, cholestatic disease
    - ALT, AST in liver, muscle, kidney
    - AST > ALT in ALD (mitochondria produce ↓ AST) fibrosis
    - Gamma-globulin
    - Albumin
    - Alkaline phosphatase (ALP or AP)
    - Gamma glutamyl transferase (GGT)
- o Hematology
    - Hemoglobin
    - White cell count
    - Platelet count
    - PPT
- o Serum antibodies
    - Nuclear
    - Smooth muscle
    - Mitochondrial
    - Liver/kidney microsomal
    - HBsAg
    - HBeAg
    - HBeAb
    - Anti-HCV and HCV RNA

- o Special tests
  - Iron, transferrin, % saturation, genetic testing
  - Ferritin concentration
  - Ceruloplasmin, as well as blood and urinary copper
  - Immunoglobulins (iGA, IgG, IgM)
  - Alpha-fetoprotein (AFP)
  - Creatinine kinase (if smooth muscle disease suspected as cause of ↑ALT/AST, fasting, LDL and HDL cholesterol, triglycerides
  - Protein electrophoresis (polyclonal ↑ gamma globulins in AIH)
  - Anti-transglutaminase
  - Note: From the above, be prepared to answer the question blood tests which may be used in primay care which suggest the cause of underlying liver disease

- • Give causes of chronically elevated aminotransferase levels without associated cholestasis and causes with cholestasis.

- ❖ Without cholestasis
  - o Medication, herbal products, illicit drugs and substance abuse
  - o Infection – HBV, HCV
  - o Drugs/toxins, alcohol
  - o NAFLD, NASH
  - o Autoimmune liver disease
  - o Genetic – hereditary hemochromatosis
    - α, AT deficiency
    - Wilson disease
  - o Celiac disease
  - o Striated muscle diseases

- ❖ With cholestasis
  - o Bile duct obstruction
  - o Idiopathic ductopenia
  - o Primary biliary cholangitis (PBC)
  - o Autoimmune cholangitis (AIC)
  - o Primary sclerosing cholangitis (PSC)
  - o Sarcoidosis
  - o Granulomatous hepatitis
  - o Hepatic tumours (primary or metastic)
  - o Medications
  - o Diet
  - o Drugs
  - o Blood products
  - o Infection

13

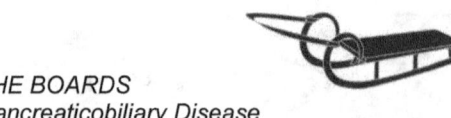

## Aminotransferases

- ALT (aka SGPT, serum glutamic pyruvic transaminase)
- AST (aka SGOT, serum glutamic oxaloacetic transaminase)
- Leak into blood when hepatocyte membrane become leaky
- Increase does not require necrosis, or reflect extent of liver damage.

- Give common causes for elevation of **aminotransferases**.
    - Marked elevation (AST, ALT > 1000 U/L))
        - Ischemia
        - Drugs/toxins
        - Viral hepatitis
        - Autoimmune hepatitis
        - Fulminant Wilson disease
        - Budd Chiari syndrome, acute
        - CBD stones / acute obstruction of biliary tree
    - Moderate elevation (8x ULN)
        - Chronic hepatitis, cirrhosis, cholestatic diseases, and replacement disease
    - Minimal elevation (2x ULN)
        - Non-alcoholic liver disease, chronic viral hepatitis (C and B), alcoholism, obesity

- Give examples of non-hepatic conditions associated with ↑ ALT or ↑ AST.
    - Thyroid
        - Hyper-/hypothyroidism
    - Muscle
        - Acute rhabdomyolysis
        - Myopathy
        - Extreme exercise
    - GI disease
        - Celiac disease
    - Macro – AST (isolated AST [not ALT], or other liver enzymes)

14

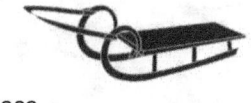

SO YOU WANT TO BE A HEPATOLOGIST!

The ALT is usually higher than AST, except with alcoholic liver disease (ALD), non-alcoholic steatohepatitis (NASH), development of the hepatic fibrosis acute rhabdomyolysis, myopathy, severe exercise, hypothyroidism or macro-AST.

- Give the explanation for AST > ALT in ALD.
    - In ALD there is ↓ pyridoxal 5' – phosphate (P5P)
    - P5P is used to synthesize ALT and AST
    - More P5P is needed to synthesize ALT and AST
    - When P5P↓, as in ALD, there will be less synthesis of ALT, so AST > ALT

- Give laboratory evaluations of conjugated hyperbilirubinemia in children.
    - Total and direct serum bilirubin
    - Alkaline phosphatase, aminotransferases, γ-glutamyl transpeptidase
    - Prothrombin time or INR, serum albumin (factor V levels, if available)
    - Complete blood cell count, differential
    - Urine culture (blood/cerebrospinal fluid, if indicated)
    - Serology for cytomegalovirus, rubella, herpes simplex, herpes type 6, toxoplasmosis, syphilis (adenovirus, Coxsackie virus, reovirus III, parvovirus B19, if available)
    - Urine for reducing substances, serum galactose-1-phosphate uridyltransferase, serum/urine amino acids and organic acids
    - Sweat chloride, genotyping for cystic fibrosis
    - $\alpha_1$-antitrypsin level and Pi phenotype
    - Urine for bile acid metabolites
    - Serum ferritin
    - TSH
    - T4, glucose, cortisol

15

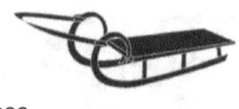

**Alkaline Phosphatase** (AP)

- o Isolated ↑ AP (normal ALT, AST; also normal GGT)
    - − Renal cell carcinoma
    - − Systemic mastocytosis
    - − Paget disease
    - − RA (rheumatoid arthritis; sometimes also ↑ GGT)

- o ↑ AP plus ↑ GGT
    - − Temporal arteritis
    - − Metastatic CRC (colorectal) cancer
    - − RA (rheumatoid arthritis; sometimes isolated ↑ AP, i.e., AP but not GGT)
    - − Granulomatous liver disease

➢ Causes of ↑ serum alkaline phosphatase (AP)

- o Mechanism of ↑ AP
    - − ↑ AP in cholestatic liver diseases because of
        - ▪ ↑ synthesis
        - ▪ ↑ leakage into serum
    - − Physiological
        - ▪ An isoenzyme of AP made by intestine ↑ after a fatty meal in persons with blood group B or O.

- Give causes of reduced serum alkaline phosphatase concentration.

| | | |
|---|---|---|
| o Endocrine | − | Hyperthyroidism |
| | − | Hypoparathyroidism |
| | − | Hypophosphatemia |
| o Stomach | − | Pernicious anemia (atropic gastritis) |
| | − | Milk alkali syndrome |
| o Bowel | − | Small bowel disease (+/- alcoholism) associated with |

- ▪ Deficiency
    - − Magnesium
    - − Vitamin C
    - − Zinc
    - − Vitamin B6
    - − Folic acid
- ▪ Excesses
    - − Vitamin D

- − Celiac disease
- − Protein-calorie malnutrition

- o Liver − WD (Wilson disease)

16

**Gamma Glutamyl Transpeptidase** (GGT)

- o Sensitive but not specific for liver disease

- Give common causes for elevation of **gamma glutamyltranspeptidase (GGT)**.
  - o Alcohol
  - o Drugs, e.g., HAART, phenytoin, barbiturates
  - o Hepatobiliary disease
    - – Replacement disease
    - – Enzyme induction
  - o GI
    - – Anorexia
  - o Endocrine
    - – Obesity
    - – Diabetes mellitus
    - – Hyperthyroidism
  - o Performance characteristics

|  | Sensitivity | Specifcity |
|---|---|---|
| – AST/ALT > 1, as an indication of cirrhosis in HCV | 44% to 75% | > 94% |
| – GGTP | | |
| ▪ As an indicator of alcohol use | 52% to 94% | Low |
| ▪ As an indicator of bile duct stones | NPV ~ 98% | |

Abbreviation: NPV, negative predictive value

- Give the laboratory tests which help distinguish between the bland versus mixed types of cholestasis.

| Laboratory Finding | Types of Cholestasis | |
|---|---|---|
| | Bland | Mixed |
| ↑ AP > 2x ULN | + | |
| ↑ ALT/AP < 2 | + | |
| ↑ ALT > 2x ULN | | + |
| ↑ ALT/AP > 5 | | + |

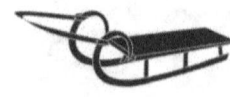

17

**Prothrombin Time**

- o Influenced by clotting factors II, V, VII, X
- o Prolonged PT with vitamin K deficiency (reduced II, VII, IX, X) and DIC
- o Serum T½ of 6 hours of factor VII, making PT useful to detect rapid changes in liver function

---

SO YOU WANT TO BE A HEPATOLOGIST!

- Give reasons why the validity of using PT or INR (intenational normalized ratio) in liver patients has been challenged.

    - o Each lab measuring INR has their own standardization of the PT based on the thromboplastin eagent that lab uses to calculate ISI (international sensitivity index), from which the INR is calculated.

    - o ".… The ISI [has been] validated only for patients taking a vitamin K antagonist

    - o Dose not reflect bleeding risk in hepatic disease
        - – Measures procoagulant clotting factors
        - – Does not measure anticoagulant clotting factors (e.g., protein C and thrombin)
        - – Protein C and antithrombin are elevated with liver disease
        - – PTT (partial thromboplastin time) used to access bleeding risk in liver disease, PT/INR used to determine if there is coagulopathy

Patients with liver disease may have a prolonged PT / ↑ INR due to deficiency of vitamin K –dependent coagulation factors (II, VII, IX, X) or DIC.

- Give the laboratory test which is used to distinguish between a deficiency of vitamin K, and DIC.

    - o Factor VII
        - – ↓ in DIC
        - – N/↑ in liver disease

---

Clinical Tips

- ↑ bilirubin, AP (alkaline phosphatase) or GGT does not necessarily indicate drug-induced liver injury (DILI), but instead may be an adaptive response through the induction of microsomal enzymes in the hepatocytes.

Please refer to Sleisenger and Fordtran's Gastrointestinal and Liver Disease. 10th Edition. Saunders/Elsevier, Philadelphia, 2016, page 1454.

- ↓ AP, ↓ AP/bilirubin ratio, and ↓ uric acid in serum → think of Wilson disease

18

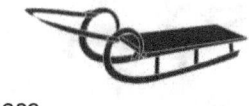

## SURGERY AND LIVER DISEASE

- Give management considerations in the **pre- and post-operative care** of the patient with advanced liver disease (based on MELD score).

  o Risk stratification
    - Child-Pugh score
    - MELD score
    - Mayo score

  o Hepatic encephalopathy (HE)
    - Correction of reversible metabolic factors (e.g., hyponatremia, hypokalemic alkalosis)
    - Oral lactulose administration, titrated to ~3-4 bowel movements per day
    - Administration of nonabsorbable antibiotics
    - Avoidance of nephrotoxic insult (e.g., ACE inhibitors, NSAIDs, narcotics, benzodiazepine)
    - Supportive care
    - Correction of reversible metabolic factors, including renal function

  o Esophageal varices
    - EGD +/- banding if not done within 1 yr, or non-specific β-blockers

  o Ascites/SBP/HRS
    - Ascites, peripheral edema
    - Oral diuretic therapy with spironolactone and/or furesomide
    - Fluid restriction (if sodium concentration is <120 mmol/l)
    - Avoidance of excessive saline administration
    - Antibiotics +/- albumin infusion for spontaneous bacterial peritonitis
    - Paracentesis with analysis of ascitic fluid for evidence of infection (SBP)

  o Diet
    - Maintenance of an adequate protein intake (1-1.5 g/kg per day)
    - Promotion of a balanced diet
    - Dietary sodium restriction (<2 g daily)

  o Coagulopathy
    - Vitamin K supplementation (oral or parenteral) (INR < 1.8)
    - ↓ fibrogen, DIC
    - Fresh, frozen plasma (FFP) transfusions
    - Intravenous administration of cryoprecipitate
    - Intravenous administration of recombinant factor VIIa
    - Platelet transfusions (< 50,000)

19

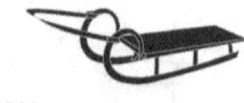

- Give anticoagulant before surgery to prevent thromboembolic disease.
  - Do not treat unless INR < 1.8 heparin

- Pain control
  - Dilaudid (0.5-1 mg q 4 h prn) or PLA
  - Acetaminophen
  - Avoid benzodiazepines, NSAIDs, narcotics
  - Consider PCA
- Assess pulmonary function (e.g., for dyspnea, $O_2$ desaturation)
  - Supplemental oxygen
  - Investigation for lung complications of cirrhosis
- Treat associated liver disease, e.g., corticosteroids, ursodeoxycholic acid, antivirals

Adapted from: Hanje AJ, and Pate T. *Nature Clinical Practice Gastroenterology & Hepatology* 2007; 4: pg. 272.

Post-operative Hepatic Dysfunction is Common. Please see Sleisenger and Fordtran's Gastrointestinal and Liver Disease. 9th Edition. Saunders/Elsevier, Philadelphia, 2010, Table 87.4, page 1449.

- Give methods to predict the influence of liver disease on **predicting post-operative mortality.**
  - Child-Pugh classification
  - ASA class
    - ASA class V best to predict 7d mortality
  - MELD (model for end-stage liver disease) score
    - MELD is best to predict mortality beyond 7 days.
  - Presence of PHT (portal hypertension)
  - Co-morbidities
  - For high risk surgery, consider performing the surgery at a centre with hepatobiliary experience, including liver transplantation (L-Tx)
  - Consider pre-operative assessment for L-Tx (liver transplantation), in case patient does not do well post-operatively

20

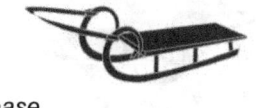

Note:

- o MELD, ASA class, and age were most important
  - www.mayoclinic.org/meld/mayomodel9.html
  - C-statistic is 0.80 (30 d) and 0.84 (90 d)
- o Emergency surgery predicted duration of hospitalization (p<0.001) but not mortality

- Give the **Child-Pugh** (CP) **classification** of liver disease.

| Parameter | 1 | 2 | 3 |
|---|---|---|---|
| o Ascites | None | Slight | Mod/severe |
| o Encephalopathy | None | Slight/mod (1-2) | Mod/severe (3-4) |
| o Bilirubin (mg/ dl) | <2 (<34) | 2-3 (34-50) | >3 (>50) |
| o Albumin (mg/ dl) | >3.5 (>35) | 2.8-3.5 (28-35) | <2.8 (<28) |
| o PT (INR) | 1-3 (<1.7) | 4-6 (1.7-2.2) | >6 (>2.2) |

| Total score | Child-Pugh classification |
|---|---|
| 5-6 | A |
| 7-9 | B |
| 10-15 | C |

Adapted from: Kim WR, et al. *Hepatology* 1999;29(6):1643-8.; and Durand F, Valla D. *J Hepatol* 2005;42.

"Life isn't about waiting for the storm to pass. It's about learning how to dance in the rain..."

Vivian Greene

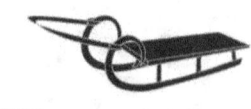

- Give the peri-operative mortality rates (MR) in persons with cirrhosis, based upon their Child-Pugh classification.

| CP Class | Surgical MR (%) |
|----------|-----------------|
| A        | 5-10            |
| B        | 30              |
| C        | 70-80           |

- 30-day perioperative mortality, 30% (total):
  - Bleeding, 10%
  - Pneumonia, 8%
  - Infection, 8%
  - Worsening Ascites, 7%

Source: Sterling RK. Evaluation and management of the surgical patient with cirrhosis: when they have to go to the operating room. *ACG Annual Scientific Meeting Symposia Sessions* 2009; 71-77.


- Give the use of the **MELD score** to predict perioperative complications.
  - Derived from creatinine, bilirubin, INR
  - Correlates with mortality rate for
    - Liver transplantation
    - Liver resection
    - Other abdominal operations
    - Cardiac surgery

  - MELD score     5-20      – 1% increase in mortality with each 1 point increase

               >20      –  2% increase in MR for each MELD point increase
    - If MELD < 11 (especially < 8), acceptable risks
    - If MELD > 20, elective surgery should be postponed
    - If MELD 12-20, complete L-TX evaluation in case of deterioration

22

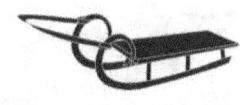

# FATTY LIVER DISEASE

➢ Pathogenesis

- Give the pathogenesis of NAFLD (non-alcoholic fatty liver disease) and NASH (non-alcoholic steatohepatitis).

- GI Tract

  o ↑ intake/absorption   - ↑ fat to liver   ▪ ↑ fat in liver

  o Fat, CHO        - CHO to liver   ▪ ↑ lipogenesis (↑ TG in liver)
                              ▪ ↑ insulin resistance

  o Bacterial toxins     - ↑ ROS       ▪ ↑ oxidative stress

- Adipocyte
  o Adipose tissue is composed of adipocytes and the stromal vascular fraction.
  o This includes macrophages and other immune cells that have a relevant role in the autocrine-paracrine regulation of adipocytes. In obesity, activation of macrophages/immune system contributes to the development of dysfunctional, insulin-resistant adipocytes that release excessive amounts of FFA and cause insulin resistance and lipoapoptosis in distant tissues (liver, muscle, pancreatic beta cells, vascular bed, other).
  o Accumulation of triglyceride-derived toxic lipid metabolites activates intracellular inflammatory pathways within hepatocytes and Kupffer and other immune cells, in resemblance to defects within adipocytes.
  o ↑ fat → insulin resistance
  o ↑ cytokines
  o Activated macrophages

  o ↑ FFA/ROS        – Actvation of macrophages/immune system → ↑ lipoptosis
                 – ↑ insulin-resistant adipocytes → ↑ FFAs

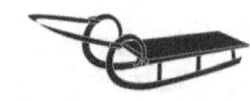

- Liver

  - Metabolism
    - ↑ insulin, ↑ insulin-resistance
    - ↑ leptin, ↑ leptin resistance
    - ↓ adiponectin

  - Mitochondria
    - ↓ β oxidation of FFA
    - ↑ synthesis of FFA
      - ↓ respiratory chain complexes
      - ↓ ATP
      - ↑ ROS, ↑ PPAR γ, ↑ TNF-α
      - ↑ DNA damage
    - ↑ SREBP1 / ↑ CHREBP → ↑ TG synthesis
    - ↓ Apo B-100 (also ↓ β oxidation) → ↓ fat transport out of liver → ↑ TG in liver

  - ↑ CYP 2E1
    - ↑ leak of electrons → ↑ ROS, ↑ RNS → ↑ NF-kB → ↑ TNF-α
    - ↓ ATP
    - ↓ antioxidant
    - ↑ membrane lipid peroxidation
    - ↑ protein/DNA oxidation
    - ↑ hepatic insulin
    - ↑ synthesis of PL, CE

- Inflammasomes (proinflammatory mulprotein complexes: redox state)
  - Nod-like receptor (NLR) protein or a PYHIN protein – sense pathogen-associated molecular pattern (PAMPs) or damage-associated molecular patterns (DAMPs)
  - Are key to the production of the proinflammatory cytokines IL-1β IL-18.
  - Reactive oxygen species (ROS) activate the NLRP3 inflammasome and their generation is triggered by many PAMPs.
  - Increased ROS generation is a proinflammatory insult in the progression of NAFLD.
  - Inflammasome-dependent processing of IL-1β and IL-18 could be important in NAFLD/NASH
  - Inflammasome-dependent processing of IL-1β and IL-18 could be important in NAFLD/NASH.

24

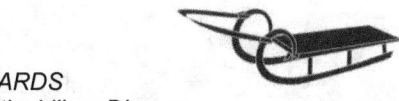

- Inflammasomes – proinflammatory multiprotein complexes consisting of a Nod-like receptor (NLR) protein or a PYHIN protein – sense pathogen-associated molecular pattern (PAMPs) or damage-associated molecular patterns (DAMPs) and are key to the production of the proinflammatory cytokines IL-1β IL-18.
  - Reactive oxygen species (ROS) activate the NLRP3 inflammasome and their generation is triggered by many DAMPs.
  - Increased ROS generation is a proinflammatory insult in the progression of NAFLD.
  - Endo-/ exotoxin-mediated release of proinflammatory cytokines

  Source: Wood NJ. Nat Rev Gastroenterol Hepatol. 2012;9(3):123.

- Dysregulated cytokine production (↑ pro- / ↓ anti-inflammatory cytokines)
  - Hepatocytes
    - IL-8, IL-18
    - Neutrophil chemotactic peptide
    - Angiogenesis factor
  - Kupffers cells
    - NF-kB → TNF-α
    - IL-10
  - Sinusoidal endothelial cells
    - Adhesion molecules
  - Stellate cells
    - TGF-β → fibrosis
  - ↑ intestinal permeability → ↑ LPS
  - ↑ LPS
  - ↑ apoptosis of hepatocytes → ↑ release of IL-8 (neutrophil chemoattractant), IL-18 (primes TNFα release, and type 1 helper T cell response)
  - ↑ TNF-α inducible IL-6, IL-8, Il-18, MCP-1 (monocyte chemoattractant protein 1)
  - As well as ↑ pro-inflammatory cytokines, there is ↓ anti-inflammatory cytokines

"hepatocyte apoptosis may sustain proinflammatory cytokine production and cell injury or death" (Sleisenger and Fordtran's Gastrointestinal and Liver Disease. 10th Edition. Saunders/Elsevier, Philadelphia, 2016, page 1230).

25

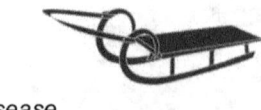

- Stellate cell activation
  - o Activation of hepatic stellate cell (HSC)
    - Pro-inflammatory cytokines
    - Angiotension
    - Oxidative stress
    - Growth factors
    - Extracellular matrix
    - PDGF (platelet-derived growth factor)
    - Connective tissue growth factor
    - Leptin-associated production of TGF-β by kupffer cells
  - o A signaling pathways regulating HSC activation
    - PDGF
      - PDF signals partially through ERK activation and also through AKT via mTOR mediated protein synthesis regulation.
      - PDGF activation also allows for influx of Ca2+ ions, which contributes to gene regulation
      - In addition to PDGF, several other growth factors can activate tyrosine receptors which lead to Akt activation and then either mTOR or JNK activation.
    - TGFβ
      - TGFB recruits Smad 2/3, leading to their phosphorylation and stimulation of fibrogenic gene expression.
    - Others
      - Emerging pathways of importance of fibrosis include contributions from
        - Adipokines (leptin)
        - Neuroendocrine signals (2-AG)
        - TLR signaling
        - Angiogenic signals (VEGF), among other
        - SREBP-1, the sterol regulatory element binding protein-1c, CHREBP, the carbohydrate regulatory element

Abbreviations: NFkB, nuclear factor kappa B; ROS, reactive oxygen species; RNS, reactive nitrogen species

Adapted from: Pellicoro A, and Faber KN. *Alim Pharm Ther* 2007; 26 (2): pg. 149-160 and Wood NJ. Nat Rev Gastroenterol Hepatol 2012; 9(3):123.

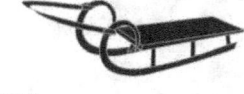

- Balance of lipolysis/lipogenesis (↑ FFA, ↓ mitochondrial function)

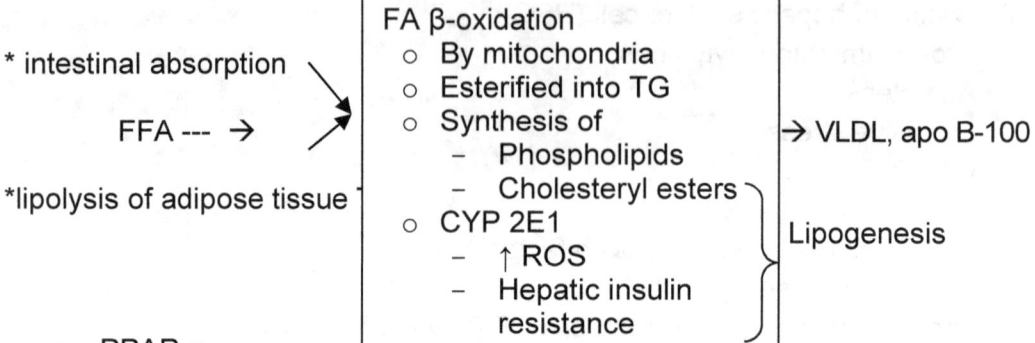

* intestinal absorption

FFA --- →

*lipolysis of adipose tissue

FA β-oxidation
- By mitochondria
- Esterified into TG
- Synthesis of
  - Phospholipids
  - Cholesteryl esters
- CYP 2E1
  - ↑ ROS
  - Hepatic insulin resistance

→ VLDL, apo B-100

Lipogenesis

- PPAR-α
  - Widely distributed among adipocytes, hepatocytes, and hepatic stellate cells, as well as macrophages and immune cells infiltrating adipose and liver tissue.
  - Function
    - FA oxidation
    - Oxidative stress
- Regulation by
  - Insulin
  - Catecholamines
  - Glucagon
  - Growth hormone
  - Leptin
  - Adiponectin

- FFA (free fatty acids)
  - Activated immune response
    - ↑ NFkB
    - ↑ IL-6
    - ↓ adiponectin
    - ↑ leptin, ↑ leptin resistance
    - Lysosomal destabilization (↑ TNF-α)
  - ↑ ROS (reactive oxygen species), ↑ CYP 2E1
  - Toxicity to mitochondrial membranes

- Mitochondrial dysfunction
  - ↓ respiratory chain complexes
  - ↑ ROS
    - ↑ TNF-α
  - ↓ ATP
  - Mitochondrial DNA damage

27

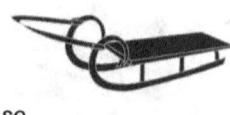

- Stellate cell
  - Activation (initiation and perpetuation)
    - Pro-inflammatory cytokines
    - Angiotension
    - Oxidative stress
    - Growth factors
    - Extracellular matrix
    - PDGF (platelet-derived growth factor)
    - Connective tissue growth factor
    - Leptin-associated production of TGF-β by kupffer cells
  - Activation of hepatic stellate cells leads to collagen deposition and the potential for cirrhosis.
  - A signaling pathways regulating HSC activation

---

SO YOU WANT TO BE A GASTROENTEROLOGIST!

- Give monogenic causes of chronic liver disease which are associated with fatty liver in children.
  - Fatty acid oxidation defects
  - Lysosomal storage diseases
  - Peroxisomal disorders

---

➢ Causes/associations

- Give conditions other than obesity, DMT2, dyslipidemia or metabolic syndrome which may also predispose to NAFLD.

| | | |
|---|---|---|
| o Endocrine | – | Hypothyroidism |
| | – | Hypopituitarism |
| | – | Hypogonadism |
| | – | Hyperuricemia |
| | – | Vitamin D deficiency |
| o Ovary | – | Polycystic ovary syndrome (PCOS) |
| o Pulmonary | – | Obstructive sleep apnea |
| o GI | – | Pancreatico-duodenal resection |
| | – | Total Parental Nutrition (TPN) |

28

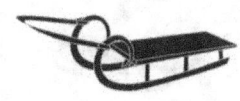

➢ Clinical

    o NAFLD is often associated with metabolic syndrome (which is diagnosed as well as with laboratory measurements) as well as with insulin resistance.

    o NAFLD, both simple steatosis as well as NASH (steatosis hepatitis with/without fibrosis) is a risk factor for HCC (hepatocellular cancer),

    o About 1/3 of persons with NAFLD and simple steatosis will progress to NASH. patients with NASH will develop cirrhosis and portal (PHT). Preventing fatty liver disease is important, but the physician needs to be able to identify the person with simple steatosis who is at risk for progression to the more serious condition, NASH.

    o It is important to assess all patients with NAFLD for their risk of progressing to NASH/cirrhosis, so that they may be managed with more than supportive care, encouragement of weight reduction and maintenance, and treatment of an associated metabolic syndrome,

- Give patient-related **predictors of progression** of NAFLD (simple steatosis) to NASH.

    o Patient
- Age > 45 years
- Female
- Ethnicity (Hispanic, Asian >White >Black)
- Type II diabetes mellitus (↑ risk of NAFLD, even in absence of metabolic syndrome)
- BMI > 35 (especially visceral obesity)
- Insulin resistance
- Hypertension
- Metabolic syndrome (insulin resistance), even in young, non-obese persons
- Stigmata of portal hypertension
- Comorbidity: alcohol, HCV infection

    o NAFLD and NASH may be distinguished using the Kleiner scoring system, also known as "NAS" (NASH activity score) (Kleiner DE, et al. *Hepatology* 2005;41:1313-21.)

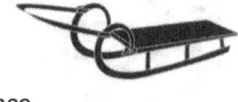

29

- o Based on:
    1. Simple steatosis
    2. Steatosis plus inflammation alone
    3. Steatosis plus ballooning
    4. Steatosis plus fibrosis (Matteoni CA, et al. *Gastroenterology* 1999:1413-9.)

- o NAFLD worsens the prognosis of liver disease associated with HCV and HH (hereditary hemochromatosis).

➢ Natural history of NAFLD

```
        20%                 ~1% / year              ~4% / year
NAFL  ⟶    NASH       ⟶     cirrhosis, HCC    ⟶   decompensation
```

- o About 2/3 of NAFLD are SS (NNFL) and 1/3 are NASH
- o Only 10-15% weight reduction reduces hepatic fat (Harrison SA, Day CP. *Gut* 2007:1760-9)
- o Agents tested to treat NAFLD, but not being of consistent benefit, include UDCA, vitamins C and E, thiazolidinediones, statins, ARBs (angiotensin receptor blockers), ghrelin-leptin modulators, and antioxidants such as SNACS-nitroso-n-acetyl cysteine. Vitamin E supplementation shows promise.
- o Bariatric surgery achieves weight reduction and benefits many parameters of NASH (Mummadi RR, et al. *Clin Gastroenterol Hepatol* 2008:1396-1402.)

Abbreviations: ARBs, angiotensin receptor blockers; NAS, NASH activity score; NNFL, non-NASH fatty liver; SS, simple steatosis
Printed with permission: Cortez-Pinto H, and Camilo ME. *Best Practice & Research Clinical Gastroenterology* 2004;18(6): pg 1097.

> Laboratory
- o ↑ALT > 2x ULN
- o ↑AST:ALT >1 [suggests fibrosis]
- o ↑ Triglycerides >1.5
- o ↑ INR
- o ↑ Bilirubin
- o ↓Platelets

30

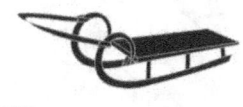

- ↓Albumin
- Indexes of insulin resistance (HOMA [homeostatic model assesssment, QUICKI, OGIS)
- ↑ Elevated ferritin levels
- ↑ Hyaluronic acid
- ↑ glucosaminoglycan
  - Produced in mesenchymal cells
  - Increased in cirrhosis because of sinusoidal capillarization
  - Fasting hyaluronan > 100 mg/L, performance characteristics for detection of cirrhosis
  - Sensitivity, 83%
  - Specificity, 78%
  - Useful if normal
- Panels of blood tess (please see later section "Detection of Hepatic Fibrosis"
  - Fibrosure
  - Fibro test
  - Fibro spect
  - NAFLD fibrosis score

➢ Diagnostic Imaging
  - Ultrasound (US)          ↑ echogenicity
  - CT              liver density = spleen
  - MRI      bright T1 – weighted imaging of liver
  - Detection of > 33% fat in liver
    - Sensitivity
      - US, 100%
      - CT, 93%  } shows lobular distribution of fat
      - MRI, 95%
    - PPV
      - US, 62%
      - CT, 76%
  - Support the diagnosis of NAFLD
  - US, CT, MRI do not predict severity: do not distinguish simple steatosis (SS) from NASH

Abbreviations: PPV, positive predictive value; NASH, non-alcoholic steatohepatitis; SS, simple steatosis

31

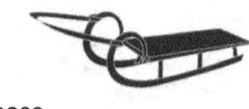

- o MRE (magnetic resonance elastography)
  - – "….superior to TE for staging liver fibrosis in patients with a variety of chronic liver disease" (Feldman M., et al. Sleisenger and Fordtran's Gastrointestinal and Liver Disease. 9th Edition. Saunders/Elsevier, Philadelphia, 2010, page 1235)
  - – Fibro Scan® (aka TE [transient elastography]) > 12.5

➢ Histopathology

- Give the pros and cons of performing a percutaneous liver biopsy in a patient with NAFLD and abnormal liver enzymes.

| Issues | Argument in Favor of Biopsy with Acceptable Risk | Reasons for not Performing a Biopsy |
|---|---|---|
| **Abnormal hepatic biochemical tests and NAFLD** | | |
| o Elevated ALT | – Confirm diagnosis | – Cause accurately identified clinically in > 90% cases without biopsy |
| o Diagnosis of NAFLD | – Patients may not have classic NAFLD risk factors | – Accurate diagnosis of NAFLD generally possible without biopsy |
| o Identify severity of NAFLD | – Only biopsy can distinguish simple steatosis from steatohepatitis | – Non-invasive markers may be developed to distinguish the two |
| o Treatment of NAFLD | – Presence of steatohepatitis or fibrosis may motivate some to undertake risk factor modification | – There is no proven therapy for NAFLD. Absence of steatohepatitis or fibrosis may remove motivation for some to undertake risk factor modification |

Printed with permission: Reddy K R. *2006 AGA Institute Postgraduate Course Syllabus:* pg. 81.

32

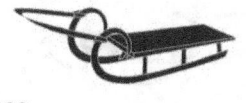

*MASTERING THE BOARDS*
*Hepatology & Pancreaticobiliary Disease*

A.B.R. Thomson

- Give liver biopsy criteria for the diagnosis of NASH.
    - Present in all or most cases
        - Diffuse or centrilobular steatosis
            - Predominantly macrovesicular
            - Degree may correlate with BMI
        - Parenchymal (lobular and portal)
            - Inflammation (+/- focal necrosis)
            - Neutrophils
            - Macronuclear cells
        - Lobular necrosis
    - Features observed with varying frequency
        - Ballooning hepatocyte degeneration
        - Pericellular fibrosis ("chicken wire fibrosis" on trichrome stain) – perivenular* (zone 3), perisinusoidal or periportal (37%-84%)
        - Mallory bodies
        - NAFLD Activity Score (see Useful background which follows)
        - Cirrhosis (7%-16% on index biopsy)
        - Glycogenated nuclei
        - Lipogranulomas
        - Stainable iron

Adapted from: Sleisenger and Fordtran's Gastrointestinal and Liver Disease.. Saunders/Elsevier, Philadelphia, 8th Edition, 2006, page 1796; 9th Edition, 2010, page 1407; 10th Edition 2016, page 1430.


**Focal Fatty Liver** (FFL)

- Patchy process of fat accumulation which may look like a hepatic mass on diagnostic imaging
- Typical appearance on CT scan which helps to distinguish FFL from metastatic lesion:
    - Density close to water
    - Not spherical in shape
    - No mass effect
- FFL may regress without treatment

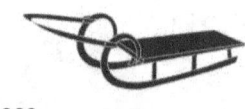

- Give causes of **macrovesicular** steatosis.
  - Liver – Wilson disease, alcohol, NAFLD/NASH, HCV-3 (acute fatty liver of pregnancy)
  - Infection – HCV-3, bacterial overgrowth, fever, viral infections
  - Drugs – corticosteroids, alcohol, estrogen, amiodarone, HAART (for HIV) tetracycline, vitamin A toxicity
  - Metabolic – hyperlipidemia, TPN, tyrosinemia, galactosemia, glycogenoses, abetalipoproteinemia, diabetes
  - Nutrition – rapid weight loss or gain, obesity, pancreatic insufficiency, Kwashiorkor, TPN, bariatric surgery, short bowel syndrome
  - Pediatric conditions - Weber-Christian
  - Ideopathic

Adapted from: Oh MK, et al. *Aliment Pharmacol Ther* 2008; 28:pg. 507.

---

Suggestion

  - Learn these few causes of microvesicular steatosis, and all the others are macrovesicular.

---

- Give causes of **microvesicular** steatosis.
  - Pregnancy—Acute fatty liver of pregnancy, HELLP syndrome
  - Infection – HBV, HCV, HDV
  - Drugs – Reye syndrome (salicylates), valoproic acid, amiodarone, AZT, DDI, tetracycline
  - Metabolic – Jamaican vomiting sickness, urea cycle and mitochondrial defects, carnitine deficiency, Wolfman disease
    - Aide de memoir: "A, B, C, D, E-J (**A**FLP; H**B**V; H**C**V; **D**rugs; H**E**LLP-Jamaican)

Adapted from: Oh, M.K. et al. *Aliment Pharmacol Ther* 2008; 28:pg. 507. Genetic abnormalities may exist in some persons with alcoholic liver disease (ALD), cholelithiasis, primary biliary cholangitis (PBC), primary sclerosing cholangitis (PSC), alpha1 anti-trypsin deficiency (α1-AT), and polycystic liver disease (PCLD)

34

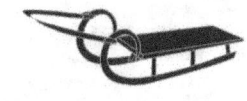

- Give the Grading and staging of the biopsy lesions of NASH (NAFLD activity score).

❖ Grades

- o Grade I, Mild
  - – Steatosis: predominantly macrovesicular, involves <33% or up to 66% of the lobules; increased BMI may correlate with degree of steatosis
  - – Ballooning: occasionally observed in zone 3 hepatocytes
  - – Lobular inflammation: scattered and mild acute (polymorphs) and chronic (mononuclear cells) inflammation
  - – Portal inflammation: none or mild

- o Grade 2, Moderate
  - – Steatosis: any degree and usually mixed macrovesicular and microvesicular
  - – Ballooning: present in zone 3 hepatocytes
  - – Lobular inflammation: polymorphs may be noted associated with ballooned hepatocytes, pericellular fibrosis; mild chronic inflammation may be seen
  - – Portal inflammation: Mild to moderate

- o Grade 3, Severe
  - – Steatosis: typically >66% (panacinar): commonly mixed steatosis
  - – Lobular inflammation: scattered acute and chronic inflammation; polymorphs may appear concentrated in zone 3 areas of ballooning and perisinusoidal fibrosis
  - – Portal inflammation: Mild to moderate

❖ Stages (fibrosis)

- o Stage 1: zone 3 perivenular perisinusoidal fibrosis, focal or extensive
- o Stage 2: as above plus focal or extensive periportal fibrosis

  ] Simple steatosis (NNFL)

- o Stage 3: bridging fibrosis, focal or extensive
- o Stage 4: cirrhosis

  ] NASH

Abbreviations: NNFL, non-NASH fatty liver

- Give the composition of **Mallory bodies**, and the hepatic conditions with which they associated.
  - Composition
    - Cytoplasmic inclusions in hepatocytes
      - "twisted rope" appearance
    - Red colour from
      - Cytokeratin intermediate filaments, and
      - Ubiquitins
  - Associations
    - ALD (alcoholic liver disease) (~66%)
    - NAFLD (non-alcoholic liver disease)
    - PBC (primary biliary cholangitis) (~25%)
    - WD (Wilson disease) (25% to 50%)
    - DILI, e.g., Amiodarone

---

Clinical Confusion – What the Experts Say About Liver Biopsy in NAFLD
"Liver biopsy is the standard means of diagnosis and the only test that can reliably differentiate simple steatosis from advanced NAFLD (i.e., non-alcoholic steatohepatitis), although non-invasive methods for assessing fibrosis are under study" (Feldman M., et al. Sleisenger and Fordtran's Gastrointestinal and Liver Disease. 9th Edition. Saunders/Elsevier, Philadelphia, 2010, page 1407).

"The correlation among clinical, laboratory, and histologic findings in NAFLD is poor, and patients with normal liver biochemical tests results can have significant liver injury on biopsy specimens" (Feldman M., et al. Sleisenger and Fordtran's Gastrointestinal and Liver Disease. 9th Edition. Saunders/Elsevier, Philadelphia, 2010, page 1407).

".....the risk of liver-related complications in NAFLD correlates, at least to some extent, with the degree of hepatocellular injury and fibrosis found on an index liver biopsy specimen" (Feldman M., et al. Sleisenger and Fordtran's Gastrointestinal and Liver Disease. 9th Edition. Saunders/Elsevier, Philadelphia, 2010, page 1408).

---

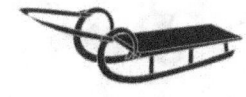

## Detection of Hepatic Fibrosis

❖ Gold standard
- Liver biopsy
  - Histological (liver biopsy) staging and grading
- Only a "bronze standard" because of considerable sampling variation (patchy changes)

❖ A panel of blood tests
- α2-microglobulin
- Apolipoproteins A-1
- Haptoglobulin
- Total bilirubin
- GGT
- ALT
- Combination of blood tests to give a predictive score (Fibrosure, Fibrospect II)
  - Hepatic fibrosis
    - First 5 above blood tests ASA "score"
  - Necroinflammatory activity
    - All above blood tests as a "score" 6 tests

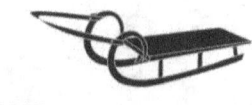

- ❖ Fibro test (aka FibroSure)
  - o Performance characteristics
    - – Sensitivity, 90%
    - – Specificity, 36%
    - – PPV, 88%
    - – NPV, 40%
    - – Validated in HBV, HCV, ALD, methotrexate in psoriasis
    - – Low cut-off (0.30)
      - ▪ NPV, 90%

- ❖ FibroSpect II
  - o A score derived from variably weighted values of the following:
    - – Hyaluronate
    - – Tissue inhibitor of metalloproteinase I
    - – α2-macroglobulin
    - – Performance characteristics for advanced fibrosis in HCV
      - ▪ PPV, 88%
      - ▪ Sensitivity, 72%
      - ▪ Specificity, 74%
  - – Severe steatosis (centrilobular, macrosteatosis)
  - – ↑ Stainable iron
  - – Signs of cirrhosis
  - – Performance characteristics for fibrosis, cut-off value
    - – High cut-off (0.70)
      - ▪ PPV, 73%
      - ▪ Specificity, 98%

- ❖ NAFLD Fibrosis Score
  - o Age
  - o BMI
  - o Blood sugar
  - o AST/ALT
  - o Platelet count

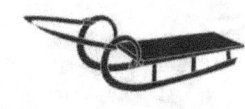

- Albumin
  - High cut-off
    - PPV, 82% to 90%
  - Low cut-off
    - NPV, 88% to 93%

Abbreviations: ALT, alanine aminotransferase; AST, aspartate aminotransferase; BMI, body mass index; HOMA, homeostatic model assessment; MDA, malondialdehyde; NPV, negative predictive value; OGIS, oral glucose insulin sensitivity index; PPV, positive predictive value; QUICKI, quantitative insulin-sensitivity check index; ULN, upper limit of normal.

Adapted from: Pinzani, et al. *Nature Clinical Practice Gastroenterology & Hepatology* February 2008; 5(2): pg 102; and Reid AE. *Sleisenger and Fordtran's Gastrointestinal and Liver Disease: Pathophysiology/ Diagnosis/ Management* 2010, pg 1408.

> Treatment

- Give a clinical approach to the patient with suspected NAFLD/NASH.
  - Abnormal liver biochemistries and/or fatty liver on abdominal ultrasound

    ↓

  - Access for
    - ALD; obesity, T2DM, dyslipidemia, metabolic syndrome (treat appropriately)
    - Exclude HAV, HBV, HCV, HH, AIH, PBC, PSC

    ↓

  - Liver biopsy with/without FibroScan

    ↓

  - Lifestyle interventions
    - ↓ body weight by at least 3% to 5%
    - Diet
      - ↓ CHO (↓ fructose), ↓ fat, ↓ calories, ↓ caffeine (coffee, unfiltered, ≤ 2 cups/d)
    - Exercise
    - Avoid heavy use of alcohol (drinkers per week: men > 14, women > 7)

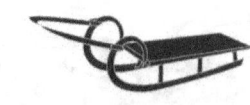

- o Insulin sensitizing agents
  - – Metformin
  - – Pioglitazone } For asscoaited metabolic syndrome
    - ▪ Weight gain; not ideal for all
- o Vitamin E 800 IU/ day
  - – Controversial use; no longer recommended in some guidelines
  - – "In patients with other types of liver disease who have co-existing NAFLD and NASH, there are no data to support the use of vitamin E or pioglitazone to improve the liver disease (Chalasani N, et al. Gastroenterology 2012; 142: 1592-1609).
  - – Note: increases risk of prostatic cancer in healthy men by 1.6 per 100 person years of vitamin E use.
- o Screen for
  - – Cirrhosis
  - – Esophageal varices
  - – Hepatic encephalopathy
  - – HCC (hepatocellular cancer)
- o Bariatric surgery
  - – ↓ fat, ↓ fibrosis
- o Consideration for liver transplantation (LT)
  - – Morbidity "obesity"
    - ▪ ↑ graft non-function
    - ▪ ↑ mortality 3 day, yr ½
    - ▪ ↑ comorbidities
    - ▪ ↑ recurrence
    - ▪ ↑ antirejection drug adverse effects

Note:

- o Patients being assessed for LT may have ascites and/or peripheral edema
  - – Corrections must be made for ascites/edema to estimate the potential LT patient's lean body mass (to exclude morbid obesity, and to thereby possibly remove this contraindication to LT).
- o Patients with NASH cirrhosis may come to liver transplantation (LT).
- o Lifelong immunosuppression will be required.
- o These immunosuppression agents may cause or worsen hepatic steatosis, or worsens components of the metabolic syndrome.

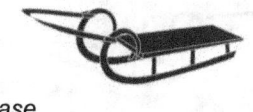

40

- Give the effects of corticosteroids, calcineurin inhibitors (CNI), and mToRi (mammalian target of rapamycin inhibitors on hepatic steatosis, weight gain, hypertension, dyslipidemia, and diabetes mellitus (DM).

| Drug class | Hepatic steatosis | Weight gain | Systemic hypertension | Dyslipidemia | New onset DM |
|---|---|---|---|---|---|
| Corticosteroids | ++ | ++ | + | + | ++ |
| CNI | - | + | ++ | ++ | ++ |
| mToRi | - | - | - | +++ | +/- |

Source: Newsome PN, et al. Gut 2012; 61: 484-500.

- Give the correction for fluid excess in estimates of lean body mass in liver patients with ascites and peripheral edema.

| Ascites | Ascites/kg | Peripheral edema / kg |
|---|---|---|
| o Minimal | 2.2 | 1 |
| o Moderate | 6 | 5 (to knees) |
| o Severe | ≥ 14 | 10 (to thighs) |

Source: Newsome PN, et al. Gut 2012; 61: 484-500.

- o Tacrolimus is preferred to cyclosporin as the CNI for LT, but it does have a major impact on the development of new onset DM or renal dysfunction; even then blood levels remain in the range of 5 to 8 ng/mL.
- o Mycophenolate permits the use of lower levels of tacrolimus.
- o mToRi may be used as first-line agent for HCC and as rescue therapy.

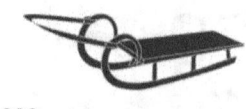

## ALCOHOLIC LIVER DISEASE (ALD)

➢ Definition

○ ALD is a disorder associated with the intake of ecessive amounts of alcohol over prolonged periods of time, leading to acute and/or chronic compensated/decompensated liver disease.

➢ Pathophysiology

○ Metabolizing enzymes
- ADH (alcohol dehydrogenase)
  ▪ Main enzyme at < 10 mM alcohol
- CYP2E1 (cytochrome P450 2E1)
  ▪ Main enzyme at > 10 mM alcohol self-inducible (alcohol increases CYP 2E1)
- Catalase
- ALDH (aldehyde dehydrogenase)

Alcohol ---$\xrightarrow{ADH}$---> Acetaldehyde

Acetaldehyde ---$\xrightarrow{ALDH}$---> Acetate

○ Role of acetaldehyde
- Acetaldehyde forms adduct with reactive residues (oxidatively modified proteins)
- Antibodies form against these adducts (e.g., MAA [malondialdehyde and acetaldehyde])

○ Methionine metabolism
- Methionine is related upon by MAT (methionine adenosyltransforate) to SAM (S-adenosyl-methionine)
  ▪ SAM usually is acted upon in the transmethylation pathway, forming SAH (S-adenosyl homocysteine)
  ▪ In ALD, there is ↓ MAT and ↓ SAM
  ▪ With SAM and ↓ transmethylation
  ▪ ↓ transmethylation - there is ↓ DNA RNA, histones, biogenic amines, phospholipids

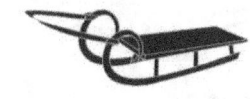

- o SAH (s-adenosyl histone)
  - – ↑ SAH and ↓ SAM/SAH ratio --→ ↓ transmethylation reactions → ↓ SAM
  - – ↓ SAM →
    - ↓ glutathione in mitochondria --→ mitochondria dysfunction
    - ↑ LPS (lipopolysaccharide)
      - – Stimulated release of TNF
      - – ↑ IL-10 from monocytic cells
    - ↑ homocysteine, ↑ SAH
  - – ↑ SAH and ↑ homocysteine
  - – ↑ hepatocyte sensitivity to TNF-mediated destruction
  - – ↑ hepatocyte sensitization from
    - ↓ glutathione in mitochondria
    - ↑ SAH
    - ↓ proteasomes
    - ↓ THF, ↓ methionine
  - – Alcohol ↓ folic and absorption and metabolism, including
    - ↓ 5-mTHF (5-methyltetrahydrofolate [THF])
- o Hypoxia
  - – Alcohol
  - – ↑ $O_2$ uptake by liver
  - – ↑ lobular O2 gradient
  - – ↑ NADH/NAD+ --→ ↑ HIF (hypoxia-inducible factor) 1 and 2 genes
  - – When alcohol ↓, HIF ↓
  - – Reperfusion injury, especially in centrilobular area
- o Mitochondria dysfunction
  - – ↑ TNF impairs function of mitochondria
  - – ↑ NADH/NAD$^+$ ---→ ↑ generation of superoxidase
  - – In ALD, ↓ transport of glutathione into mitochondria
  - – Glutathione-depleted mitochondria -→ ↑ sensitive to damage by TNF
  - – ↑ depolarization leads to
    - ↑ membrane permeability
    - ↑ apoptosis of hepatocytes

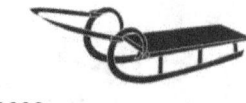

- o Redox state (oxidative-reduction state)
  - – Alcohol --→ ↑ CYP 2E1 --→ leaking of electrons --→ ↑ oxidative stress
  - – ↓ ATP
    - ▪ ↓ metabolism of
      - – Carbohydrate
      - – Fat (e.g., steatosis)
  - – ↑ oxidants: ↑ ROS (reactive oxygen species), ↑ RNS (reactive nitrogen species), ↑ oxidative stress
  - – ↓ antioxidants
  - – ↑ cell injury
    - ▪ ↑ membrane lipid peroxidation
    - ▪ ↑protein and DNA oxidation
  - – ↑ NF-kB (nuclear factor kappa B) --→ ↑ TNF
- o Dysregulated proteasome system
  - – ↓ removal of proteins damaged by oxidative stress
- o Dysregulated cytokines production
  - – Hepatocytes
    - ▪ IL-8, IL-18
    - ▪ Neutrophil chemotactic peptide
    - ▪ Angiogenesis factor
  - – Kupffer cells
    - ▪ NF-kB → TNF-α
    - ▪ IL-10
  - – Sinusoidal endothelial cells
    - ▪ Adhesion molecules
  - – Stellate cells
    - ▪ TGF-β → fibrosis
  - – ↑ intestinal permeability → ↑ LPS
  - – ↑ apoptosis of hepatocytes → ↑ release of IL-8 (neutrophil chemoattractant), IL-18 (primes TNFα release, and type 1 helper T cell response)
    - ▪ ↑ TNF-α inducible IL-6, IL-8, Il-18, MCP-1 (monocyte chemoattractant protein 1)
  - – As well as ↑ pro-inflammatory cytokines, there is ↓ anti-inflammatory cytokines
- o Apoptosis

Sleisenger and Fordtran's Gastrointestinal and Liver Disease. 9th Edition. Saunders/Elsevier, Philadelphia, 2010, page 1387; 10th Edition, 2016, pages 1431-1432.

44

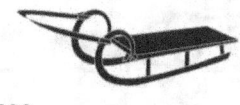

- o Autoimmune changes
  - – Mutation in CTLA-4G (cytotoxic T lymphocyte-associated antigen 4G) allele actives T cell function
  - – Hydroxyethyl radical from breakdown of alcohol modifies CYP 2E1
  - – Modifies CYP2E1 plus CTTA-4G mutation → ↑ anti-CYP2E1 autoantibodies
  - – Activation of HSC and Hepatic Fibrosis

---

**SO YOU WANT TO BE A HEPATOLOGIST!**

Women are at greater risk than men in developing alcohol-related liver injury, and for this injury to progress faster to more severe forms of ALD. "Although rates of metabolism and elimination of alcohol have been reported to be more rapid in women than men, when adjusted for liver volume, elimination rates are similar between genders" (Feldman M., et al. Sleisenger and Fordtran's Gastrointestinal and Liver Disease. 9th Edition. Saunders/Elsevier, Philadelphia, 2010, page 1388).

- • Give factors which are greater in women as than in men which may explain then greater risk of ALD in women than in men.
  - o LPS (endotoxemia)
  - o Lipid peroxidation
  - o Monocyte chemotactic protein mRNA
  - o NF-kB activation
  - o Polymorphism in the promoter regions of TNF-α and IL-10

---

- ➢ Histopathology
- o Steatosis
  - – Centrilobular
  - – Perivenular
  - – Microvesicular
  - – If combination of macro- plus microvesicular, then there is an ↑ risk of cirrhosis
- o Ballooning degeneration
- o Mallory bodies in damaged hepatocytes
- o Necroinflammatory reaction around damaged
  - – Polymorphonuclear leukocytes

45

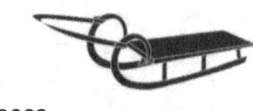

- o Central vein
  - – Sclerosing hyaline necrosis
- o Micronodular fibrosis, perisinusoidal
  - – Macronodular cirrhosis
- o Hepatic siderosis occurs in ~20% of ALD patients
- o Conditions which may mimic ALD
  - – NAFLD (non-alcoholic fatty liver disease)
  - – HH (hereditary hemochromatosis)
  - – BCS (Budd-Chiari syndrome)
  - – Amiodarone hepatotoxicity

- Give a comparison of viral vs alcoholic hepatitis, based on histology and physical, laboratory tests and liver histology.

|  | Viral Hepatitis | Alcoholic Hepatitis |
|---|---|---|
| o History | – Risk factors | ▪ Significant alcoholic intake |
| o Physical examination | – Mild hepatomegaly<br>– Extrahepatic stigmata not prominent | ▪ Moderate to marked hepatomegaly<br>▪ Florid stigamata, |
| o Laboratory tests | – AST variable | ▪ AST < 300 |
| o Liver histology | – Mononuclear cells<br>– Portal tract centred<br>– Ground glass cells (HBV)<br>– Special stains (HBV)<br>– Fat, esp. with HCV | ▪ Polymorphs<br>▪ Pericentral, diffuse<br>▪ Mallory hyaline<br>▪ Macrovesicular fat<br>- |

"Try not to become a man of success but a man of value."

Albert Einstein

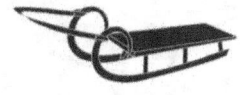

- ➤ Prognosis

- Give the 5 year survival rates of persons with alcoholic liver disease (ALD).

| Stages of ALD | 5 year Survival Rates |
|---|---|
| o Overall | 50% |
| o Steatosis | 75% |
| o Hepatitis | 50% |
| o Cirrhosis plus hepatitis | 35% |

- Give the 1 month survival rate of persons with acute alcoholic hepatitis (AH).

| Complications Associated with AH | 1-mon Survival Rate |
|---|---|
| o Alcoholic hepatitis plus HE | 50% |
| o Alcohol hepatitis plus HRS | 75% |

Abbreviations: HE, hepatic encephalopathy; HRS, hepatorenal syndrome; MR, mortality rate

- Give the 5 year survival rates of alcoholic cirrhosis.

| | Compensation | CTP Score | 5 year Survival Rate |
|---|---|---|---|
| o | Compensated | 5-7 | 60% |
| o | Decompensated | Ascites | < 50% |
| | | Variceal bleeding | |
| | | HE | ~20% |
| | | SBP | ~50% |
| | | HRS | Median, < 2 weeks |

- Give the 2 year survival rate in persons with ALD who practice abstinence from alcohol.

| After Hospital Admission for ALD | 2 year Survival Rate |
|---|---|
| o Abstinence | ~ 75% |
| o No abstinence | ~25% |

Abbreviations: CTP, Child-Turcotte-Pugh; HE, hepatic encephalopathy; HRS, hepatorenal syndrome; SBP, spontaneous bacterial peritonitis;

47

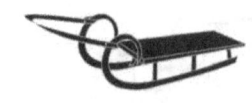

- Give **prognostic scoring systems** used for patients with alcoholic hepatitis (AH), the components used to calculate the scores, and the value of the score which reflects a poor prognosis.

| Name of Prognostic Test | Components | Poor Prognosis Score |
|---|---|---|
| o  MADDREY Score | MDF = 4.6 (patients PT – control PT) + total bilirubin (mg/dL) | ≥ 32 |
| o  MELD score* | MELD score = $3.8 \log_e$ (bilirubin (mg/dL) + 11.2 $\log_e$ (INR) + 9.6 $\log_e$ (creatinine) mg/dL | > 18 |

| | 1 | 2 | 3 |
|---|---|---|---|
| Age | < 50 | ≥ 50 | - |
| WBC | < 15 | ≥ 15 | |
| Urea (mmol/L) | < 15 | ≥ 5 | - |
| PT ratio | < 15 | 1.5 – 2.0 | > 2 |
| Bilirubin | < 7.3 | 7.3 – 14.6 | > 14.6 |
| | | | > 8 (day 1 or 7) |

*MELD, Model for End-Stage Liver Disease, available online calculator: www.mayoclinic.org/meld/mayomodel7.html

Source: O'Shea RS, et al. Alcoholic liver disease. Hepatology. 2010;51(1):307-28

- Give conditions which may accelerate the progression of ALD.
  - o HCV
    - – Look for focal lymphoid aggregates
    - – Portal inflammation
    - – Periportal or bridging fibrosis
    - – HCV + ALD have 10x ↑ risk of cirrhosis, and ↑ risk of HCC
  - o Obesity
  - o Smoking

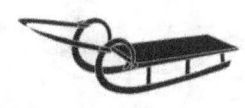

## SO YOU WANT TO BE A HEPATOLOGIST!

A male alcoholic with cirrhosis develops feminization.

- Give the mechanisms responsible for the shift of sex hormones from androgens to estrogens.

    o ↑ SHBC (sex hormone binding globulin) →
    - ↑ bound testosterone (T) ↓ free T
    - ↓ bound estrogen (E), ↑ free E

    o ↓ production of dehydroepiandrosterone → ↓ production of testosterone

    o Alcohol toxicity
    - On Leydig cells
    - On hypothalamic-pituitary-gonadal axis
        ▪ ↓ LH (luteinizing hormone)
        ▪ ↓ responsiveness to GRH (gonadotropin-releasing hormone)

On the basis of your knowledge of disordered coagulation and the balance between pro- and anticoagulant factors which develop in patients with cirrhosis.

- Give possible criticisms to the inclusion of the INR in the calculation of the MELD score.
    o Interlaboratory variability
    - The substantial interlaboratory variability with use of the standard international sensitivity index (ISI) to normalize varying sensitivities of thromboplastin reagents
    - …. This variability may result in as much as 25% difference in mean INR for a single patient sample assayed with different reagents"

➢ Laboratory

- Give laboratory abnormalities commonly seen in persons with alcoholic hepatitis.
    o Hematology
    - Macrocytic anemia (↑ MCV)
    - ↑ WBC
    - ↓ platelets

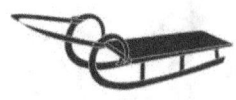

- o  Tests of liver function and injury
  - −  ↓ albumin
  - −  ↑ bilirubin
  - −  ↑ INR
  - −  ↑ AST/ALT (ratio of 1.5 to 2.5 and total increase <10-fold)
  - −  ↑ GGT
  - −  ↑ alkaline phosphatase (mild)
- o  General chemistry
  - −  ↑ blood sugar
  - −  ↑ uric acid
  - −  ↑ triglycerides
  - −  Ketosis
- o  Genetic testing
  - −  Genotypes of the aldehyde dehydrogenase (ALDH2-*2 allele) and the P4502EI (C2 allele)
  - −  Polymorphism of TNF2 at position -238 (G→A)
  - −  A→ e mutation in exon 1 of the Cytotoxic T-lymphocyte antigen-4 (CTLA-4) gene

Abbreviations: ALT, alanine aminotransferase; AST, aspartate aminotransferase; GGT, γ-glutamyltransferase; MCV, mean corpuscular volume.

Printed with permission:  Shah VH. *Mayo Clinic Gastroenterology and Hepatology Board Review* 2008: pg. 331.

XXXXXXXXXXXXXXXXXXXXXXXXXXXXXXXXXXXXXXXXXXXXXXXXXXXXXXXXXXXXXXXXXXXX

SO YOU WANT TO BE A HEPATOLOGIST!

The most sensitive and specific tests for recent alcohol use in the concentration of alcohol in the blood, urine, or breath.

- •  Give the disadvantage of using these measurements to prove recent alcohol take, and indicate how this has been addressed.
  - o  The concentration of alcohol in blood, urine or breath is influenced by the short half-life of alcohol in this body pools.
  - o  Biomarkers of recent alcohol abuse may have a longer T½, and thereby overcome the short half-life of alcohol
  - o  The most specific of these markers is CDT (carbohydrate-deficient transferrin)
  - o  The specificity of CDT increases markedly when CDT is combined with the measurement of GGTP.

XXXXXXXXXXXXXXXXXXXXXXXXXXXXXXXXXXXXXXXXXXXXXXXXXXXXXXXXXXXXXXXXXXXX

50

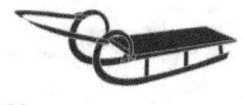

➤ Treatment

- Give treatments for ALD (not specifically acute alcoholic hepatitis) which have proven to be of benefit.
  - o Risk assessment
    - – MDF score (> 32)
    - – MELD score (> 20)
  - o Manage alcohol withdrawal and alcoholism
  - o Abstinence
    - – Baclofen (GABA [gamma aminobutyric acid] agonist), naloxone
    - – Psychological and addiction services support
  - o Treat associated alcohol withdrawal
    - – Monitoring
    - – Hydration
    - – Sedation (Ativan)
  - o Smoking cessation
  - o Obesity reduction

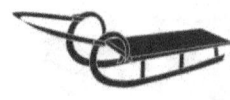

- Correction of malnutrition (protein/calorie)
  - Aggressive nutritional support
  - Enteral nutrition
- Treat complications of cirrhosis, e.g., esophageal varices, hepatic encephalopathy, ascites, spontaneous bacterial peritonitis, hepatorenal syndrome
- Screen for hepatocellular cancer
- Update appropriate vaccination
- Appropriate-for-age cancer screening
- Acute alcoholic hepatitis
- Glucocorticosteroids for DF > 32, and with **no**
  - GI bleeding needing blood transfusion
  - Active infection
  - Hepatorenal syndrome
  - 40 mg prednisone od; reassess at day 7 using Lille score to determine if it is beneficial to continue corticosteroids
  - If patient responds, then (↑ 1 yr survival
- Other agents have been subjected to experimental use in AH.
  - Pentoxifylline (non-selective phosphodiesterase inhibitor)
    - Recent studies signal the possibility that this may do harm, and it is not standard of care.
- Liver transplantation (LT)
  - Some centres report lower rates, especially in those who continue to drink or smoke (↑ risk of post-operative cancer of pharynx, esophagus, stomach)
  - AH
    - One centre (Paris) reported benefit in a group of highly selected patients; this study is being repeated in USA.
- Most liver transplantation centres require a 6 mon period of abstinence before considering patient with ALD to be a possible LT candidate.
- Even with 6 mon abstinence, a sizable proportion of previous abstinent ALD patient will resume alcohol intake after LT, allow it in often only modest amounts.

52

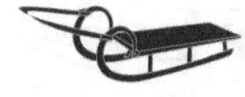

## AUTOIMMUNE HEPATITIS (AIH)

➢ Definition: "AIH is a disorder of unknown cause characterized by unresolving inflammation of the liver and by the presence of interface [limiting plate of the portal tract is disrupted by a lymphoplasmacytic infiltrate] on histologic examination, … hypergammaglobulinemia" (Sleisenger and Fordtran's Gastrointestinal and Liver Disease. 10th Edition. Saunders/Elsevier, Philadelphia, 2016, page 1493), and autoantibodies".

➢ Demography

- o Varies world-wide
- o In North America, incidence ~ $2/10^5$ / year
- o Prevalence ~ $17/10^5$

---

**SO YOU WANT TO BE A HEPATOLOGIST!**

- Give the comparison of non-hereditary versus hereditary AIH (aka APECED*).

| Feature | Non-hereditary | Hereditary |
|---|---|---|
| o Gender effect | F > M | F = M |
| o Gene mutation | No | ▪ Single-gene mutation on chromosome 21q22.3 of AIRE (autoimmune regulator)<br>▪ Autosomal recessive, complete gene penetrance |
| o HLA predisposition | HLA-DR3 (DRB1*0304) | No |
| o Response to therapy | – 65% achieve remission within 3 years<br>– Therapy improves 10-year survival rate to 93% | ▪ Severe AIH<br>▪ Poor response to usual theerapy |

Abbreviation: APECED, autoimmune polyendocrinopathycandidiasis – ectodermal dystrophy

---

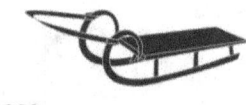

*MASTERING THE BOARDS*
*Hepatology & Pancreaticobiliary Disease*

A.B.R. Thomson

➢ Pathophysiology

• Give the immunopathophysiology of primary/idiopathic AIH.

  o Unknown and possible environment antigenic peptide (molecular mimicry) --→ inciting antigen fits in the antigen-binding groove of the class II DR molecule of the MHC antigen presenting cells (in USA/Canada, DRB1 gene, susceptibility alleles DRB1*0301 and DRB1*0401)

  o The DR molecule-antigen complex of the APC (antigen-presenting cell) interacts with the antigen receptor of CD4+ T-helper cells (1st signal).

  o The CD28 molecule on the surface of CD4+ t-helper cell binds to the B7 ligand on the surface of the APC" (2nd signal) (Feldman M., et al. Sleisenger and Fordtran's Gastrointestinal and Liver Disease. 9th Edition. Saunders/Elsevier, Philadelphia, 2010, page 1464).

  o CD4+ T-helper cells differentiate into Th1 or Th2 T-cells

  o The cytokine milieu of Th1 and Th2 cytokines is regulated

  o This balance between Th1 and Th2 may be disturbed by
    – ↓ NKT (intrahepatic natural killer T cells)
    – ↓ regulation of CD8+ T cell proliferation by
    – T-reg (T-regulatory CD4+ CD25+) cells

54

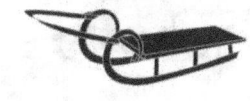

- o Hepatocyte damage is caused by
    - – Cell-mediated cytotoxicity (regulated by type 1 cytokines), or
    - – Antibody-dependent cell-mediated cytotoxicity (regulated by type 2 cytokines), or by
    - – Both mechanisms
- o Th1 (type 1 cytokine) pathway of activated CD4+ t-helper cells is stimulated by polymorphism of
    - – TNF A*2 (TNF gene)
    - – TNF receptor superfamily gene (FAS)
    - – CTLA4 (the cytotoxic T lymphocyte antigen 4 gene)
    - – TNFRSF6 (FAS gene phenotype at position – 670)
- o These polymorphisms and Th1 T-cells
    - – Sensitize cytotoxic T cells
    - – ↑ cell-mediated cytotoxicity
    - – ↑ apoptosis of hepatocytes
- o The cytokine pathways are increase by ↓ activity of T-reg (T-regulatory) cells

- o Th2 (type 2 cytokine) pathway of activated CD4+ T-helper cells causes differentiation of B cells into plasma cells
    - – Plasma cells → ↑ production of immunoglobulin
    - – Immunoglobulins → antibody-mediated cellular toxicity

---

SO, IF YOU HAVEN'T GIVEN UP AND THROWN IN THE TOWEL, AND YOU STILL WANT TO BE A SUPER-STAR HEPATOLOGIST!

- • Give infectious agents which have homology with epitopes of CYP2D6, and are recognized by anti-LKM1.

Organisms showing molecular mimicry / molecular footprint / share motif with anti-LKM1 include

- o HCV
- o CMV
- o HSV

"These molecular mimicries may result in cross-reactivity antibodies and support the hypothesis that repeated viral infections may break self-tolerance and cause disease."

---

55

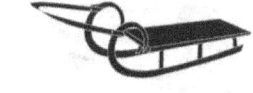

- Give prescription **medications**, OTC preparations or herbs which may induce or unmask an AIH-like syndrome.

  o Antibiotics
    – Minocycline
    – Nitrofurantoin
    – Rifampin
    – Interferon
    – INH

  o Metabolic
    – Orlistat
    – Statins
    – Propyl thiouracil

  o Antihypertensives
    – Alpha methyldopa

  o Herbs
    – St. John's Wort
    – Chapannal leaf
    – Black cohosh

  o Immune
    – Anti-TNF therapy

Abbreviation: OTC, over-the-counter

Printed with permission: Heathcote EJ. *2007 AGA Institute Spring Postgraduate Course Syllabus*: 96.

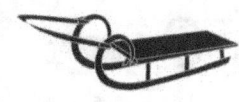

- ➤ Types/laboratory
- Give a classification of autoimmune hepatitis (AIH) based on autoantibody profiles of patients.
  - o Type 1 AIH
    - Sudden onset of symptoms in 40%, including fulminant hepatic failure
    - 38% have associate "autoimmune" disorders
    - F:M ratio of 3.6:1
    - Usual age of presentation, 50 years
    - Serum antibodies
      - ANA (anti-nuclear antibody)
      - SMA (smooth muscle antibodies
      - ANA plus SMA
      - Anti-actin
      - PANCA (perinuclear anti-neutrophil cytoplasmic antibodies; aka ANNA, anti-neutrophil nuclear antigens)
      - ↑ IgG
  - o Type 2 AIH
    - Usually diagnosed in children aged 2 to 4 years positive for anti-LKM1 (liver-kidney microsome) 1 expression of anti-LKM1 is associated with DB1*07 anti-LKM1 reduce the activity of CYP2D6
  - o Type 3 (M, 30) ASLA/LP+
  - o Overlap syndrome AMA-neg. PBC, PSC, AMA-

Adapted from: Czaja AJ. *Sleisenger and Fordtran's Gastrointestinal and Liver Disease* 2006. pg. 1872-1875; and 2010, pg. 1467.

- Give a comparison of type 1 vs type 2 AIH.

| Feature | Type 1 AIH | Type 2 AIH |
|---|---|---|
| o Characteristic autoantibodies | ANA | Anti-LKM-1 antibody |
| | ASMA | Anti-LC-1 antibody |
| | Anti-actin antibody | |
| | Anti-SLA/LP antibodies | |
| | 25% of patients ANA negative | |

57

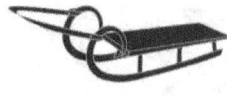

| Feature | Type 1 AIH | Type 2 AIH |
|---|---|---|
| o Geographical variation | Worldwide | Worldwide (especially high in Germany (~20% of all AIH) |
| o Age at presentation | All ages | Usually childhood and young adulthood |
| o Sex (F:M) | 3:1 | 10:1 |
| o Clinical phenotype | Variable | Generally severe |
| o Histopathological features at presentation | Broad range: mild disease to cirrhosis | Generally advanced, ↑ inflammation/cirrhosis common |
| o Treatment failure | Rare | Common |
| o Relapse after drug withdrawal | Variable | Common |
| o Need for long-term maintenance | Variable | Approximately 100% |

- o Note:
    - Immunofluorescence is the traditional method for measuring the repertoire of conventional autoantibodies in AIH
    - Many laboratories (especially those in the USA) are increasingly using ELISA-based methods, especially for anti-LKM antibodies.
    - In relation to anti-LKM-1 antibodies, these may be erroneously reported as detectable anti-mitochondral antibodies.

Abbreviations: ANA, antinuclear antibody; ASMA, anti-smooth muscle antibody; anti-LC, anti-liver cytosol; anti-LKM, liver kidney microsomal antibody; anti-SLA/LP, soluble liver antigen/liver pancreas antigen.

Printed with permission: Gleeson D, Heneghan MA; British Society of Gastroenterology. British Society of Gastroenterology (BSG) guidelines for management of autoimmune hepatitis. Gut. 2011;60(12):1611-29, Table2.

Please see: Swan MG. Chapter 58. In: Therapeutic Choices. Grey J, Ed. 6th Edition, Canadian Pharmacists Association: Ottawa, ON, 2011, Table 5: Autoimmune Hepatitis, page 778.

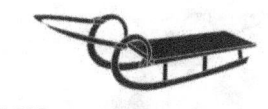

- ➤ Clinical
  - ○ Asymptomatic ~ 40% (70% may later become symptomatic)
  - ○ Spontaneous resolution ~ 15%
  - ○ Compensated cirrhosis ~ 40%
  - ○ Esophageal varices (EV) ~ 55%

- Give clinical presentations of AIH.
  - ○ Acute hepatitis
  - ○ Fulminant hepatitis
  - ○ Asymptomatic chronic hepatitis +/- cirrhosis
  - ○ Symptomatic chronic hepatitis +/- cirrhosis
  - ○ "Burned out" decompensated cirrhosis +/-
  - ○ *De novo* or recurrent AIH after liver transplantation (alloimmune)
  - ○ AIH with overlapping PBC/PSC/AMA-neg PBC
  - ○ Suspected from liver disease associated with other conditions
  - ○ HCC (hepatocellular cancer)

- Give immune disorders which are associated with AIH.

  | | |
  |---|---|
  | ○ Skin, eye | – Iritis |
  | | – Gingivitis |
  | | – Dermatitis herpetiformis |
  | | – Erythema nodosum |
  | | – Lichen planus |
  | | – Pyoderma gangrenosum |
  | ○ CNS/PNS | – Peripheral neuropathy |
  | | – Myasthenia gravis |
  | ○ Thyroid | – Autoimmune thyroiditis |
  | | – Graves disease |
  | ○ Heart, lung | – Pleuritis |
  | | – Fibrosing alveolitis |
  | | – Pericarditis |

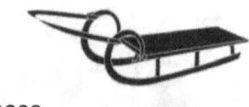

- o Pancreas
  - Insulin-dependent diabetes
  - Autoimmune pancreatitis
- o Gut, liver
  - Celiac disease
  - Ulcerative colitis
  - Autoimmune sclerosing cholangitis
  - Pernicious anemia (PA)
  - Autoimmune cholangitis (PSC)
- o Kidney
  - Glomerulonephritis (immune complex)
- o Blood
  - Coombs- positive hemolytic anemia
  - Cryoglobulinemia
  - Idiopathic thrombocytopenic purpura (ITP)
  - Pernicious anemia + ITP (Evan syndrome)
  - Neutropenia
- o MSK
  - Rheumatoid arthritis
  - Sjögren syndrome
  - Synovitis
  - Systemic lupus erythematous
  - Focal myositis

Abbreviation: MSK, musculoskeletal system

Printed with permission: Czaja AJ. *Mayo Clinic Gastroenterology and Hepatology Board Review* 2008: pg. 398.

---

Clinical Cautions

- o The presence of symptoms of AIH does not refect the hepatic histology – "histological findings, including the frequency of cirrhosis, are similar in asymptomatic and symptomatic patients….."
- o "the asymptomatic state does not preclude the need for glucocorticoid therapy if other objective manifestations of disease activity are present or emerge, and close surveillance of these patients for worsening inflammation is justified".
- o Untreated asymptomatic mild AIH still progress, and there are no clinical indices that predict the course of the disease".

(Sleisenger and Fordtran's Gastrointestinal and Liver Disease. 9th Edition. Saunders/Elsevier, Philadelphia, 2010, page 1471).

---

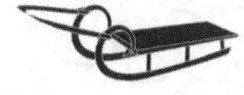

> Diagnosis

- o The diagnosis of AIH is based on exclusion and probabilities expressed through the use of **scoring systems**.

- o Other causes of chronic liver disease with similar features need to be excluded, including conditions which overlap with AIH (PBC, PSC, AIH with cholestatic features, autoantibody-negative AIH).

- o There are scoring systems which may be used to assist in making a definite or a probable diagnosis: Please see Sleisenger and Fordtran's Gastrointestinal and Liver Disease. 9th Edition. Saunders/Elsevier, Philadelphia, 2010, Table 88.1 and 88.2, page 1463; 10th Edition, 2016, Table 90.2 and 90.3, page 1499.

- • Give the **definite and probable criteria** for the diagnosis of AIH.

| Definite AIH | Probable AIH |
|---|---|
| o Exclude other causes of chronic liver disease | |
| – Normal AAT phenotype | – Partial AAT deficiency |
| – Normal ceruloplasmin level | – Abnormal copper or ceruloplasmin level but Wilson disease excluded |
| – Normal iron and ferritin levels | – Nonspecific iron or ferritin abnormalities |
| – No active hepatitis A, B, or C infection | – No active hepatitis A, B, or C infection |
| – Daily alcohol <25 g | – Daily alcohol <50 g |
| – No recent hepatotoxic drugs | – No recent hepatotoxic drugs |
| – Predominant serum aminotransferase abnormality | – Predominant serum aminotransferase abnormality |
| o Suggestive laboratory tests | |
| – Globulin, $\gamma$-globulin, or IgG level $\geq$1.5 times normal | – Hypergammaglobulinemia of any degree |
| – ANA, SMA, or anti-LKM1 $\geq$1:80 in adults and $\geq$1:20 in children; no AMA | – ANA, SMA, or anti-LKM1$\geq$1:40 in adults; other autoantibodies |

*MASTERING THE BOARDS*
*Hepatology & Pancreaticobiliary Disease*

A.B.R. Thomson

| Definite AIH | Probable AIH |
| --- | --- |

o Liver biopsy

- Interface hepatitis–moderate to severe
- No biliary lesions, granulomas, or prominent changes suggestive of another liver disease

- Interface hepatitis–moderate to severe
- No biliary lesions, granulomas, or prominent changes suggestive of another disease

Printed with permission: Czaja AJ. *Mayo Clinic Gastroenterology and Hepatology Board Review* 2008: pg. 392.

o **Simplified scoring system** for diagnosis of autoimmune hepatitis

| Category | Variable | Score |
| --- | --- | --- |
| o Autoantibodies | | |
| – Antinuclear antibodies (ANA) | 1:40 | +1 |
| – Smooth muscle antibodies | >1:80 | +2 |
| – Antibodies to liver kidney microsome type 1 | >1:40 | +2 |
| – Antibodies to soluble liver antigen | Positive | +2 |
| o Immunoglobulin level | | |
| – Immunoglobulin G | >Upper limit of normal | +1 |
| | >1.1 times upper limit of normal | +2 |
| o Histologic findings | | |
| – Morphologic features | Compatible with autoimmune hepatitis | +1 |
| | Typical of autoimmune hepatitis | +2 |
| o Viral disease | | |
| – Absence of viral hepatitis | No viral markers | +2 |
| o Pre-treatment aggregate score | | |
| – Definite diagnosis | | >7 |
| – Probable diagnosis | | 6 |

Adapted from: Hennes EM, Zeniya M, Czaja AJ, et al. Simplified diagnostic criteria for autoimmune hepatitis. *Hepatology* 2008;48:169-76.

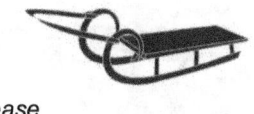

Clinical Words of Wisdom – the need for liver biopsies in AIH

- o "evaluation of liver tissue [doing a liver biopsy] before drug withdrawal is essential to establish remission because histologic activity may be present in 55% of patients who satisfy other requirements for remission".

- o "…histological improvement lags behind clinical and histologic resolution by three to eight months….."

- o "……complete resolution of the clinical and histological manifestations of the disease [AIH] does not preclude relapse after drug withdrawal" (Sleisenger and Fordtran's Gastrointestinal and Liver Disease. 9th Edition. Saunders/Elsevier, Philadelphia, 2010, page 1473; 10th Edition, 2016, page 1508).

- o **Revised** original scoring system for the diagnosis of autoimmune hepatitis

| Category | Variable | Score |
|---|---|---|
| o Gender | Female | +2 |
| o AP/AST | >3 | -2 |
| | <1.5 | +2 |
| o Gamma globulin or IgG level above normal | >2.0 | +3 |
| | 1.5-2.0 | +2 |
| | 1.0-1.5 | +1 |
| | >1.0 | 0 |
| o ANA, SMA, or anti-LKM1 titer | >1:80 | +3 |
| | 1:80 | +2 |
| | 1:40 | +1 |
| | <1:40 | 0 |
| o AMA | Positive | -4 |
| o Viral markers | Positive | -3 |
| | Negative | +3 |
| o Drug history | Yes | -4 |
| | No | +1 |
| o Alcohol | <25 g/day | +2 |
| | >60 g/day | -2 |

63

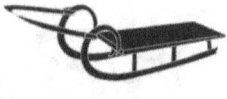

| Category | Variable | Score |
|---|---|---|
| o HLA | – DR3 or DR4 | +1 |
| o Immune disease | – Thyroiditis, ulcerative colitis, synovitis, others | +2 |
| o Other liver define autoantibodies | – Anti SLA, anti actin, anti LC1, Panca | +2 |
| o Histologic features | – Interface hepatitis | +3 |
| | – Plasmacytic infiltrate | +1 |
| | – Rosettes | +1 |
| | | -5 |
| | – None of above | -3 |
| | – Biliary changes | -3 |
| | – Other features | |
| o Treatment response | – Complete | +2 |
| | – Relapse | +3 |

o Pre-treatment aggregate score
  – Definite diagnosis >15
  – Probable diagnosis 10-15

o Post treatment aggregate score
  – Definite diagnosis >17
  – Probable diagnosis 12-17

Adapted from: Alvarez F, Berg PA, Bianchi FB, et al. International Autoimmune Hepatitis Group report: Review of criteria for diagnosis of autoimmune hepatitis. *J Hepatol* 1999; 31: 929-38.

➤ Prognosis

• Give the factors associated with clinically significant endpoints in autoimmune hepatitis (AIH).

| Endpoint | ↑ Relapse (off treatment) | Progressive Fibrosis / Cirrhosis | Liver-related Death / Transplantation |
|---|---|---|---|
| o Frequency | 50–90% | 10–50% | 10–20% |
| o Factors | | | |

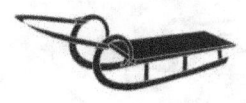

| Endpoint | ↑ Relapse (off treatment) | Progressive Fibrosis / Cirrhosis | Liver-related Death / Transplantation |
|---|---|---|---|
| ○ Frequency | 50–90% | 10–50% | 10–20% |
| − At presentation | Long symptom duration<br><br>↑ serum globulin<br><br>LKM antibody positive<br><br>SLA/LP positive or no immune markers | ↓ albumin and coagulopathy<br><br>Confluent necrosis on biopsy | Females<br><br>African-American men<br><br>Type 2 AIH and SLA positive AIH<br><br>Cirrhosis<br><br>Confluent necrosis |
| ○ On treatment | Short treatment duration<br><br>Long time to remission | Persistent AST elevation (failure of AST to halve in 6 months)<br><br>Failure to achieve remission over 2 years<br><br>Persistent inflammation on liver biopsy | Poor response, long time to achieve remission, persistent serum AST elevation |
| ○ Pretreatment withdrawal | Raised serum ALT or AST<br><br>Raised serum globulin IgG<br><br>Liver biopsy with any inflammation, or with portal tract plasma cells | | |
| ○ Subsequently | | Multiple relapses | Multiple relapses<br><br>Development of cirrhosis |

Abbreviations: ALT, alanine aminotransferase; AST, aspartate aminotransferase; LKM-1, liver kidney microsomal-1 antibody; SLA/LP, soluble liver antigen/liver pancreas antigen.

Printed with permission: Gleeson D, Heneghan MA; British Society of Gastroenterology. British Society of Gastroenterology (BSG) guidelines for management of autoimmune hepatitis. Gut. 2011;60(12):1611-29, Table 6.

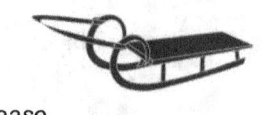

*MASTERING THE BOARDS*
*Hepatology & Pancreaticobiliary Disease*

A.B.R. Thomson

- ➢ Treatment
  - o Predictors of response to treatment of autoimmune hepatitis (AIH)
    - – Low levels of anti-α-actinin at baseline are independent predictors of response.
    - – Autoantibodies against filamentous-actin and α-actinin.
    - – Can be used as predictors of response to treatment in patients with AIH 1
    - – HLA-DR3 negative

Please see Feldman M., et al. Sleisenger and Fordtran's Gastrointestinal and Liver Disease. 9th Edition. Saunders/Elsevier, Philadelphia, 2010, Table 88.4, page 1467, for a summary of the "Variant Forms of Autoimmune Hepatitis"; also see 10th Edition, 2016, pages 1500-1501.

  - o The **Mayo Clinic treatment schedules** for adults with severe autoimmune hepatitis

| Treatment duration (weeks) | Combination therapy | | Prednisone monotherapy (mg daily) |
| --- | --- | --- | --- |
| | Prednisone (mg daily) | Azathioprine (mg daily) | |
| 1 | 30 | 50 | 60 |
| 1 | 20 | 50 | 40 |
| 2 | 15 | 50 | 30 |
| Maintenance until end point | 10 | 50 | 20 |

Printed with permission: Loza AJM, and Czaja AJ. *Nature Clinical Practice Gastroenterology & Hepatology* 2007; 4(4): pg. 204.

  - o Treatment choices depending upon response to initial treatment
    - – Continue prednisone or prednisone plus azathioprine until
    - – Remission
      - ▪ "......absence of symptoms, resolution of all laboratory indices of active inflammation and histologic improvement of normal liver tissue or inactive cirrhosis" (Sleisenger and Fordtran's Gastrointestinal and Liver Disease. 9th Edition. Saunders/Elsevier, Philadelphia, 2010, page 1473).
    - – Treatment failure
      - ▪ "worsening of the serum AST or bilirubin levels by at least 67% of previous values, progressive histological activity, or onset of ascites or encephalopathy"

66

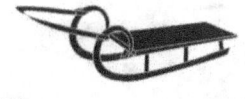

- Incomplete response: "….improvement that is insufficient to satisfy remission criteria" (Feldman M., et al. Sleisenger and Fordtran's Gastrointestinal and Liver Disease. 9th Edition. Saunders/Elsevier, Philadelphia, 2010, page 1474).
- Drug toxicity
- Relapse
  - Occurs in 50% in 6 months
  - ~ 75% in 3 years
  - Defined as "… the reappearance of histologic disease after discontinuation of drug therapy" after previous achieved remission
  - Rational for maintenance therapy: repeated relapse and re-treatment leads to
    - ↑ cirrhosis
    - ↑ hepatic failure
    - ↑ need for liver transplantation
    - ↑ drug adverse effects
    - ↑ mortality

| Clinical Event | Treatments Choices | | | |
|---|---|---|---|---|
| | 1st | 2nd | 3rd | 4t |
| ○ Treatment failure | Prednisone (30 mg daily) and Azathioprine (150 mg daily), or prednisone alone (60 mg daily) | Prednisone (30 mg daily) Plus Mercaptopurine (1.5 mg/kg body weight daily) | Cyclosporin (5-6 mg/kg body weight daily) or prednisone (30 mg daily) plus Mycophenoate mofetil (2 g daily) | Tacrolimus (4 mg twice daily) |
| ○ Drug toxicity | Azathioprine (2 mg/kg body weight daily) if prednisone intolerant | Prednisone (20 mg daily) if Azathioprine intolerant | Budesonide (3 mg twice daily) | UDCA (13-15 mg/kg body weight daily) |
| ○ Incomplete Response | Prednisone maintenance (≤ 10 mg daily) if serum AST level < three times normal value | Azathioprine maintenance (2 mg/kg body weight daily) if serum AST level <threetimes normal value) | Budesonide Maintenance (3 mg twice daily) | UDCA Maintenance (13-15 mg/kg body weight daily) |

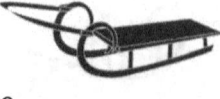

| Clinical Event | Treatments Choices | | | |
|---|---|---|---|---|
| | 1st | 2nd | 3rd | 4t |
| o Relapse | Azathioprine maintenance (2 mg/kg body weight daily) if serum AST level <three times normal value | Prednisone Maintenance reduced to (< 10 mg daily) if serum AST level <three times normal value | Mycophenolate mofetil maintenance (2 g daily) | Cyclosporin Maintenance (5-6 mg/kg body weight daily) |

Abbreviations: AST, aspartate aminotransferase; UDCA, ursodeoxycholic aid

Printed with permission: Loza A, et al. *Nature Clinical Practice Gastroenterology & Hepatology* 2007; 4(4): pg. 206.

- o Liver transplantion

Clinical Tip – Early Failure of Treatment and Need for Liver Transplantation.

- – Profile of patient who needs to be considered early for liver transplantation include:
  - ▪ Decompensated patients with biopsy evidence of multilobular necrosis, in whom
  - ▪ Hyperbilirubinemia does not improve, and
  - ▪ At least one other laboratory test does not return to normal

- Give the complications of liver transplantation (LT) which are more common for AIH than compared with non-autoimmune liver disease.

  - o Acute rejection

  - o Chronic rejection

  - o Steroid-resistant rejection

  - o Difficult in stopping steroids

- ➤ **AIH overlap** (variant) **syndromes**
  - o AIH plus PBC
    - – Low titres of PBC-specific M2 mitochondrial antigens
    - – AMA may come and go in 18% of persons with AIH

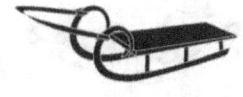

- o AIH plus PSC/PSC in adults, 41% of AIH who have
  - – Cholestatic 'la' findings
  - – Associated IBD (especially UC)
  - – Failure to respond to steroids
  - – Have cholangiographic changes of PSC
  - – 54% of persons with PSC have features supporting a diagnosis of AIH (definite, or probable)
  - – The duct changes in AIH plus PSC may be only in the small ducts ("small duct PSC")
  - – In children with AIH
  - – Large duct small duct PSC
  - – AMI-positive PBC
  - – AMA-negative PBC
  - – Autoimmune cholangitis

- o Autoantibody negative AIH
  - – No antibodies, but
  - – Usually abnormal
    - HLA (HLA-D3 or DR4)
    - Interface hepatitis

- Give the difference in the treatment of AMA-positive and –negative AIH (autoimmune hepatitis).

  - o AIH ⇌ PBC in 10% to 15%, causing 2 overlap syndromes

  - o AMA-positive AIH  steroids, azathioprine (treat as per guideline for AIH, type I; may also be ANA-positive)

  - o AMA- negative PBC  (aka autoimmune cholangiopathy) steroids, UDCA (ursodeoxycholic acid)

Please see: Swan MG. Chapter 58. In: Therapeutic Choices. Grey J, Ed. 6th Edition, Canadian Pharmacists Association: Ottawa, ON, 2011, Table 3: Hepatic Encephalopathy, page 775.

  - o AIH plus HCV infection
    - – About 10% of persons with AIH also have HCV infection, and about half of HCV patients have features suggestive or AIH, such as
      - Autoantibodies
      - Other immune diseases, or
      - Both of above
    - – The treatment of AIH will affect the HCV, and vice versa. Treatment is usually focused on the predominant component, AIH or HCV.
    - – It is often best to first treat the AIH, because if interferon is used in the treatment of HCV, it would worsen the AIH.

69

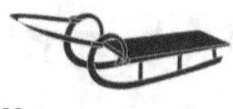

- Give the features which help to distinguish between autoimmune predominant AIH, or AIH plus HCV (HCV predominant).

| Feature | AIH predominant | HCV predominant |
|---|---|---|
| o Associated diseases | – "autoimmune" disorders in 38% | "immune complex" |
| o Autoantibodies | – Multiple | One |
| o Symptomatic cryoglobulinemia | – Rare | Common |
| o AST, IgG | ↑↑ | ↑ |
| o Histology** | – Panacinar hepatitis<br>– Interface hepatitis<br>– Portal plasma cells | – Steatosis<br>– Portal lymphoid aggregates |
| o Immune complex disorders | – Vasculitis<br>– Glomerulonephritis | |

- Give the treatments of the overlap/variant of AIH.

| Variant Syndrome | Salient Features | Empiric Treatment Strategies |
|---|---|---|
| o AIH and primary biliary cholangitis (PBC) | – AMA positivity<br>– Cholestatic and hepatitic tests<br>– Increased serum IgM and IgG levels | ▪ Corticosteroids if serum ALP is ≤ twice ULN<br>▪ Add ursodeoxycholic acid (UDCA) if serum ALP is > twice ULN and/or florid duct lesions in liver tissue |
| o AIH and primary sclerosing cholangitis (PSC) | – Ulcerative colitis<br>– ↑↑↑ risk of CRC<br>– Pruritus<br>– Cholestatic and hepatic tests<br>– ALP:AST>1.5 | ▪ Corticosteroids |

| Variant syndrome | Salient Features | Empiric Treatment Strategies |
|---|---|---|
| o AIH and cholangitis (possibly AMA-negative biliary sclerosis) | – Abnormal cholangiogram<br>– Fatigue<br>– Pruritus<br>– Cholestatic and hepatitic tests<br>– AMA negative<br>– ANA and/or SMA positive<br>– Normal cholangiogram | ▪ Prednisone, ursodeoxycholic acid, or both, depending on hepatic and cholestatic components |

Abbreviations: ALP, Alkaline phosphatase; AMA, antimitochondrial antibodies; ANA, antinuclear antibodies; AST, aspartate aminotransferase; CRC, colorectal cancer; SMA, smooth muscle antibodies; ULN, upper limit of normal.

Adapted from: *Sleisenger & Fordtran's Gastrointestinal and Liver Disease: Pathophysiology/Diagnosis/Management* 10th Edition. Saunders/Elsevier, Philadelphia, 2016, Table 90-4, page 1504.

- Give **preventative measures** about which to advise patients with AIH treated with prednisone +/- azathioprine.

❖ General

  o Monitor for weight gain

  o Supplement with calcium, vitamin D, +/- bisphosphonates

  o Monitor blood sugar, lipids, fat soluble vitamins

  o Monitor CBC, ALT (if on Azathioprine)

  o Annual checks for BP, cataract, glaucoma, BMD, Pap' smear, esophageal varices

  o Check stools for ova/parasites after foreign travel

  o "Stop" order on Rx

  o Screening mammography, colonoscopy

  o Access for depression

  o Stress high doses of steroids, if necessary

  o Wear medical alert bracelet.

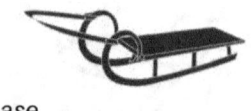

- o Avoid stopping steroids suddenly (Addisonian crisis, recurrence of AIH)
- o Avoid unplanned pregnancy; consider avoiding pregnancy if portal hypertension is marked; contraception
- o Drug interactions
- o Immunizations (see below)

❖ Specific

- o If cirrhotic: avoid sedation, NSAIDs, anesthesia, interferon
- o If cirrhotic, screen for HCC
- o Avoid vaccination with varicella, MMR, yellow fever
- o Vaccination for H. influenza, HAV, HBV, pneumococcus (hyposplenism)
- o Assess for esophageal varices for primary prevention with banding or beta blockers (avoid use in pregnancy – fetal hypoglycemia)
- o Assess for Ascites and spontaneous bacterial peritonitis (SBP)

Adapted from: Heathcote J. *Am J Gastroenterol* 2006;101:S630–S632.


➢ Prognosis

- o Death from bleeding EV (esophageal varices) ~ 20%
- o Relapse may occur after drug withdrawal
- o The clinical course is influenced by the level of ALT and gamma globulins, serology (anti-soluble liver antigen (SLA), anti-asialoglycoprotein receptor (ASGPR), anti-chromatin), liver biopsy (bridging or multilobular necrosis, or cirrhosis), HLA status, and response to treatment. Each of the above is associated on adverse outcome.
- o The MELD (model for end-stage liver disease) score predicts survival
    - – Based on degree of impaired liver function, not affected by cause or presence of cirrhosis
    - – MELD ≥ 12 (at presentation), 97% of these persons will fail steroid therapy

For the details of these prognostic factors and outcome, please see Sleisenger and Fordtran's Gastrointestinal and Liver Disease. 9th Edition. Saunders/Elsevier, Philadelphia, 2010, Table 88.5, page 1469.

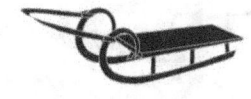

**PRIMARY BILIARY CHOLANGITIS** (PBC; previously called primary biliary cirrhosis)

➢ Definition: PBC is an autoimmune liver disease characterized by specific antibodies, a characteristic liver biopsy (inflammatory distraction of the intralobular bile ducts), and progressing to chronic cholestasis, biliary cirrhosis, and complications related to portal hypertension and liver failure.

➢ Demography

  o F >> M, 9:1

  o Age of diagnosis
    – Usually 30 to 60 years

  o Incidence
    – $3/10^5$

  o Prevalence
    – $40/10^5$

➢ Pathogenesis

• Give the pathoimmunology of PBC (primary biliary cholangitis).

  o Immune-mediated response to an unknown antigen (molecular mimicry)

  o Activation of CD4+ and CD8+ T lymphocytes, B cells, and NK cells

  o Aberrant polyclonal activation of B cells (↑ IgG, IgM)

  o Breakdown of tolerance against mitochondrial antigens → production of autoantibodies against proteins on the inner membrane of mitochondria
    – AMA (anti-mitochondrial antibody, in 95% of PBC patients) directed against the E2 component of
      ▪ PDC E2 (pyruvate dehydrogenase complex)
      ▪ PDC E1a subunit of PDC
      ▪ E3 BP subunit of PDC
      ▪ BCO-ADC-E2 (branched-chain of 2-oxo-acid dehydrogenase complex)
      ▪ Molecular target is gene gp120 or nucleoprotein p62
      ▪ Anti-gp 210
        – AMA+PBC, 25%
        – Sensitivity AMA-PBC, 50%
        – Specificity, AMA+PBC, 99%, AMA-PBC, 25%

73

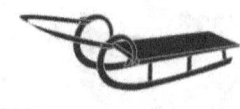

- Gp 210 and p62 associated with poor prognosis
- Gp 201 protein and AMA persist in serum after liver transplantation for PBC
  - Clinically for AMA, immunoblotting and ELISA (enzyme-linked immunosorbent) assays have excellent performance characteristics for AMA: > 90% for both sensitivity and specificity.
  - These methods may detect AMA in persons who were negative by direct immunofluorescence testing
- PDC-E2-specific CD4+ lymphocytes interact with duct cells in the small intrahepatic bile ducts
- This interaction of CD4+ and CD8+ T cells is facilitated by ICAM-1 (intracellular adhesion molecule 1)
- Other antibodies:
  - ANA (antinuclear antibodies)
    - In 50% of AMA+PBC, and 85% of AMA-PSC
    - Anti-MNA (anti-multiple nuclear dot)antibodies
    - Molecular target, sp 100 (soluble protein)
  - Anti-centromere antibodies
  - Antinuclear envelop antibodies
- Other autoantibodies
  - Rheumatoid factor, 70%
  - Anti-smooth muscle, 16%
  - Anti-thyroid, 41%
- HLA class II molecular phenotype may be associated with PBC

➢ Clinical
- Time course from no symptoms (asymptomatic) to symptoms
  - 40% in 5 to 7 years
  - 95% in 20 years
- Development of esophageal varices (EV) ~ 30%
  - Bleeding of EV in 3 years ~ 12%
- Metabolic bone disease
- No portal hypertension
  - Cirrhotic or non-cirrhotic

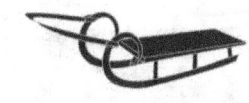

- Give the reason why patients with PBC but no cirrhosis may develop portal hypertension.

  o NRH (nodular regenerative hyperplasia) may be associated with PBC, and causes presinusoidal portal hypertension

- Give the reason why PBC patients with hypercholesterolemia do not have early onset of atherosclerotic disease.

  o The hypercholesterolemia in PBC is from HDL and not from LDL-cholesterol, so the risk of artherosclerosis is not increased.

---

Clinical Curiosities in PBC

o The commonly observed symptom of fatigue is an independent predictor of mortality, especially mortality from cardiac death.

o Gallstones occur in about 1/3 of persons with PBC.

o Recurrence of PBC after liver transplantation "does not seem to decreases survival" (Sleisenger and Fordtran's Gastrointestinal and Liver Disease. 10th Edition. Saunders/Elsevier, Philadelphia, 2016, page 1523).

---

➢ Genetics

  o MHC class II HLA-DR8 allele

  o CTLA-4 gene

  o IL-I

"Your greatest invention lies in your hands, it is

your future."

Apoorve Dubey

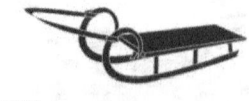

*MASTERING THE BOARDS*
*Hepatology & Pancreaticobiliary Disease*

A.B.R. Thomson

➢ Laboratory

o Suggested flow chart for investigating patients with cholestatic liver disease

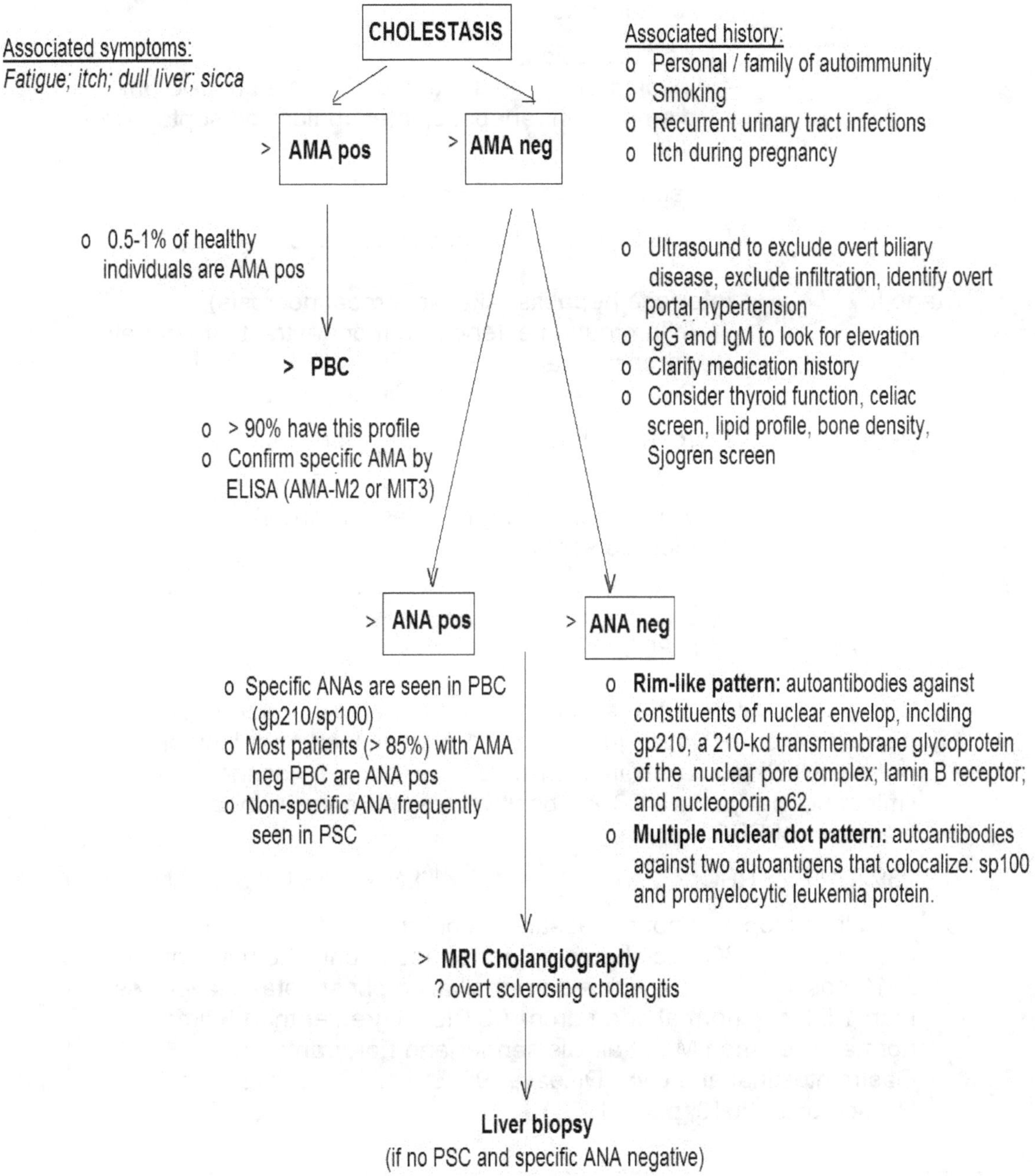

**CHOLESTASIS**

Associated symptoms:
*Fatigue; itch; dull liver; sicca*

Associated history:
o Personal / family of autoimmunity
o Smoking
o Recurrent urinary tract infections
o Itch during pregnancy

> **AMA pos**  > **AMA neg**

o 0.5-1% of healthy individuals are AMA pos

o Ultrasound to exclude overt biliary disease, exclude infiltration, identify overt portal hypertension
o IgG and IgM to look for elevation
o Clarify medication history
o Consider thyroid function, celiac screen, lipid profile, bone density, Sjogren screen

> **PBC**

o > 90% have this profile
o Confirm specific AMA by ELISA (AMA-M2 or MIT3)

> **ANA pos**  > **ANA neg**

o Specific ANAs are seen in PBC (gp210/sp100)
o Most patients (> 85%) with AMA neg PBC are ANA pos
o Non-specific ANA frequently seen in PSC

o **Rim-like pattern:** autoantibodies against constituents of nuclear envelop, inclding gp210, a 210-kd transmembrane glycoprotein of the nuclear pore complex; lamin B receptor; and nucleoporin p62.
o **Multiple nuclear dot pattern:** autoantibodies against two autoantigens that colocalize: sp100 and promyelocytic leukemia protein.

> **MRI Cholangiography**
? overt sclerosing cholangitis

**Liver biopsy**
(if no PSC and specific ANA negative)

Printed with permission: Hirchfield GM, et al. BPRCG 2011; 25: 701-712.

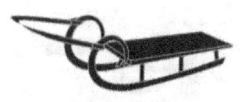

➤ Pathology

• Give the histopathology used to determine Ludwig's 4 stage classification of PBC.

Stage I
- o Focal areas of inflammation (lymphocytes) confined to the portal space
- o Florid duct lesion
  - – Inflammatory destruction of the small (< 100 μm diameter) intrahepatic, interlobular and septal bile ducts
- o Development of ductopenia
- o Reactive proliferative of bile ductules

Stage II
- o Interface hepatitis (aka piecemeal necrosis):
  - – Inflammation extends from portal tract into hepatic parenchyma
  - – Some destruction of the limiting plate

Stage III
- o Fibrosis, with no regenerating modules

Stage IV
- o Fibrosis
  - – With regenerating nodules (cirrhosis)
  - – Fibrous septa

---

Clinical Tip: Liver Biopsy in PBC

- o "In a patient with AMA in serum, the combination of a serum alkaline phosphatase [AP] level greater than 1.5 times the upper limit of normal [ULN] plus a serum AST level less than 5 times the upper limit of normal yields a 98.2% positive predictive value for a diagnosis of PBC".

- o 98% PPV for PBC: AMA+, ↑ AP > 1.5 x ULN + ↑ AST < 5 x ULN

- o "….a liver biopsy is not necessary to confirm the diagnosis in most patients with PBC and should be performed in only the mimicry of AMA-positive patients with a serum alkaline phosphatase level less than 1.5 times normal or a serum AST level greater than 5 times normal" (Feldman M., et al. Sleisenger and Fordtran's Gastrointestinal and Liver Disease. 9th Edition. Saunders/Elsevier, Philadelphia, 2010, page 1481).

---

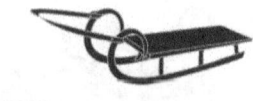

➤ Differential diagnosis

• Give examples of chronic benign biliary disorders involving the intrahepatic, extrahepatic, and combined intra- and extrahepatic ducts (big duct abnormalities), which may mimic PBC.

   o Congenital
- – Alagille syndrome (and nonsyndromatic)
- – Cystic fibrosis
- – Duct plate abnormalities
- – Choledochal cysts

   o Infectious
- – Cytomegalovirus
- – Biliary sepsis
- – Parasites
- – HIV (intrahepatic), AIDS cholangiopathy (extrahepatic)

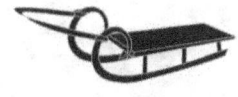

- o Infiltrative
  - – Cholangiocarcinoma
  - – Histiocytosis X
  - – Lymphoma
  - – Mastocytosis

- o Ischemic
  - – Thrombosis of hepatic artery
  - – Paroxysmal nocturnal hemoglobulinuria (PNH)
  - – Vasculitis
  - – Henoch-Schönlein disease
  - – Ischemic strictures (post liver transplantation)

- o Immune
  - – PSC, secondary sclerosing cholangitis
  - – Sarcoid autoimmune cholangiopathy
  - – Graft vs host disease
  - – Allograft rejection

- o Drugs and toxins
  - – Drugs
  - – Floxuridine
  - – TPN-associated cholestasis

- o Idiopathic
  - – Caroli syndrome

Abbreviation: PNH, paroxysmal nocturnal hemoglobulinuria; TPN, total parenteral nutrition

- Give the comparison of contrast PBC and AIH under the following headings.

| Finding | PBC | AIH |
| --- | --- | --- |
| o Gender | F>M | F>M |
| o Prominent symptoms | Pruritus | Fatigue |
| o Laboratory | AMA+, ↑ IgM (if associated autoimmune syndromes) | AMA-, ↑ IgG, ASA+, Anti-DNA+ |
| o Pathology | | |
| - Ducts | Florid duct damage | Minimal duct damage |
| - Hepatocytes | Intact lobules | Interface hepatitis (zone 1) |
| - Infiltration | Lymphoid aggregates | Lymphocytes and plasma cells |

Abbreviation: AIH, autoimmune hepatitis; ASA, anti-smooth muscle antibody; PBC, primary biliary cholangitis

79

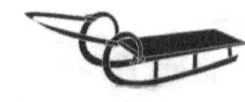

## AMA-Negative PBC

- o Symptoms, biochemistry, liver histology, clinical course, therapy and indications for liver transplantation are similar to AMA + PBC
- o Human leukocyte antigen (HLA) alleles may be different in AMA- versus AMA + PBC, with possible loss of protective allele
- o No difference in Treg (regulatory T cells or t cell subgroups)
- o Serology
  - – Most have ANA or anti-smooth muscle antibodies
  - – 50% have anti-gp 210

➤ Prognosis

- • Give the predictors for survival in PBC.

  | | |
  |---|---|
  | o Patient | – Older age |
  | | – Symptoms |
  | | – Complications |
  | |    ▪ Hepatomegaly |
  | |    ▪ Ascites, edema |
  | |    ▪ GE variceal bleeding |
  | o Laboratory | – ↑ AP, bilirubin, INR |
  | | – ↓ albumin |
  | o Histopathology | – Cholestasis |
  | | – Mallory hyaline |
  | | – Fibrosis |
  | | – Cirrhosis |

Abbreviation: AP, alkaline phosphatase

Please refer to Sleisenger and Fordtran's Gastrointestinal and Liver Disease. 9th Edition. Saunders/Elsevier, Philadelphia, 2016, Box 91-1, page 1517.

- o Prognosis (useful to select optimal timing for liver transplantation)
  - – Simple: total serum bilirubin > 10 mg/mL
    - ▪ Life expectancy then is only 2 years
  - – Sophisticated: Mayo Risk score for PBC: Please see http://www.mayoclinic.org/gi-risk/mayomodel2.html

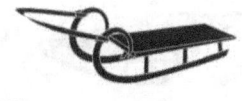

➢ Treatment
- o UDCA (ursodeoxycholic acid)
  - Used routinely in patients with stage 1 to 3 PBC
  - 7-β epimer of chenodeoxycholic acid
  - 13-15 mg/kg per day, with meals, taken od, or divided inti bid
  - Take 2 hr before or after bile acid binding agents, e.g., cholestyramine
- o Budesonide
  - Non-systemic steroid
  - 6 mg po od
  - Used in stages 1 to 3 PBC
    - Alone, or with UDC (requires more clinical data)
    - Avoid use in stage 4 ($\downarrow$ metabolism of budesonide → ↑adverse effects)
- o Nutrition
  - Fat soluble vitamins
- o Treat associated
  - Pruritis
  - Steatorrhea
  - Proximal renal tubular disease (type II)
- o Pruritus
  - The mechanism of the development of pruritus in PBC is unknown; the pruritic factor is not bile acids themselves,
  - However, binding bile acids with cholestyramine and increasing their fecal excretion by diluting the bile acid pool with more hydrophobic UDCA may improve the pruritus.
  - The antibiotic Rifampin induces CYP, and this presumably reduce itching by acting on the release of endogenous opiates. It is not clear what is the mechanism of the known anti-pruritic effect of
  - Antihistamines, 5-HT3 antagonists, serotonin reuptake inhibitors, or phenobarbital

Adapted from: *Sleisenger & Fordtran's Gastrointestinal and Liver Disease: Pathophysiology/ Diagnosis/ Management* 2006; pg.1894.; also Glasova H and Beuers U. *J Gastroenterol Hepatol* 2002; 17(9): 938-48.

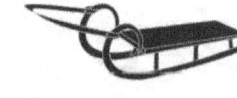

- Give beneficial outcomes for the use of UDCA in PBC.

**Stages at diagnosis of PBC**

|                | 1  | 2  | 3  |
|----------------|----|----|----|
| After 5 years  | 4  | 12 | 59 |
| After 10 years | 17 | 27 | 76 |

|                                        | UDCA |
|----------------------------------------|:----:|
| o Mayo risk score                      | ↓    |
| o Biochemistry                         | ↓    |
| o Liver biopsy progression to cirrhosis| ↓    |
| o Cirrhosis development                | ↓    |
| o Gastroesophageal varices             | ↓    |
| o Ascites                              | ↓    |
| o Liver transplantation                | ↓    |
| o HCC risk                             | ↓    |
| o Death                                | ↓    |

➢ Liver transplantation (LT)

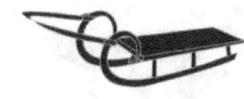

*MASTERING THE BOARDS*
*Hepatology & Pancreaticobiliary Disease*

A.B.R. Thomson

- The number of LT performed for PBC is falling, not because of a ↓ incidence or prevalence, but instead because of the favourable outcomes with UDCA

- Survival rates for LT for PBC
  - 1 year    > 90%
  - 5 year    > 80%

- Organ allocation in PBC is established by risk stratification with the MELD (Model for End-stage Liver Disease) score

- See: http://mayoclini.org/meld/mayomodel6.html

- Risk of recurrence of PBC after LT
  - Median time ~ 4 years
  - ↑ with time: ~ 40% in 10 years post LT
  - ↑ risk of recurrence with
    - ↑ age
    - Males
    - Use of tacrolimus

- Give the diagnostic criteria for recurrent PBC after liver transplantation (LT) for PBC, as well as the important differential diagnostic considerations.

| Diagnostic Criteria for Recurrent PBC | Differential Diagnostic Considerations |
| --- | --- |
| o LT for confirmed diagnosis of PBC | ▪ HCV infection with lymphocytic cholangitis |

83

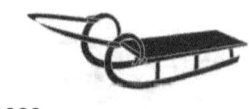

o Persistence of serum AMA

o Compatible Histopathology
  - Portal inflammation
  - Lymphocytic inflammatory infiltrates
  - Lymphocytic cholangitis
  - Epithelioid granulomas

- Drug-induced liver injury (DILI)
- Acute cellular rejection
- Biliary obstruction
- Graft-vs-Host Disease (GVHD)

➤ Exclusion of differential diagnostic considerations

Interpretation: 2 of 4 diagnostic criteria = probable; 3 of 4 = definite

Printed with permission: Ilyas JA, et al. Liver transplantation in autoimmune liver diseases. Best Pract Res Clin Gastroenterol. 2011;25(6):765-82.

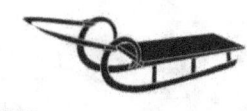

84

## PRIMARY SCLEROSING CHOLANGITIS (PSC)

➢ Definition

  o Chronic cholestatic liver disease characterized by inflammation and fibrosis of the extrahepatic and intrahepatic bile ducts than can progress to cirrhosis.

➢ Demography

  o Incidence – $1/10^5$ per year

  o Prevalence – $10/10^5$

  o The prevalence of PSC is ~21 and ~6 per 100,000 men and women, respectively.

➢ Genetics

  o HLA A1-B8-DRB1*0301-DQA-1*0501-DQB1*0201, and DRB*1301-DQA-1*0103-DQB1*0603

  o Genetic polymorphisms: TNF α; stromelysin, matrix metallopeptidase 3; MHC class I polypeptide-related sequence A, chemokine C-C motif receptor 5; intracellular adhesion molecule-1, CD54

➢ Laboratory

• Give serum autoantibodies which are most prevalent in PSC.

| Antibody | Prevalence |
|---|---|
| o Anti-neutrophil cytoplasmic antibody (ANCA) | 50%–80% |
| o Anti-nuclear antibody (ANA) | 7%–77% |
| o Anti-cardiolipin antibody (ACA) | 4%–66% |
| o Anti-endothelial cell antibody (AEA) | 35% |
| o Anti-smooth muscle antibody | 13%–20% |
| o Thyroperoxidase | 7%–16% |
| o Rheumatoid factor | 15% |
| o Thyroglobulin | 4% |

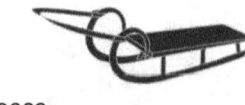

*MASTERING THE BOARDS*
*Hepatology & Pancreaticobiliary Disease*

A.B.R. Thomson

➢ Diagnostic Imaging

• Give the features on diagnostic imaging that distinguish between the cholestatic conditions PSC and PBC (primary biliary cholangitis).

| PSC | PBC |
|---|---|
| o Usually intra- and extrahepatic ducts tapered and narrow | – Intrahepatic ducts smoothly tapered and narrow |
| o Diffuse segmental strictures | ▪ Lymphocytic interface may be hard to distinguish from AIH (autoimmune hepatitis) |
| o Dominant strictures | ▪ Diffusely thickened, fibrotic wall |
| o Intrahepatic duct "pruning" (↓ arborisation) → "beading" | ▪ Inflammation of duct epithelium and glands |
| | ▪ Hyperplasia of biliary glands |
| | ▪ Neural proliferation |
| | ▪ Atrophy of biliary epithelium |

Abbreviations: AMA, antimitochondrial antibodies; anti-BEC, anti-(human) biliary epithelial cells; ANA, antinuclear antibodies; pANCA, perinuclear antineutrophil cytoplasmic antibodies

➢ Pathology
o Liver biopsy necessary to make diagnosis because ERCP likely normal

➢ Endoscopy
o Large-duct PSC (95%) 80% is associated with IBD.
    – If large-duct PSC is not associated with IBD, test for ↑ IgG4 to diagnose autoimmune cholangitis.
    – Diagnosis may be made by ERCP/MRCP.
    – Small-duct PSC (5%)
    – Small-duct PSC is a variant in which only the intrahepatic ducts are induced.
        ▪ Small-duct PSC $\xrightarrow{20\%}$ large-duct PSC $\xrightarrow{10\%}$ cholangiocarcinoma
o PSC + gallbladder polyps → elective cholecystectomy for high risk of malignant degeneration of even small gallbladder polyps
o "onion skin" lesion: (fibro-obliterative process)
    – Destruction of the bile duct
    – Ductopenia
    – Replacement of destroyed duct with fibrous tissue

86

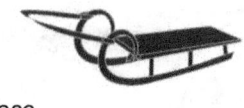

- Small interlobular/septal bile duct branches: fibro-obliterative cholangitis
- Periductular inflammation
- Atrophy
- Stages
    - Stage I (portal stage)
        - Portal tracts
            - Inflammation
            - Fibrosis
            - Cholangitis
    - Stage II (periportal stage)
        - ↑ inflammation interface hepatitis
        - ↑ fibrosis
        - Piecemeal necrosis
        - Ductular proliferation
        - Cholangitis
    - Stage III (septal stage)
        - Fibrosis which bridges from one portal tract to the next
    - Stage IV (cirrhosis)

➢ Differential diagnosis

- Give a classification of the secondary causes/ associations of secondary sclerosing cholangitis (SSC), and provide examples.
    - GI disease associations
        - Colon
            - Ulcerative Colitis
            - Crohn colitis or ileocolitis
        - Liver
            - Hepatic allograft rejection
            - Hepatic graft-versus-host disease ( after bone marrow transplantation)
            - Cystic fibrosis
            - Overlap with primary biliary cholangitis (PBC)
            - May be difficult to distinguish from AIH (PSC may have lymphocytic interface hepatitis)

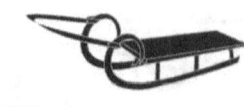

- Bile ducts
  - Cholangiocarcinoma
  - Choledocholithiasis
  - Stricture
  - Biliary parasites
  - Recurrent pyogenic cholangitis
  - Fungal infection
  - Cholangitis
- Pancreas
  - Chronic pancreatitis
  - IgG4-associated cholangitis (IAC), with or without IgG4-associated pancreatitis
- Post-liver transplantation (fibro-intimal hyperplasia)
- Systemic diseases with fibrosis
  - Retroperitoneal fibrosis
  - Riedel thyroiditis
  - Mediastinal Fibrosis
  - Pseudotumour of the orbit
  - Inflammatory pseudotumour
  - Peyronie disease
  - Chronic sclerosing sialadenitis

- Autoimmune or collagen vascular disorders
  - Systemic lupus erythematosus
  - Systemic sclerosis
  - Type I diabetes mellitus
  - Rheumatoid arthritis
  - Sjögren syndrome
  - Autoimmune hemolytic anemia
- Kidney
  - Membranous nephropathy
  - Rapidly progressive glomerulonephritis
- Infections
  - Biliary TB
  - HIV (CD4+ T lymphocytes < 100/mm$^3$)
    - AIDS cholangiopathy
    - Cryptosporidium
    - Microsporidium
    - CMV

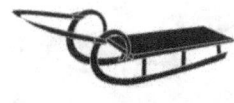

- Inflammation
  - Sarcoidosis
  - Hypereosinophilic syndrome
- Immunodeficiency diseases
  - Congenital immunodeficiency
  - Combined immunodeficiency
  - Dysgammaglobulinemia
    - X-linked agammaglobulinemia
  - Acquired immunodeficiency
    - Selective immunoglobulin A deficiency
    - Acquired immunodeficiency syndrome (HIV/AIDS)
    - Angioimmunoblastic lymphadenopathy
- Congenital abnormalities
  - Caroli disease
  - Choledochal cyst
- Iatrogenic (drugs)
  - Hepatic arterial infusion of chemotherapy, intraductal formaldehyde or hypertonic saline (used for echinococcal cyst removal)
  - Intra-arterial floxuridine (FUDR, causing ischemia and toxic vasculitis)
  - Formaldehyde (for hydratid cyst)
  - Intra-arterial floxuridine
- Ischemic
  - Vascular injury from liver surgery
  - Hepatic allograft arterial occlusion
  - Paroxysmal nocturnal hemoglobinuria
  - Prolonged circulatory failure (shock)
  - Systemic vasculitis
- Infiltration
  - Benign
    - Mastocytosis
    - Histiocytosis X
    - Biliary papillomatosis
  - Malignant
    - Cholangiocarcinoma
    - Hepatocellular carcinoma (HCC)
    - Metastatic cancer
    - Lymphoma

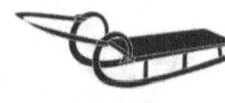

Adapted from: Sleisenger and Fordtran's Gastrointestinal and Liver Disease. 10th Edition. Saunders/Elsevier, Philadelphia, 2016, Box 68-1, page 1167.

---

**SO YOU WANT TO BE A GASTROENTEROLOGIST!**

An Asian Canadian with no previous biliary tract surgery presents with recurrent episodes of fever, RUQ pain and jaundice (Charcot triad). He is negative for AMA, ANA, ASMA, pANCA and HIV. MRCP shows multiple filling defects and a stricture/dilation of the left hepatic duct.
- Give the likely diagnosis.

    o RPC (recurrent pyogenic cholangitis) may be confused with PSC, but the demography, negative serology, and the findings on MRCP of defects in the left rather than the right hepatic duct make this diagnosis likely.

- In the context of investigating a person with PSC and possible cholangiocarcinoma, give reasons for false-negative and false-positive CA 19-9 elevations, as well as a false-positive PET scans.

    o CA 19-9
    - False negative
        - Negative Lewis antigen status
    - False positive
        - Choledocholithiasis
        - Bacterial cholangitis
    o PET scan
    - False positive
    - Bacterial tract inflammation

---

**PSC and Inflammatory Bowel Disease** (IBD)

➢ Demography
- o 80% of PSC have IBD
- o 3% of IBD have PSC
- o Associated with ulcerative colitis (UC) and Crohn colitis, but not Crohn disease of just the small bowel

90

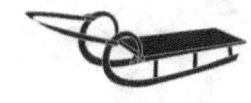

➢ Clinical
  o Cholestasis, biliary cirrhosis
  o Complications
    – Inflammatory bowel disease (especially ulcerative colitis)
    – Biliary and gallbladder tumours

- Give characteristics of inflammatory bowel disease (IBD) associated with primary sclerosing cholangitis (PSC).

  o Site
    – More extensive colitis
    – More R-sided colitis of inflammatory activity
    – More CRC, puchitis, backwash ileitis
    – Rectal sparing
    – ↑ backwash ileitis

  o Activity
    – Often mild clinical course
    – Clinical course of PSC + IBD
      ▪ Independent
      ▪ Colectomy does not affect PSC

  o Complication
    – ↑↑↑ risk of colorectal neoplasia
    – ↑ risk of pouchitis in patients undergoing proctocolectomy with IPAA
    – ↑ risk of peristomal varices in patients undergoing proctocolectomy with ileostomy
    – After liver transplantation  for PSC
      ▪ UC may still develop
      ▪ HGD/CRC may develop
        –HGD may already have been present
        –HGD may develop following diagnosis of UC
    – UC → panproctocolectomy → PSC may develop de novo
    – PSC → liver transplantation → UC may develop de novo, or PSC may recur
    – Necessary to perform annual colonoscopy in UC + PSC

Abbreviations: CRC, colorectal cancer; HGD, high grade dysplasia

Adapted from: Chapman R, et al. Hepatology. 2010;51(2):660-78.

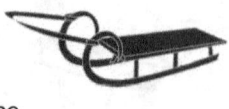

- Give **biliary tract complications** in PSC.

❖ Gallbladder

- o Gallbladder tumours (in 41%)
  - − Current guidelines recommend an annual screening ultrasound for gallbladder cancer in patients with PSC, and a cholecystectomy once a gallbladder polyp is detected regardless of size.
- o Gallbladder polyps → cancer
  - − Gallbladder polyps < 8 mm on ultrasound have a low likelihood of being malignant in non-PSC persons.
- o Cholelithiasis (in~ 25%)

❖ Biliary tree

- o Choledocholithiasis in ~25%)
  - − Use the Child-Pugh score to risk-stratify patients with PSC who undergo a cholecystectomy.
  - − Primary sclerosis cholangitis (PSC) with or without cirrhosis have a high morbidity rate following a cholecystectomy that is comparable to patients with cirrhosis from other causes.
- o Cholangitis
- o Multiple strictures
- o Single/strictures
- o "dominant" stricture (> 1.5 cm)
  - − Intrahepatic > 10 mm in length
  - − Extrahepatic, > 15 mm)
- o Cholangiocarcinoma (in ~ 10%)
- o Cirrhosis, and its complications

Adapted from: Eaton JE, et al. Am J Gastroenterol 2012; 107: 431-439.

- Give cause of rectal sparing in UC.
  - o PSC + UC
  - o Crohn colitis
  - o Rectal therapy

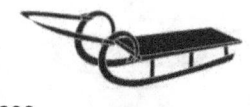

➢ Prognosis

o This ↑↑ mortality in PBC (medial survival time after diagnosis, 10-12 years) is attributed

- To complications from cirrhosis as well as the high incidence of malignancies associated with PSC
- Colorectal cancer
- Cholangiocarcinoma
- Gallbladder cancer

| | Years | | |
|---|---|---|---|
| | 1 | 2 | 5 |
| o % progression beyond Stage | | | |
| – II → III/IV | 42% | 66% | 93% |
| – II → IV | 14% | 25% | 52 |

o Asymptomatic PSC
- Median survival free of liver failure, 71%

o Symptomatic PSC
- 6 years survival rate, 60%
- "…may facilitate selection for timing of liver transplantation (Feldman M., et al. Sleisenger and Fordtran's Gastrointestinal and Liver Disease. 9th Edition. Saunders/Elsevier, Philadelphia, 2016, Table 68-1, page 1172).

o Prognostic models (multivariant)
- Please see Sleisenger and Fordtran's Gastrointestinal and Liver Disease. 10th Edition. Saunders/Elsevier, Philadelphia, 2010, Table 68.2, page 1159 for "Independent Predictors of Survival and Prognostic Sclerosing Cholangitis".

o After development of cholangiocarcinoma
- Median survival, 5 months (in ~10%)
- With appropriate indication and surgical resection by hepatic segmentectomy or lobectomy, 5 year survival rate ~25%.

Please see Sleisenger and Fordtran's Gastrointestinal and Liver Disease. 9th Edition. Saunders/Elsevier, Philadelphia, 2010, Table 69.5, page 1176.

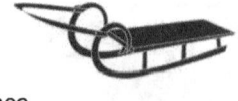

> Treatment
  - o Suppportive for complications
  - o UDCA **no** longer recommended in PSC, unless for overlap syndrome (PSC plus PBC)
  - o Endoscopic stenting of strictures
  - o Annual screening
    - – Colon
    - – Bile ducts
    - – Gallbladder
  - o Liver transplantation

---

Clinical Gem

.....endoscopic management of a dominant stricture may alter the course of PSC [for the better]" (Feldman M., et al. Sleisenger and Fordtran's Gastrointestinal and Liver Disease. 9th Edition. Saunders/Elsevier, Philadelphia, 2010, page 1166)

---

- Give the clinical scenarios and diagnostic considerations > 90 days after OLT (orthoptic liver transplantation) for recurrent primary sclerosing cholangitis (PSC).

| Clinical Scenario | Diagnostic Considerations |
|---|---|
| o OLT for confirmed diagnosis of PSC | ▪ Hepatic artery thrombosis or stenosis |
| o Cholangiographic evidence of:<br>– Intrahepatic and/or extrahepatic strictures*<br>– Beading and irregularity of bile ducts | ▪ Solitary anastomotic stricture<br>▪ Ischemic strictures<br>▪ Bacterial or fungal cholangitis with strictures |
| o Compatible Histopathology<br>– Fibrous cholangitis and/or<br>– Fibro-obliterative lesions with or without ductopenia, fibrosis or cirrhosis<br>– Interface hepatitis | ▪ Chronic ductopenic rejection<br>▪ ABO incompatibility between donor and recipient<br>▪ CMV infection<br>▪ Cryptosporidium |

Printed with permission: Ilyas JA, et al. Best Pract Res Clin Gastroenterol 2011;25(6):765-82; and Eaton JE, et al. Am J Gastroenterol 2012; 10: 431-439.

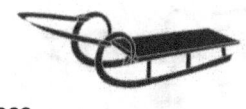

# METABOLIC BONE DISEASE

- ➢ Terminology
  - o Osteoporosis (OP)
    - – Defective bone formation
  - o Osteomalacia
    - – Defective bone mineralization

- ➢ Demography
  - o At diagnosis, 20% of PBC patients already have osteoporosis
  - o Cumulative risk of fragility fractures – 10% to 20%
  - o Presence and severity of OP increased with progression from stage 1 and 2 to stages 3 and 4 PBC
  - o After liver transplantation (LT) for PBC
    - – 50% develop a pathologic fracture within 1 month

- ➢ Causes/associations

- • Give the factors that ↑ risk of bone disease in patients with chronic cholestatic liver disease.
  - o ↓ physical activity
  - o ↓ body mass index (BMI)
  - o ↑ age
  - o Smoking
  - o Female sex
  - o ↓ sunlight exposure
  - o Family history

- ➢ Pathophysiology
  - o ↓ Intake
  - o ↓ Absorption due to cholestasis
    - – Vitamin D and K deficiency
    - – ↓ calcium availability (steatorrhea)
    - – ↑ serum bilirubin
    - – Genetically abnormal vitamin D receptor genotype
  - o ↑ Requirements
    - – Menopause/hypogonadism

95

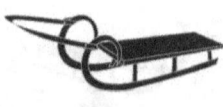

## NON-VIRAL INFECTIOUS CAUSES OF HEPATITIS

There are certain "buzz words" which are meant to signal a likely cause of infectious hepatitis.

- Give "buzz words" which when applied to the patient with acute hepatitis, suggest typhoid fever from infection with either Salmonella typhi or Salmonella paratyphi.

  o Hepatitis plus
    - "Stepwise fever"
      - Stepwise increase temperature
    - "Temperature-pulse dissociation"
      - Pulse rate does not increase as much as expected for the temperature (i.e., relative bradycardia)
    - "Rose spots on skin"
      - Salmon-pink macules on skin of trunks

  o Other clues that acute hepatitis might represent typhoid fever.
    - RLQ tenderness (ileitis/cecitis)
    - ALT/LDH < 4 (↑ ALT, ↑↑ LDH)
    - ↑ AP (AP increased more than in most patients with hepatitis)
    - ↑↑ WBC, with "left shift"

  o Treatment
    - Fluoroquinolone

A young woman presents with RUQ pain and tenderness, fever and abnormal liver enzymes. The CT of the upper abdomen shows only non-specific hepatic changes.

- In this context, give the meaning of the "**Fitz-Hugh Curtis (FHC) syndrome**" and "violin string". perihepatic adhesions on laparoscopy.

  o Fitz Hugh Curtis syndrome is a gonococcal or chlamydial infection of the female pelvic organs which involves the surface of peritoneum, causing the perihepatic fibrinous exudate (violin string adhesions).

  o In diagnosis would be suspected in a sexually active women with a painful pelvic examination.

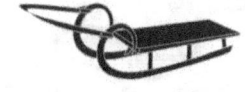

# VIRAL HEPATITIS

- Give the name of common viral infections of the liver.
  - The "viral alphabet soup" (HAV, HBV, HCV, HDV, HEV*)
  - EBV (Epstein-Barr virus)
  - CMV (cytomegalovirus)
  - HSV* (herpes simplex virus)

- Give a comparison of viral hepatitis (A, B, C, D, E) under the headings - virus type, mode of transmission, incubation period, serological diagnosis, risk of fulminant hepatitis and risk of chronicity.

| | Virus type | Trans-mission | Incuba-tion (days) | Serologic diagnosis | Fulminant hepatitis | Risk of chronicity |
|---|---|---|---|---|---|---|
| **➤ Fecal/oral** | | | | | | |
|    o HAV | RNA | | 20-35 | HAV-IgM | 0.1-2.0% | No |
|    o HEV | RNA | | 10-50 | Anti-HEV | 1-2% 15-20% Pregnant | No |
| **➤ Percutaneous** | | | | | | |
|    o HBV* | DNA | -IVDU | 60-110 | HBsAg | 0.1-0.5% | Adults < 5% Preschoolers 25% Neonates >90% |
|    o HCV** | RNA | -Sexual (MSM, prostitute services, promiscuity) | 35-70 | Anti-HCV | <1% | > 80% |
|    o HDV | RNA | -IVDU (IV drug use ) (even once), pre-1990 blood transfusions -Sexual promiscuity | 60-110 | Anti-HDV | | Usual in a superinfection with HBV; rare by itself |

\* Also perinatal

\*\* Pre-1990 blood transfusion

Abbreviation: MSM, mem who have sex with men

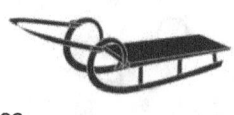

*MASTERING THE BOARDS*
*Hepatology & Pancreaticobiliary Disease*

A.B.R. Thomson

- Give which two of the viral causes of hepatitis have a higher mortality during pregnancy.
  - HEV
  - HSV

- Give the prevention, vaccination, post-exposure prophylaxis and treatment which is recommended for exposure to HAV, HBV and HCV.
  - Prevention
    - Good sanitation and hygiene
    - Avoid high risk behavior
    - For HBV, condoms are advised for multiple sex partners, anal intercourse, and intercourse during menses
  - Vaccination
    - HAV
    - HBV
    - HCV
      - No vaccine
  - Post-exposure prophylaxis)
    - HAV
      - Children ≥ 2 years of age in communities with high rates of Hep A
      - Chronic liver disease
      - All household and sexual contacts
      - Immune serum globulin 0.02 mL/kg IM if within 2 weeks of exposure
        - Vaccinate
      - No treatment for casual school or work contacts
    - HBV
      - When HBC reactivation ("flare", decompensation) may occur – use of chemotherapy, prednisone, anti-TNF therapy
    - HCV
      - Needlestick injury:
      - Test for HCV-RNA, AST, bilirubin at baseline, then at 4 and 12 weeks—of positive, treat with PEG-IFN and Ribavirin
      - Perinatal: Rare transmission—more likely if mother is immunosuppressed

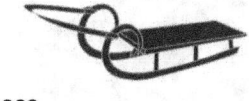

98

- Treatment when infected
  - Supportive care. Most cases resolve spontaneously. Hospitalization rarely needed. Prophylaxis and prevention of secondary spread is perhaps the most important aspect of treatment.
  - Activity—symptom guided return to work: no activity limitations.
  - Diet—fatty foods poorly tolerated, exclude ETOH, no other dietary restrictions.
  - Drugs—no role of corticosteroids—may increase the risk of a chronic carrier state, avoid sedatives, tranquilizers.

Adapted from: Grover PT, and Ma M. *First Principles of Gastroenterology* 2005: 547-552.

Please see: Peltekian KM, Hirsch G. Chapter 59. In: Therapeutic Choices. Grey J, Ed. 6th Edition, Canadian Pharmacists Association 2011, Table 6, page 797-8.

## **Hepatitis A Virus** (HAV) **Infection**

- Demography
  - Transmission is by fecal-oral route
    - Person-to-person
    - Contaminated food or water
  - Males >> females
    - Injection illicit drugs
    - Non-injection illicit drugs
    - MSM (men who have sex with men)

- Clinical presentations
  - Acute hepatitis
  - Fulminant hepatitis failure (FHF)
    - Week 1 of HAV, 55%
    - Week 4 of HAV, 90%
    - Clinical alert
  - Relapsing or "prolonged" but not chronic course
  - HAV may trigger onset of AIH (autoimmune hepatitis)

- Diagnosis
  - About one third of adults with acute HAV will have hyperbilirubinemia
  - Relapse of ↑ ALT may occur weeks after the acute symptoms have reduced, if glucocorticosteroids were inappropriately given.

99

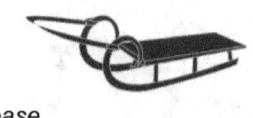

- o IgM-anti HAV
    - – Once symptoms occur, IgM-anti HAV is positive in serum
    - – Usually becomes negative by 4 months
    - – Sometimes becomes negative after 12 months
- o IgG-anti-HAV
    - – Marker of previous HAV infection

➤ Prognosis

- o HAV has one serotype, and four genotypes (I, II, III, and IV).
- o Hospitalization, 25%
- o Death
    - – Overall, 0.3%
    - – > 49 years, 1.8%
    - – Also high in patients with chronic liver disease

---

Clinical Alert: IgM anti-HAV and low HAV RNA

".... Detection of IgM anti-HAV coupled with non-detection or finding of low-titer HAV RNA in patients with severe acute hepatitis [HAV] may signal an ominous prognosis and the need for early referral for liver transplantation" (Sleisenger and Fordtran's Gastrointestinal and Liver Disease. 9th Edition. Saunders/Elsevier, Philadelphia, 2010, page 1283).

---

➤ Prevention

- o Sanitation
- o Lifestyle considerations
- o HAV vaccine
    - – Comparable to SIG for post-exposure protection against HAV
- o Serum immune globulin (SIG)
    - – Lasts ~ 20 year
    - – Reduced response when HIV > 400 copies/mL, and CD4+ < 25/mm$^3$
- o For persons with chronic liver disease
    - – Pre-exposure prophylaxis

For Groups at High Risk of Hepatitis a virus Infection, please see Sleisenger and Fordtran's Gastrointestinal and Liver Disease. 10th Edition. Saunders/Elsevier, Philadelphia, 2016, Table 78.1, page 1306).

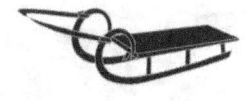

**Hepatitis B Virus** (HBV) **Infection**

➤ Demography

- Give the geographic site for the most common distribution of Hepatitis B genotypes A-H.

    A.      Northwestern Europe, North America, Central Africa

    B,C.    Southeast Asia, including China, Japan, and Taiwan (prevalence is increasing in North America)

    D.      Southern Europe, Middle East, India

    E.      West Africa

    F.      Central and South America, United States (Native Americans), Polynesia

    G.      United States, France

    H.      Central and South America

Please see: Sleisenger and Fordtran's Gastrointestinal and Liver Disease. 10th Edition. Saunders/Elsevier, Philadelphia, 2016, Box 79-1page 1313.

- o HBV progression

    Acute HBV → chronic HBV:
    - – Neonate    90    asymptomatic enteric disease
    - – Children    50
    - – Adults      10    usually symptomatic, unless healthy carriers

Source: *Clin Liver Disease* 10; 14: 75-91; *Hepatology* 07; 45:1056-75

- o Spontaneous HBeAg seroconversion, ~10%
- o 5-year cumulation risk of progression of HBeAg – positive chronic hepatitis B to cirrhosis, ~10%
- o HBV-associated compensated cirrhosis progressing to decompensation, 16%
- o 5-year cumulative risk of developing HCC, 14%

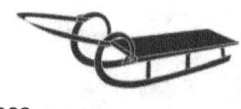

> Molecular biology

- Give the **molecular biology** of HBV infection.

  o HBV is a DNA virus which goes through an RNA intermediate, and requires an active viral reverse transcriptase/polymerase enzyme.

  o High daily point mutation rate, low replication fidelity

  o The 5 gene encodes HBsAg, a viral surface, envelop protein

  o Liver damage from HBV is immune-mediated (not a direct hepatocyte cytopathic effect of HBV).

  o Cellular immune response – innate and adaptive

  o Viral clearance by CTLs (cytotoxic T lymphocytes)

102

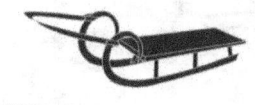

- CD4+ T cells produce antiviral cytokines which reduce the production of neutralizing antibody.
- The core gene has
  - Precore region → HbeAg
  - Core region → core proteins
- HBV DNA polymerase reverse transcriptase pregenomic RNA into a negative-strand HBV DNA ("needed for encapsidation of viral RNA into a negative strand of viral DNA (reverse transcription) and conversion of this first HBV DNA strand into a second DNA strand of positive polarity (Sleisenger and Fordtran's Gastrointestinal and Liver Disease. 10th Edition. Saunders/Elsevier, Philadelphia, 2016, page 1314).
- The negative-strand HBV DNA is a template for the synthesis of a positive-strand.
- The positive strand is incorporated into the maturing nucleocapsid.
- The nucleocapsids are coated with the surface protein (HBsAg) in the ER.
- From the ER, the enveloped nucleocapsid bud off from the hepatocyte membrane, and enter the circulation.

➢ Pathogenesis

- Give the mode of transmission and the approximate lifetime risk of HBV infection in persons who reside in different geographical areas.

| Geographical Area | Lifetime Risk of HBV Infection | Mode of Transmission |
|---|---|---|
| o NA, WE, SA, Au | < 20% | – Horizontal person-to-person, young adults<br>– Sexual |
| o SE, EE, ME, IS fUSSR, NAFR | 20% to 40% | – Infancy<br>– Early childhood |
| o SEA, CHINA, AFRICA | 60% to 80% | – Perinatal<br>– Horizontal, young children |

Abbreviations: Au, Australia; EE, Eastern Europe; fUSSR, former USSR; IS, Indian Subcontinent; ME, Middle East; NAFR, Northern Africa; NA, North America; SEA, South East Asia; SA, South America; SE, Southern Europe; WE, Western Europe

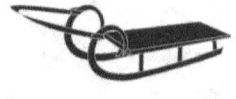

➢ Clinical

• Stages (based on serology)
   ○ Immune tolerant
      – Normal ALT level
      – Minimal or no inflammation or fibrosis
      – High levels of HBV DNA
      – HBeAg+
   ○ Immune reactive
      – May be high levels of HBV DNA, but HBeAg may cause an immune tolerant phase, with inflammation of the liver
      – ALT normal or near normal
   ○ When HBV is acquired early in life such as from vertical transmission, and in those who have a high-normal ALT, they may already have entered the immune clearance phase.
   ○ Liver biopsy "….can be a useful tool to distinguish persons in the immune clearance phase despite normal or near-normal ALT levels but with active liver disease from active liver disease". (Sleisenger and Fordtran's Gastrointestinal and Liver Disease. 9th Edition. Saunders/Elsevier, Philadelphia, 2010, page 1294).
   ○ Immune active
      – Liver inflammation and fibrosis
      – ↑ HBV DNA (lower than in immune tolerant)
      – HBeAg + or –
      – ↑ ALT
      – Active T cell response to virus
   ○ Inactive
      – Normal ALT
      – Healing liver histology
      – Resolving liver fibrosis
      – Low or absent HBV DNA
      – Strong T cell response to virus
   ○ Recovery
      – Lower risk of developing HCC
      – Loss of HBsAg

Adapted from: McMahon BJ, et al. Clin Gastro Hep 2012; 10: 218-219.

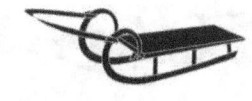

- Clinical presentations
  - Active hepatitis
    - Circulating HBsAg – anti-HBs complexes activate complement
    - HBsAg – anti-HBs complexes are deposited in wall of the blood vessels of the skin synovium
    - Serum sickness-like prodrome, with 1/3 of patients developing jaundice
    - Low levels of HBV may persist in the serum
  - Fulminant hepatitis
    - Due to "massive immune-mediated lysis of infected hepatocytes"
    - Usual-onset
      - Within 4 weeks of symptoms of HBV
    - May develop late-onset liver failure after several months of onset of HBV symptoms
    - Survival
      - Spontaneous, 20%
      - With liver transplant, 50%
    - May be associated with "flares" (exacerbations of disease)
      - ↑ ALT (2x the baseline value)
      - IgM anti-HBe
      - Associated with histological progression of disease
  - Chronic active HBV carrier (active HBsAgcarrier)
    - HBV replication
      - PCR-based, +
      - Non-PCR-based testing, +
    - AST, ALT
      - Intermittent or persistent increases
    - Liver biopsy
      - Chronic hepatitis
  - Chronic inactive HBV (inactive HBsAg carrier)
    - HBsAg positive for > 6 mon
    - HBeAg negative, anti-HBe positive
    - HBV-DNA <$10^5$ copies/mL  (<20,000 lk, low risk of HCC)
    - Persistently normal ALT/AST (low risk of progression)
    - Liver biopsy showing no inflammation
    - No evidence of on-going replication (inactive chronic HBV infection)

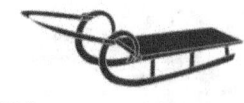

- o Progression
  - – Infection
    - ▪ Vertical, 95%
    - ▪ Horizontal, < 5%
  - – HBV infection → carrier state, < 5%
  - – Cirrhosis, 5 year survival rate
    - ▪ Compensated, 84%
    - ▪ Decompensated, 14%
- o Resolved hepatitis B
  - – Previous known history of acute or chronic hepatitis B
  - – HBsAg negative
  - – HBeAg negative
  - – HBcAb positive/HBsAb positive
  - – Undetectable HBV-DNA
  - – Normal ALT

Adapted from: Keeffe EB, et al. *Clin Gastroenterol Hepatol* 2006;4(8):936-62.

- o Reactivation
  - – A proportion of these with inactive carrier state undergo spontaneous or immunosuppression-mediated reactivation of replication of HBV DNA
  - – ↑ HBV DNA in serum
  - – ↑ ALT
  - – Necroinflammation recurs
  - – Seroconversion of HBeAg$^{+/-}$
  - – During or after HBeAg seroconversion (anti-HBe → HBeAg$^+$), precore or core promoter mutants appear
  - – Precore or core promoter mutants ↓ HBeAg production
  - – Optimal time for treatment
- o Immune clearance
  - – ↓ HBV DNA
  - – ↑ ALT
  - – HBeAg$^+$
  - – Hepatic necroinflammation (immune-mediated lysis of HBV-infected hepatocytes)
  - – Optimal time for treatment

106

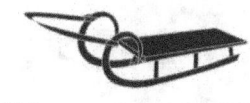

- Associations with HBV
  - Fibrosing cholestatic hepatitis
    - Reactivation of HBV from immunosuppressants given for organ transplantation ↑↑↑ HBsAg and HBeAg in liver tissue
  - Infection with other hepatotrophic viruses (A, C, D)
  - Extrahepatic manifestations
    - Fever, arthralgias (proximal interphalangeal pints), angioneurotic edema
    - PAN (polyarteritis nodosa)
    - HBV-associated renal disease
      - Glomerulonephropathy
      - Membranous glomerulonephritis
      - Membranoproliferative glomerulonephritis
      - Immune-complex glomerulonephritis
      - Nephrotic syndrome
      - Renal failure
      - Cryoglobulinemia

➢ Laboratory

- Give the laboratory assessment prior to therapy of HBV, and explain why.
  - HBsAg – if positive, measure
  - HBeAg and anti-HBe
  - Measure HBV DNA if ↑ ALT
  - ALT, ALP, bilirubin, albumin, PT INR, CBC, HIV, anti-HCV

Printed with permission: Grover PT, and Bain V. *First Principles of Gastroenterology* 2005:547-556.

- Give markers of HBV infection, and what they signify.
  - HBsAg – appears first and if persists for > 6 months, the patient is chronically infected (exposed, chronic infection)
  - HBsAb – implies recovery or immunity to HBV, either naturally occurring or after vaccination
  - HBcAb-IgM – past or present HBV infection (newer and more sensitive assays may also be positive during reactivation of chronic infections)
  - HBeAg – indicates active infection/replication of HBV
    - Absence cannot be taken as absence of viral replication (i.e., precore mutant, e.g., eAg negative)

107

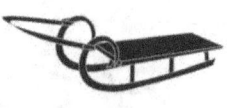

- o Anti-HBe
  - – Presence indicates seroconversion
  - – Can also be found in active disease in patients with HBeAg negative chronic hepatitis. (not replicating – precore mutant)
- o HBV-DNA
  - – Detectable in serum
  - – Measure of the level of viral replication. (infected;reflects risk of HCC)

Printed with permission:  Balart LA. *2007 ACG Annual Postgraduate Course*: 198.

- o The CDC now recommends HBV diagnostic testing in all persons going on immunosuppressants or undergoing cancer chemotherapy
- o Natural clearance of HBV occurs in 5% of neonates and 95% of adults infected with HBV
- o Baseline HBV DNA levels in patients 30-65 years old are directly related to the likelihood of developing HCC 10 years later

- Give the laboratory features which suggest each of the 5 stages of HBV.

| Stage | HBeAg | HBV DNA | ALT/AST | Progression to Fibrosis |
|---|---|---|---|---|
| o Immune tolerant | + | ↑↑ | N/low | Very low |
| o Immunoreactive (HBeAg - positive necroinfllammation | + | ↑ | ↑/ fluctuating | low |
| o Inactive HBV carrier state | Negative (zero conversion to anti-HBe antibody) | < 2000 IU/mL<br><br>Low/ undetectable | N | Low |
| o After seroconversion, or after years of immunoreactive phase | Negative | ↑/↓ | ↑/↓ | High |
| o HBs antigen negative | Negative | HBV DNA in liver but not detectable in blood | N | Low |

Abbreviation: CHB, chronic hepatitis B infection

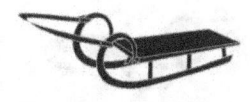

- Give the clinical laboratory and histopathology characteristics of the **different stages** of chronic hepatitis B infection.

| Features | Immune tolerant | Immune reactive | Low replicative stage | e- Ag negative reactivation |
|---|---|---|---|---|
| o ALT | Normal | Elevated | Normal | Fluctuates (fluctuating viremia) |
| o HBV-DNA by PCR | >20,000 IU/ml | >20,000 IU/ml | <2,000 IU/ml | >2,000 IU/ml |
| o e-antigen | (+) | (+) | (-) | (-) |
| o e-antibody | (-) | (-) | (+) | (+) |
| o Liver biopsy | Inactive | Active/+ fibrosis | Inactive | Active/+ fibrosis |
| o Course | No progression of disease for about 3-6 months | HBeAg seroconversion with treatement | - | 8-10% develops cirrhosis each year, compared with 2-6% of HBeAg positive patients |
| o Treatment | No | Yes | No | Yes |

Adapted from: Herrera JL. *2009 ACG Annual Postgraduate Course:*161- 166.

---

SO YOU WANT TO BE A HEPATOLOGIST!

In acute HBV, HBsAg disappears, and several weeks later anti-HBs appears.

- Give the serological test used during this "**window period**" to prove acute HBV infection.

  - During the window period when HBsAg disappears and anti-HBs appears, the presence of serum IgM-anti-Hbe confirms a recent HBV infection.

In both acute and in chronic HBV infection, there may be both HBsAg as well as anti-HBs in the serum.

- Give the explanation for this possibly surprising finding.

  - There may be two subtypes of HBsAg, one which causes the liver disease, and one minor HBsAg against which the low concentration of anti-HBs is formed.

---

109

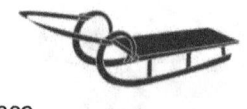

SO YOU WANT TO BE A HEPATOLOGIST!

In non-endemic areas for HBV, there may be isolated anti-HBe in the serum of the health general population.

- Give reasons for anti-HBe being in the serum of healthy persons
  - Acute HBV
    - IgM anti-HBe
    - Recovery
    - Exacerbation of HBV in chronic carrier
    - Progression
  - Recovery from acute HBV
  - Exacerbations of HBV in chronic carrier
  - Progression of acute HBV
  - Chronic HBV → HBsAg is undetectable
  - Acute HBV window period
  - Chronic
    - Short term
    - Long term
    - IgM anti-HBe
    - Window period (HBs Ag$^+$ → HbsAg$^-$, and development of anti-HBs)
    - Small amounts of HBV DNA in serum, liver and peripheral mononuclear cells; anti-HBs undetectable)
  - Technical factors relating to sensitivity of HBsAg assay
  - Coinfection of HBV plus HCV (60%)
  - False-positive test
  - HBV DNA in serum

110

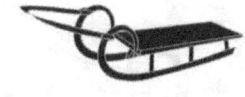

- ➢ Histopathology

- • Give the hepatic histopathological features of HBV infection.

  - o Ground-glass hepatocytes
    - – HBsAg in the ER of infected hepatocytes
    - – Cysteine in HBsAg stained by orcein, Victoria blue, aldehyde fuchsin indicate viral replication
    - – Also there may be core antigen in cytoplasm and hepatocyte nuclei
    - – After treatment cytoplasmic core antigen disappears, but persistence of nuclear core antigen indicates presence of HBV cccDNA template
  - o Peripheral infiltration with mononuclear cells
  - o Interface hepatitis (disruption of hepatocytes of the limiting plate)
  - o Fibrous tissue extending from peripheral areas
  - o Active septa mononuclear cells between fibrous extensions from portal tracts and hepatocyte parenchyma

- ➢ Prevention (HBV vaccination)
  - o Neutralizing antibody anti-HBs is produced against the "a" epitope of HBsAg by HBsAg-specific helper T cells and by T cell-dependent B cells.
  - o Protective levels of anti-HBs occur in > 90% of persons who are vaccinated with HBsAg.
  - o If a person who has been anti-HBc has had a mild.
  - o Subclinical HBV infection, either because
  - o After HBV vaccination, subclinical HBV infection may occur, either because
    - – Over time the litre of anti-HBs may have fallen to levels which are no longer protective (25% to 50% of vaccinated persons develop non-protective levels of anti-HBs over 5 to 10 years)
    - – Initial hyporesponders, with the development of low and non-protective concentrations of anti-HBS
  - o Booster doses of vaccine are needed
    - – In hemodialysis patients
    - – In persons who are immunocompetent
  - o Some persons with low or no anti-HBS after vaccination appear to be protected
  - o HBV anti-core[+] can reactivate with Prednisone, azathioprine, anti-TNF therapy

111

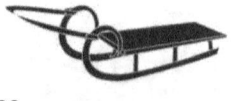

- Patients on infliximab are at risk for vaccine-preventable disease, including hepatitis B virus (HBV).

- Older age, lower albumin levels, and the presence of pancolitis were risk factors for the absence of protective antibodies against HBV.

- A significant minority of previously vaccinated patients do not respond to an HBV booster, indicating that they are not at risk for HBV infection.

Source: Mosses J, et al. Am J Gastroenterol 2012; 107: 133-138.

---

**SO YOU WANT TO BE A HEPATOLOGIST!**

- Give causes of ground-glass hepatocytes.
  - Chronic HBV
  - DILI (drug-induced liver injury)
  - Fibrinogen storage disease
  - Glycogenesis, type IV

---

- Give high-risk groups for whom hepatitis B virus (HBV) vaccination should be considered.
  - Health care workers
  - Hemodialysis patients
  - Household contacts and sexual partners of HBV carriers or patients with acute hepatitis B
    Injection drug users
  - Inmates of correctional facilities: International travellers to areas endemic for HBV who may have intimate contact with the local population or take part in medical activities
  - Men who have sex with men (MSM)
  - Patients who are likely to require multiple transfusions with blood or blood products
  - Patients with chronic liver disease (other than chronic hepatitis B)
    Potential organ transplant recipients
  - Public safety workers with likelihood of exposure to blood
  - Sexually active heterosexual men and women, if they have more than one partner
  - Staff and clients of institutions for developmentally disabled persons

Printed with permission: *Sleisenger and Fordtran's Gastrointestinal and Liver Disease: Pathophysiology/ Diagnosis/ Management*. 9th edition, 2010, page 1308.

112

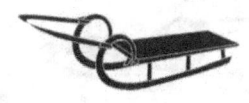

# SO YOU WANT TO BE A HEPATOLOGIST!

- Give reasons why a person immunized with HBs-Ag vaccine may not develop an adequate anti-HBs response.

  - Persons
    - Very young, or old (> 50 yrs)
    - Obese
    - Smoking
    - Chronic liver disease
    - Immunosuppressed
      - Transplantation
      - Chemotherapy
      - Immunodeficient HIV positive
    - Co-infection
      - HIV
      - HCV
    - Administration of vaccine into buttock muscles
    - Genetic factors
      - HLA
        - Alleles DR3, DR7, DQ2
        - No HLA-A2
  - Vaccine-frozen   – Wrong dose or timing of vaccine
  - Virus   – Mutant HBV virus strains (HBV escapes mutants)

- Give the **immunoprophylaxis** for HBV in adults accidentally exposed to possibly infectious blood (within the last 7 days), or sexual contacts (within the past 14 days).
  - Check donor blood for HBsAg; check victim's blood for HBsAg and HBcAb
  - Give at once 0.06 mL/kg HBIG plus first dose of hepatitis B vaccine

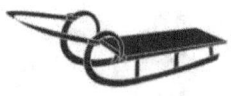

| | HBsAg | HBcAb | Further action to victim |
|---|---|---|---|
| – Victim | -ve | +ve | None: Immune |
| – "Donor" (source) | +ve | -ve | Continue vaccine course |
| | -ve | -ve | None, or continue vaccine course if victim is at risk of further hepatitis B exposure |

Adapted from: Sherlock S, and Dolley J. *Diseases of the Liver and Biliary System* (Eleventh Edition) 2002. pg. 285-303.

Please see *Sleisenger and Fordtran's Gastrointestinal and Liver Disease: Pathophysiology/ Diagnosis/ Management*. Ninth edition, 2010, for the following additional information: Table 78.6, "High-Risk Groups for Whom Hepatitis B Virus (HBV) Vaccination Should be Considered", page 1308.

- Give the reason why it is important to distinguish between inactive HBV carrier state (stage III) from HBe-Ag negative CHB.

| | Prognosis | Risk of complications |
|---|---|---|
| ○ Inactive HBV carrier | Good | Low |
| ○ HBe-Ag negative CHB | Poor | High |

➢ Treatment

- Give goals of treatment of HBeAg⁺ and HBeAg⁻ HBV infection.

E-antigen (+)          HB E-antigen (-) (+)

- ○ Loss of E-antigen (seroconversion, off treatment)
  - – e-Ag seroconversion is not possible if the patient is infected with the e-Ag mutant of the HB virus)
  - – HBsAg seroconversion (occurs in < 10%, and is often not seen for 4-5 years after therapy has been completed and e-Ag has occurred

- ○ Appearance of anti-HBe antibody

- ○ ↑ loss of HBsAgConversion to inactive status

- ○ Normalization in serum liver aminotransferase

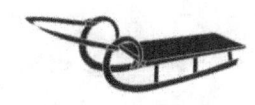

- ○ ↓↓ detectable HBV DNA
  - – Keep the HBV DNA levels as low as possible
    - ▪ ↑ immunological response to HBV
    - ▪ ↓ HLA class I antigen expression on surface of hepatocytes
    - ▪ ↑ CD8+ CTL activity
    - ▪ ↓ HBV ccc DNA ("the genomic template for viral transcription)
    - ▪ No drug resistance
    - ▪ Associated with seroconversion (HBeAg+ → HBeAg-)
      - –Genotype A~ 50%
      - –B, C, D ~ 25%
  - – Does not completely eliminate HBV infection, since the HBV (a DNA virus) becomes integrated within the hepatocyte genome as CCC, (covalently closed circular) DNA
- ○ Improvement in liver hepatic necroinflammation
- ○ Improve the patient's quality of life
- ○ Prevention of progression of the disease to cirrhosis, HCC, decompensation.
- ○ ↓ risk of hepatocellular carcinoma (HCC)
- ○ ↓ HBs Ag

Printed with permission:  Shiffman ML. *2008 AGA Annual Postgraduate Course Syllabus*: pg. 166.

---

The importance of HBeAg status

- ➢ HBeAg
  - ○ Represents
    - – ↑ viral replication
    - – Active liver disease
    - – Need for antiviral therapy

---

115

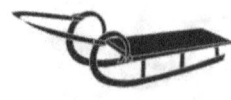

- Give the comparisons of HBeAg positive vs HBeAg negative HBV infection.

| Comparisons | HBeAg Positive | HBeAg Negative |
|---|---|---|
| o Epidemiology | – Most common type in North America | ▪ Higher incidence in Asia, Europe and other Mediterranean countries |
| o Rate of progression to cirrhosis | – Lower rate of progression to cirrhosis (10-20% /yr) (immune tolerance) | ▪ Higher rate of progression to cirrhosis |
| o Monitoring of treatment response | – HBeAg seroconversion to anti-HBV positive (also, possibly seroconversion to HBs Ag negative)<br>– Normalization of liver enzymes and marked reduction in HBV DNA | ▪ Normalization of liver enzymes and marked reduction in HBV DNA |

SO YOU WANT TO BE A HEPATOLOGIST!

Adults who are HBeAg-positive usually have active HBV, whereas children who are HBeAg-positive do not.
- Give the explanation why HBeAg$^+$ in children is not usually associated with active hepatitis.

  o The secretion of HBeAg may be reduced by
    – Precore or core promoter mutations
    – Low levels of wild-type HBV

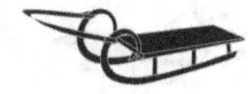

➢ Indications

- Give the indications for initiation of HBV therapy.
  - ○ ↑ HBV DNA (> 2000 IU/mL)
  - ○ ↑ ALT (> ULN)
  - ○ Moderate/severe necroinflammation, and/or
  - ○ ≥ moderate fibrosis
  - ○ When to start HBV therapy without liver biopsy
    - − HBeAg-negative, ↑ ALT (2x ULN), HBV DNA > 2000 IU/mL; or
    - − HBeAg-positive
  - ○ When to start HBV therapy with normal ALT.
    - − ↑ HBV DNA, necroinflammation changes and fibrosis on a liver biopsy
    - − Compensated cirrhosis, even if HBV DNA undetectable
    - − Decompensated cirrhosis plus detectable HBV DNA
  - ○ When to start HBV therapy for acute BV infection
  - ○ Chronic HBV
    - − HBeAg⁺
      - ▪ 90% have HBV DNA > 105 copies/mL
    - − HBeAg⁻
      - ▪ Lower serum HBV DNA levels, especially if ALT is normal
      - ▪ Higher HBV DNA in HBeAg⁻ with ↑ ALT
  - ○ Seroconversion (HBeAg⁺ → HBeAg⁻, anti-HBe) usually associated with ↓ HBV DNA

- Give when anti-HBV therapy should be given for acute HBV.
  - ○ Active HBV:
    - − HBeAg (+), HBV DNA >500,000 copies/mL (20,000 Iμ/ml), and elevated ALT > 2 X ULN
  - ○ Active hepatitis with variable degrees of fibrosis on liver biopsy
  - ○ Pre-core mutations of HBV:
    - − Includes patients with all features above, except eAg(-)
  - ○ Inactive HBV:
    - − Patients with inactive HBV, and HBV DNA < 500,000 copies/mL are NOT currently considered candidates for HBV therapy, unless they have evidence of cirrhosis on liver biopsy. These patients are at low risk to develop fibrosis progression or HCC.

117

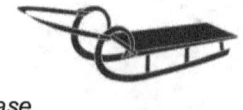

- HBV acute infection, when HBeAg lasts beyond 12 wks
  - HBV therapy may reduce the 5% risk of development of chronic HBV
- Fulminant HBV
  - INR > 1.5 plus clinically deep jaundice
  - Anti-HBV useful since patient may need a liver transplantation
- ↑ risk of progression (fibrosis progression, cirrhosis and HCC)
- Immune tolerant

- Give the pre-treatment **baseline evaluation** of the patient with HBV infection.
  - Revised normal ALT levels (30 IU/L for men, and 19 IU/L for women) should be used as criteria for treatment
  - Baseline evaluation should include HBV genotype, particularly if peginterferon therapy considered
  - Preferred first line treatment options: adefovir, entecavir, peginterferon alfa-2a, and possibly telbivudine (Lamivudine not first-line choice secondary to high rate of resistance to Interferon alfa-2b
  - Liver biopsy should be considered for patients with normal ALT levels, especially if age >35-40 years

- Give the **general management strategy** of the person with HBV.
  - Treatment strategies
    - PEG-IFN or NA monotherapy for finite duration
    - NA for long-term duration
  - PEG-IFN or NA monotherapy used for finite duration
    - PEG-IFN (in the absence of contraindications) for HBeAg- positive and -negative patients for 48 weeks

Caution: do not combine PEG-IFN with lamivudine or telbivudine (development of severe neuropathy)

  - Entecavir or tenofovir for 12 months after seroconversion in about 2/3 of these initially HBeAg-positive HBV patients
  - NA for long-term duration
  - Entecavir or tenofovir monotherapy for
    - HBeAg-positive patients who failed to seroconvert or HBeAg-negative patients
    - All HBV cirrhosis

118

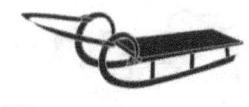

- o Monitoring and applying stopping rules
- Give the potential management strategies for HBV by on-treatment virologic response categories.
  - o Virological response - HBV DNA < 2000 IU/mL at 0, 6 and 12 months after the end of therapy
  - o Sustained virological response - HBV DNA < 2000 IU/mL at 12 months after the end of therapy
  - o Virological break through
    - $\uparrow$ HBV DNA 1 $\log_{10}$ IU/mL compared to lowest previous level of HBV DNA on Rx
    - Characterized by $\uparrow$ ALT
    - Due to
      - Poor adherence to therapy, or
      - HBV resistance (due to therapy associated selection of HBV resistant variants)

| Category | Strategy* |
|---|---|
| o Primary treatment failure at week 12 | - If noncompliant, counsel patient on importance of adherence to prescribed drug regimen<br>- If compliant, change therapy to more potent drug or possibly a drug combination |
| o Complete virologic response at week 24 | - Continue therapy with same drug; monitoring may be extended to 6-month intervals |
| o Partial virologic response at week 24 | - If drug has a low genetic barrier to resistance, add a second drug that is not cross-resistant<br>- If drug has a high genetic barrier to resistance, repeat monitoring at 3-month intervals and continue beyond 48 weeks<br>- If drug has a delayed antiviral effect e.g., adefovir, repeat monitoring at 3-month intervals and if response becomes complete at 48 weeks, continue therapy; but if response remains partial or becomes inadequate at 48 weeks, add a more potent drug |
| o Inadequate virologic response at week 24 | - Add another drug (preferably one that is more efficacious, or if such a drug is not available, then add one that is not cross-resistant)<br>- Repeat monitoring at 3-month intervals |

- Monitoring after 48 weeks may be extended from 3 to 6 months if response becomes complete

*patients with advanced disease should be monitored at 3-month intervals while on treatment, regardless of virologic response

Printed with permission:  Keeffe EB. *2007 AGA Institute Postgraduate Course*: pg. 77.

- Give factors that are predictive of a viral response (VR) to treatment of HBV infection.
  - Patient
    - Immunocompetent
  - HBV
    - Adult-acquired infection
    - Low HBV-DNA level
      - ↑ response to interferin
      - HBV recurrence with liver transplantation
    - Absence of HDV or HIV co-infection
    - HBeAg +ve
  - Biopsy
    - Active liver disease—ALT > 5x upper limit of normal (ULN), active hepatitis on biopsy
  - Specific treatment algorithms
    - HBeAg+
    - HBeAg-

Adapted from: Keeffe EB, et al. *Clin Gastroenterol Hepatol* 2006;4(8):936-62.

- Give the recommendations regarding monitoring and stopping HBV treatment.

❖ PEG-IFN
  - HBeAg-positive
    - On treatment
      - Every 6 and 12 months: anti-HBe antibodies, serum HBV DNA, ALT, HBsAg at 12 months
    - Off treatment
      - Every 12 months: HBeAg, anti-HBe antibodies, serum HBV DNA, ALT, HBsAg

120

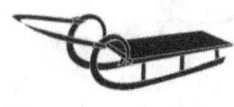

- HBeAG seroconversion (HBeAg-positive → negative
  - Test HBsAg every 12 months (seroreversion)
- No HBeAg seroconversion (serum HBsAg > 20,000 IU/mL, or no ↓ HBsAg at 3 months
  - Stop PEG-IFN
- o HBeAg-negative
  - On treatment, at month 3 if ↓ HBV DNA ≥ 2 $\log_{10}$ IU/mL, and no ↓ HBsAg
    - Stop PEG-IFN (especially genotype D)

- ❖ NA (nuceos[t]ide
  - o On treatment every 6 months HBeAg, anti-HBe, HBV DNA, serum creatinine
    - Measure HBsAg every 12 months after HBe seroconversion
    - Stop NA 12 months after anti-HBe seroconversion, or
    - Stop NA until loss of HBsAg (with or without antibodies to HBsAg), especially if there is severe fibrosis or cirrhosis.

- • Give when HBV therapy should be reassessed or stopped.
  - o HBeAg+: HBeAg seroconversion and – HBV DNA
  - o HBeAg-: ? Long term therapy
  - o Inadequate VR (<2,000 IU/mL) at week 24
  - o Development of antiviral drug resistance

Abbreviation: VR, viral response

Printed with permission: Keeffe EB. *2007 AGA Institute Postgraduate Course*: 75.

- o If HBV DNA reappears during treatment of HBV, resistance to the drug has likely occurred.
- o In fulminant HBV, the HBsAg may have disappeared, but the diagnosis can be made by finding HBV.

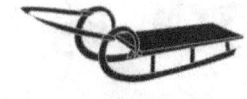

122

**Drug choices**

- o IFN (interferon)
    - – PEG-IFN (pegylated IFN)
- o Nucleosides
    - – Lamivudine
    - – Telbivudine
    - – Emtricitabine
    - – Entecavir
- o Nucleotides
    - – Adefovir
    - – Tenofovir

- • Give the recommendations for treatment strategy (treatment algorithm) of **HBeAg-positive compensated patients**, based on their HBV DNA and ALT.

| HBV DNA | ALT | Treatment Strategy |
|---|---|---|
| o <20,000 IU/mL | Normal | - No treatment<br>- Monitor every 6-12 months<br>- Consider therapy in patients with known significant histological disease even if low-level replication |
| o ≥20,000 IU/mL | Normal | - Low rate of HBeAg seroconversion for all treatments<br>- Monitor every 3-12 months<br>- Younger patients often immune tolerant<br>- Consider biopsy; particularly if older than age 35-40 years; treat if significant disease. In the absence of biopsy, observe for rise in ALT levels.<br>- If treated, adefovir, entecavir, peginterferon alfa-2a, or possibly telbivudine preferred. |
| o ≥20,000 Iµ/ml | Elevated | - Adefovir, entecavir, peginterferon alfa-2a, or possibly telbivudine are preferred<br>- If "high" HBV DNA: adefovir, entecavir or telbivudine preferred over peginterferon alfa-2a. |

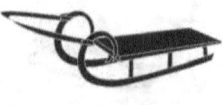

- o HBV disease
  - "acute" > 20,000 HBV DNA IU/ml
  - "inactive" < 20,000 HBV DNA IU/ml

- Give the recommendations for treatment strategy of HBeAg-negative compensated patients, based on their HBV DNA and ALT.

| HBV DNA | ALT | Treatment strategy |
|---------|-----|--------------------|
| o <2,000 IU/mL | Normal | - No treatment: majority inactive HBsAg carriers<br>- Monitor every 6-12 months |
| o ≥2,000 IU/mL | Normal | - Consider biopsy; treat long term if disease present. In the absence of biopsy, observe for rise in serum ALT levels (ALT often fluctuates).<br>- If treated, adefovir, entecavir, peginterferon alfa-2a, or possibly telbivudine preferred. |
| o ≥2,000 IU/mL | Elevated | - Adefovir, entecavir, peginterferon alfa-2a, or possibly telbivudine are preferred<br>- Long term treatment required for oral agents |

Printed with permission: Keeffe EB, et al. *Clin Gastroenterol Hepatol* 2006;4(8):936-62.

➢ Useful background

Results of main studies for the treatment of chronic hepatitis B at 6 months following 48 all 52 weeks of pegylated interferon alpha (PEG-IFNα), and at 48 all 52 weeks of nucleos(t)ide analog (NA) therapy.

| HBeAg Positive | PEG-IFN | | Nuclesoside Analogs | | | Nucleotide Analog | |
|----------------|---------|---------|------|------|------|------|------|
| | PEG-IFN-2a | PEG-IFN-2b | LAM | TEL | ENT | ADE | TEN |
| Dose | 180 µg | 180 µg | 100 µg | 600 mg | 0.5 mg | 10 mg | 245 mg |
| Anti-HBe seroconversion (%) | 32 | 29 | 16-18 | 22 | 21 | 12-18 | 21 |
| HBV DNA < 60-80 IU/mL (%) | 14 | 7 | 36-44 | 60 | 67 | 13-21 | 76 |

124

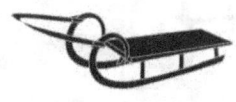

| HBeAg Negative | PEG-IFN | Nuclesoside Analogs | | | Nucleotide Analog | |
|---|---|---|---|---|---|---|
| | | LAM | TEL | ENT | ADE | TEN |
| ALT normalisation (%) | 41 | 32 | 41-72 | 77 | 68 | 48-54 | 68 |
| HBsAg loss (%) | 3 | 7 | 0-1 | 0.5 | 2 | 0 | 3 |
| Dose | | 180 µg | 100 µg | 600 mg | 0.5 mg | 10 mg | 245 mg |
| HBV DNA < 60-80 IU/mL (%) | 19 | 72-73 | 88 | 90 | 51-63 | 93 |
| ALT normalisation (%) | 59 | 71-79 | 74 | 78 | 72-77 | 76 |
| HBsAg loss (%) | 4 | 0 | 0 | 0 | 0 | 0 |
| Drug resistance 1 / 5 years | 0/0 | 24/70 | 41 | 0.2/1.2 | 0/29 | 0/0 |

Abbreviations: ADE, adefovir; ENT, entecavir; LAM, lamivudine; TEL, telbividine; TEN, tenofovir

Printed with permission: European Association for the Study of the Liver. EASL clinical practice guidelines: Management of chronic hepatitis B virus infection. J Hepatol. 2012;57(1):167-85.

"Great thoughts speak only to the thoughtful mind, but great actions speak to all mankind."

Emily P. Bissell

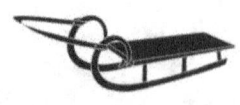

- Comparisons between current nucleos(t)ide analogues in treatment-naïve patients with chronic hepatitis B , in terms of (by reduction and undetectable) HBV-DNA (PCR) and HBeAg seroconversion and drug resistance

| | Lamivudine | | Adefovir | | Entetavir | | Telbivudine | | Tenotovir | |
|---|---|---|---|---|---|---|---|---|---|---|
| | e(+) | e (-) | e(+) | e (-) | e(+) | e (-) | e(+) | e (-) | e(+) | e (-) |
| HBV-DNA (PCR) Log reduction: | | | | | | | | | | |
| Year 1 | 5.4 | 4.5 | 3.6 | 3.7 | 6.9 | 5.0 | 5.7 | 4.4 | 6.5 | 4.5 |
| | | | | | | | | | | |
| Undetectable: | | | | | | | | | | |
| Year 1 | 40% | 7.3% | 21% | 61% | 6.7% | 9% | 60% | 88% | 76% | 93% |
| Year 2 | 39% | 52% | NA | 71% | 74% | NA | 5.6% | 82% | 78% | 99% |
| Year 3 | 20% | 40% | NA | 77% | NA | NA | NA | NA | NA | NA |
| Year 4 | NA | 34% | NA | 73% | NA | NA | NA | NA | NA | NA |
| | | | | | | | | | | |
| HBeAg Seroconversion | | | | | | | | | | |
| Year 1 | 20% | NP | 13%[a] | NP | 21% | NP | 23% | NP | 23% | NP |
| Year 2 | 26% | NP | 29%[a] | NP | 31% | NP | 30% | NP | 26% | NP |
| Year 3 | 40% | NP | 37%[a] | NP | NA | NP | NA | NP | NA | NP |
| Year 4 | 47% | NP | 35%[a] | NP | 47% | NP | NA | NP | NA | NP |
| | | | | | | | | | | |
| Drug resistance | | | | | | | | | | |
| Year 1 | 11- | 6-27% | 0% | 0% | 0% | 0% | 5% | 2% | 0% | 0% |
| Year 2 | 14% | 26- | NA | 3% | 0% | NP | 25% | 11% | 0% | 0% |
| Year 3 | 40% | 54% | NA | 11% | 1.2% | NP | NA | NA | NA | NA |
| Year 4 | 56% | | 20% | 29% | 1.2% | NP | NA | NA | NA | NA |

Abbreviations: HBV, hepatitis B virus; PCR, polymerase chain reaction; E, hepatitis B e antigen; NA, not available; NP, not applicable

[a]Cumulative incidence

Printed with permission: Chien RN and Liaw YF. *Best Practise Res Clin Gastroenterol* 2008;22:1081-1092.

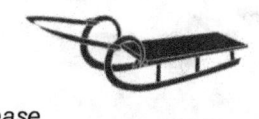

Note:

- o The dose of NAs (NTs and NSs) must be reduced if creatinine clearance < 50 mL/min.

- o All HBV positive patients must be screened for HIV before starting their HBV treatment with lamivudine, entercavir or tenofovir, since these drugs have activity against HIV and should not be used as more therapy for HBV for fear of causing HIV resistance.
  - – PEG-IFN, adefovir and telbivudine are not active against HIV.

- o PEG-IFN has advantages over nucleos(t)ide (NA) because of
  - – The absence of resistance
  - – The possibility of seroconversion (HBsAg-positive → negative) in about 25% of patients
  - – The ~4% change of loss of HBsAg in persons who achieve and maintain undetectable HBV DNA (by sensitive testing).
  - – IFN therapy responders enjoy a ~ 50% reduction in cirrhotic complications and 80% reduction in liver- related mortality.

- o Overview of response rates in HBeAg positive and HBeAg negative patients with currently available antiviral drugs.

| Antiviral Therapy | HBeAg Positive HBeAg Seroconversion | | HBeAg Negative Undetectable HBV DNA | |
|---|---|---|---|---|
| | End of Therapy | Post Treatment | End of Therapy | Post Treatment |
| o Alpha interferon | 35% | 30% | 60% | 35% |
| o Peginterferon | 40% | 35% | 63% | 19% |
| o Lamivudine | 19% | 12% | 65% | 10% |
| o Adefovir | 12% | NA | 51% | NA |
| o Adefovir in lamivudine resistance | 20% | NA | 19% | NA |
| o Entecavir | 21% | NA | 90% | NA |
| o Entecavir in lamivudine resistance | 8% | NA | 26% | NA |
| o Telbivudine | 22% | NA | 88% | NA |
| o Tenofovir | 21% | NA | 92% | NA |

Abbreviation: NA, not applicable

Printed with permission: Buster, et al. *Best Practise Res Clin Gastroenterol* 2008;22:1093-1108.

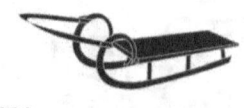

# INTERFERON

- Give the advantages and disadvantages of interferon for the treatment of chronic HBV infection.

| Agent | Advantages | Disadvantages |
|-------|------------|---------------|
| o Interferon | - HBsAg loss<br>- Short treatment duration<br>- No drug resistance | ▪ Parenteral administration<br>▪ Frequent side effects |
| o Peg-IFN | - HBsAg loss<br>- Fixed duration of treatment<br>- No drug resistance | ▪ Parenteral administration<br>▪ Frequent side effects but less than interferon |

- Give the early and late adverse effects of interferon.
  - o Early
    - Flu-like illness; headaches, nausea
    - Tenderness at site of infection
  - o Late
    - General
      - ▪ Fatigue
      - ▪ Irritability Anxiety and depression
    - Eyes
      - ▪ ↑ retinopathy DM
      - ▪ Optic tract neuropathy
    - CNS
      - ▪ CNS (neuropsychiatric)
    - MSK
      - ▪ Muscle aches
    - Skin
      - ▪ Alopecia
      - ▪ Lichen planus worsens
    - GI
      - ▪ Weight loss
      - ▪ Diarrhea
      - ▪ Anorexia
      - ▪ IBD worsens
    - Endocrine
      - ▪ Autoimmune autoantibodies
      - ▪ Worsening thyroid disease
      - ▪ Autoimmune diseases worsen
    - Pregnancy class C
    - Bone marrow suppression ▪ Bacterial Infections

Adapted from: Grover PT, and Bain V. *First Principles of Gastroenterology* 2005: 547-563.

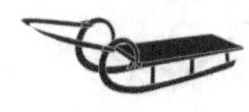

- Give **contraindications** to the use of IFN/PEG-IFN.
    - ○ Decompensated HBV cirrhosis (↑ risk of bacteremia and ↑ decompensation)
    - ○ Autoimmune disease
    - ○ Uncontrolled severe depression/psychosis
    - ○ Pregnancy
    - ○ Renal transplant patients (↑ risk of rejection)

## Nucleoside (NS) / nucleotide (NT) analogs (NA)

- Give the advantages and disadvantages of nucleosides and nucleotide analogs for the treatment of chronic HBV infection.

| Agent | Advantages | Disadvantages |
|---|---|---|
| ○ Lamivudine | - Oral administration<br>- Excellent tolerance<br>- Use in ESLD<br>- Use in adefovir failures | ▪ Drug resistance: common (~20%/year, and up to 70% with 4-5 years of therapy) |
| ○ Adefovir | - Oral administration<br>- Excellent tolerance<br>- Use in ESLD<br>- Use in lamivudine failures | ▪ Less potent, with suboptimal responses not uncommon<br>▪ Drug resistance: delayed and less common (0% at year 1, 2% at year 2, 7% at year 3, 15% at year 4, and 29% at year 5 of therapy) |
| ○ Entecavir | - Oral administration<br>- Excellent tolerance<br>- High potency in lowering HBV DNA levels<br>- Use in adefovir failures | ▪ Drug resistance: rare in nucleoside naïve patients (0.1% at year 1, 0.4% at year 2 and 1.1% at year 3), but common in patients with lamivudine resistance (6% at year 1, 14% at year 2, and 32% at year 3) |
| ○ Telbivudine | - Oral administration<br>- Excellent tolerance<br>- High potency in lowering HBV DNA levels | ▪ Drug resistance: intermediate rates (5% at year 1, and 21.6% at year 2 in HBeAg-positive patients, and 8.6% in HBeAg-negative patients) |

Abbreviation: ESLD, end-stage liver disease

Printed with permission: Keeffe EB. *2007 AGA Institute Postgraduate Course*: 76.

- ○ "Competitive inhibitors of reverse transcriptase and DNA polymerase".
- ○ "Replace natural nucleoside during the synthesis of the first or second strand (or both) of HBV DNA".

129

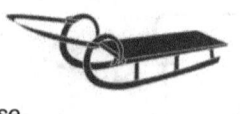

- Lamivudine
  - High rate of viral mutation and viral resistance
- ~40% at 2 years, 65% at 5 year
- Higher rate of resistance with treatment of co-infection with treatment of co-infection with HIV.
- HBV viral suppression
  - Lam < adefovir (Ade) < enterocovir < telbivudine (Tel) < tenofovir (Ten)
- HBV resistance
  - Ten > The > Ent >Ade
  - Rate of resistance
    - Lam    69% / 5 yrs  ⎤
    - Ade    30% / 4 yrs  ⎥  don't use
    - Ten    rare          ⎦

- Give pros and cons of Lamivudine versus interferon (IFN) for the treatment of HBV.

| Favoring Lamivudine | Favoring IFN |
|---|---|
| o  Needle phobia | –  Young Asian |
| o  HIV co-infection | –  Genotype A |
| o  Other immunosuppression (e.g., transplantation) | –  Recent infection |
| o  Patients with depression | –  AST > 100 |
| o  Low WBC count | –  Low serum HBV-DNA |
| o  Low platelet count | –  Active liver biopsy |
| o  Autoimmune disease | –  eAg+ |
| o  Decompensated cirrhosis | –  Possibility of seroconversion (eAg+→eAb+) |
| o  Vertical transmission | –  Marginal benefit to baby |
| o  Cost concerns | –  Contraindicated with depression, renal failure |
| o  Pregnancy, may be used | |
| o  Has 70% resistance rate at 5 years. It acts as an immunomodulatory agent resulting in loss of circulating HBeAg and HBV DNA in 30-40% of cases, and to a lesser extent as an antiviral agent resulting in loss of HBsAg in less than 5% of cases. | |
| o  Cross resistance with tenofovir | |

Adapted from: Grover PT, and Bain V. *First Principles of Gastroenterology* 2005:547-552.

130

- o **Adefovir dipovoxil**
  - Acyclic phosphate nucleotide analog of adenosine monophosphate
  - ↓ HBV polymerase and reverse transcriptase
- o **Entercavir**
  - Deoxyguanine nucleotide analog which selectively inhibits replication of HBV
  - ↓ priming of HBV DNA polymerase
  - ↓ synthesis of 192 nd strand of HBV DNA
  - Low rates of resistance (1.2% after 5 years), and
  - 20% rate of eAg seroconversion after 48 weeks
- o Development of resistance is associated with flares.
- o **Telebuvidine**
  - L. nucleoside analog of thymidine
  - Because telbivudine develops resistance mutations at the same site as for lamivudine, telbivudine is not effective in persons who have lamivudine resistance
- o **Tenofovir disoproxil fumarate**
  - Chemically similar to adefovir mechanism of action similar to adefovir (a cyclic nucleotide inhibitor of HBV polymerase and reverse transcriptase
  - Resistance does not occur
  - The diagnosis of chronic HBV infection in an HIV patient is an indication to start tenofovir-based HAAR therapy
  - Tenofovir is a selective inhibitor of HBV-DNA polymerase, and is active in HBV

- Give the management of nucleoside and nucleotide resistance.
  - o Nucleoside resistance
    - Lamivudine, telbivudine, entecavir → tenofovir or adefovir (nucleotide analogues)
    - Note: nephrogenic potential is adefovir > tenofovir; in fact, tenofovir may actually improve renal function
  - o Nucleotide resistance
    - Adefovir
      - Naïve → tenofovir or entecavir (preferred for ↑↑ HBV DNA levels)
      - Prior lamivudine resistance → tenofovir plus telbivudine or entecavir (nucleoside analogues)
    - Tenofovir
      - Naïve → lamivudine, telbivudine, entecavir
      - Prior lamivudine resistance→ entecavir

131

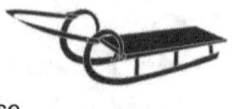

- Give the recommendations for treatment of **HBV-associated cirrhotic patients** (HBeAg positive or negative).

| HBV DNA | Cirrhosis | Treatment Strategy |
|---|---|---|
| o  <2,000 | Compensated | – May choose to treat or observe<br>– Adefovir or entecavir preferred |
| o  ≥2,000 | Compensated | – Adefovir or entecavir are first-line options<br>– Long-term treatment required, and combination therapy may be preferred |
| o  <200 or ≥200 | Decompensated | – Combination with lamivudine, or possibly entecavir, plus adefovir preferred<br>– Long-term treatment required, and combination therapy may be preferred<br>– Wait list for liver transplantation |

- Give the management options of **rescue therapy** for HBV when there is resistance to lamivudine, adefovir, entecavir or telbivudine.

| Resistant Drug | Rescue Therapy |
|---|---|
| o  Lamivudine | – Continue lamivudine and add adefovir or tenofovir<br>– Switch to emtricitabine/tenofovir |
| o  Adefovir | – Continue Adefovir and add lamivudine<br>– Switch to or add entecavir (if no prior LAM-R)<br>– Switch to emtricitabine/tenofovir |
| o  Entecavir | – Switch to or add adefovir or tenofovir |
| o  Telbivudine | – Continue telbivudine and add adefovir or tenofovir<br>– Switch to emtricitabine/tenofovir |

Abbreviation: LAM-R, resitance to LAM

Printed with permission:  Keeffe EB, et al. A *Clin Gastroenterol Hepatol* 2008;6(12):1315-41.

132

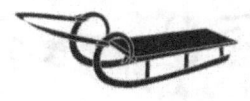

## Mutants and Mutations

- o HBsAg mutants
  - – Vaccine escape
    - ▪ In persons for whom HBIG does not present HBV, about half of these "escapes" are due to alterations in the "a" determinants of the HBsAg, leading to immune escape.
  - – May influence HBV recurrence after liver transplantation.
- o Mutations in the Precore, Basal Core Promoter and Core Genes
  - – More common in HBe-Ag-negative persons
  - – Stop the synthesis of HbeAg
  - – ↑ development of fulminant HBV
  - – ↑ risk of HCC
  - – ↓ response to interferon
- o Mutations in HBV DNA polymerase
  - – "HBV reverse transcriptase function of the polymerase gene is highly preserved…." (Sleisenger and Fordtran's Gastrointestinal and Liver Disease. 9th Edition. Saunders/Elsevier, Philadelphia, 2010, page 1291).

---

**SO YOU WANT TO BE A HEPATOLOGIST!**

- o Viral resistance may occur weeks to months before a virologic breakthrough

- In the context of HBV, define "**virologic breakthrough**".

- o Virologic breakthrough
  - – "> 1 $\log_{10}$ (10-fold) increase in serum HBV DNA levels above the previous nadir" (Sleisenger and Fordtran's Gastrointestinal and Liver Disease. 9th Edition. Saunders/Elsevier, Philadelphia, 2010, Table 78.3, page 1304).

- Virologic rebound may follow virologic breakthrough; define "virologic rebound".
  - o Virologic rebound HBV DNA > $10^5$ (20,000 IU/mL)

---

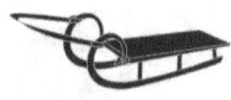

## Special Conditions in Treating HBV Infection

- o **Chronic renal failure, dialysis and renal transplantation**
  - – The dose of NAs (NTs and NSs) must be reduced if creatinine clearance < 50 mL/min.
  - – Vaccinate HBV surrogate patients with renal transplant, requiring renal dialysis, or end-stage renal disease
  - – HBV positive, renal impairment
    - ▪ NA dose reduction, except for tenofovir
    - ▪ Avoid PEG-IFN renal transplant patient (↑ risk of rejection)
    - ▪ Monitor creatinine clearance
    - ▪ Treat co-existing hypertension and diabetes mellitus

- o **HIV co-infection**
  - – All HBV positive patients must be screened for HIV before starting their HBV treatment with lamivudine, entercavir or tenofovir, since these drugs have activity against HIV and should not be used as more therapy for HBV for fear of causing HIV resistance.
  - – PEG-IFN, adefovir and telbivudine are not active against HIV.
  - – Tenofovir, emtricitabine or lamivudine, plus a third day which is active against HIV

- o **HCV co-infection**
  - – Treat HCV, monitor HBV DNA and treat HBV activation with NAs (activity of HBV is often suppressed in presence of HCV).

- o **Post-LT** (liver transplantation)
  - – Entecavir monotherapy prophylaxis, or
  - – Tenofovir plus emtricitabine with or without HBIG (hepatitis B immunoglobulin)
  - – Lamivudine plus adefovir plus HBIG

- o **Acute liver failure** (ALF) for severe acute HBV infection
  - – Start entecavir or tenofovir
  - – Assess for possible need for liver transplantation
  - – Continue entecavir or tenofovir for at least
    - ▪ 3 months after seroconversion of HBsAG (HBsAg → anti-HBs)
    - ▪ 12 months after seroconversion of HbeAg (HBeAg > anti-HBe)

134

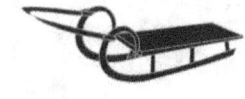

- o **Woman with cirrhosis** / advanced fibrosis, "planned pregnancy" (2-method contraception, PEG-IFN for 12 months
  - If couple not cooperative with 2-month contraception, or IFN otherwise contraindicated, use NA with FDA B category drug
- o Unexpected pregnancy
  - If on PEG-IFN → telbivudine or tenofovir (FDA X → B class Rx)
  - If an lamivudine, adefovir or entecavir → tenofovir or telbivudine (FDA C → B class Rx)
  - If HBV infection newly diagnosed, use the usual (non-pregnant) indications for HBV Rx for possible hepatic flare, during or after pregnancy
  - To prevent vertical transmission to newborn child
    - NA to reduce viral loads (especially for mothers HBeAg-positive, and/or serum HBV DNA > $10^{-7}$ IU/mL
    - HBIG plus HBV vaccination
  - Safety of NA for mother who wishes to breastfeed is unknown
  - FDA category
    - B tenofovir (preferred), telbivudine
    - C lamivudine, adefovir, entecavir
    - **X PEG-IFN – Do not use**

## "Flares" of the Acute Hepatitis

- Give causes of "flares" of acute hepatitis (reactivation, decompensation) in persons with chronic HBV, as related to the HBV.

| Cause of Flares | Comment |
|---|---|
| o Spontaneous | - Seroconversion HBeAg+ →HBeAg- <br> - Reappearance of IgM anti-HBC (often during the second to third month may herald virologic response <br> - Anti-HBe → HBeAg (seroconversion) <br>    • Type II polyclonal IgG, plus monoclonal IgM <br>    • Type III polyclonal IgG, plus rheumatoid factor |
| o Drugs <br>   – Immuno-suppressives | - During withdrawal of immunosuppressants; requires preemptive antiviral therapy <br> - Withdrawal of immunosuppression <br>    • Extrahepatic manifestations <br>    • Active state of immune clearance with anti-HBs or anti-HBe → HBsAg <br>    • Immunosuppressants <br>    • Biologicals <br>    • Chemotherapy |

135

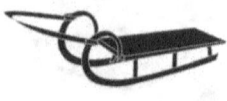

| Cause of Flares | Comment |
|---|---|
| o Lamivudine | - Development of YMDA mutants<br>- Severe consequences in patients with advanced liver disease |
| o Adefovir, entecavir | - On withdrawal, flares are caused by rapid reemergence of wild-type HBV; can have severe consequences in patients with advanced liver disease |
| o HIV treatment | - Flares also can occur with immune reconstitution or secondary to antiretroviral drug hepatotoxictity |
| o Genotypic variation<br>   – Precore and core promoter mutants | - Fluctuations in serum ALT levels are common with precore and core promoter mutants<br>- HAV, HCV, HDV, HIV |
| o Superimposed infection | |
| o Other hepatitis viruses | - HBV replication |
| o Alcohol use | |

- o Reactivation of HBV infection
    - – ↑ HBV-DNA
    - – ↑ IgM anti-HBe
    - – ↑ ALT, AST
    - – Acute lobular hepatitis, plus anti-HBe
    - – Acute lobular hepatitis, plus previous histological changes of chronic hepatitis

Adapted from: Poterucha JJ. *Mayo Clinic Gastroenterology and Hepatology Board Review* 2008, pg.298; Sleisenger and Fordtran's Gastrointestinal and Liver Disease. 10th Edition. Saunders/Elsevier, Philadelphia, 2016, page 1454.

---

**SO YOU WANT TO BE A HEPATOLOGIST!**

- Give the reason why anti-HBV therapy during pregnancy is not usually indicated.

    - o When "newborn child of an HBV-positive mother is given HBV vaccination plus injection of HBIG, breakthrough HBV infection in the child occurs in < 5%

    - o Lamivudine may be discontinued during pregnancy
        - – HBC, FDA category B
        - – HBC plus HIV, FDA category C

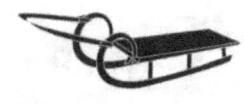

- o **Before starting immunosuppressive therapy or chemotherapy**
  - – HBe-Ag-positive
    - ▪ NA before, during and for 12 months after immunosuppressive therapy or (preferable entecavir or tenofonir) chemotherapy, regardless of serum HBV DNA level
  - – HBeAg-negative patients with detectable HBV DNA –treat as per above
  - – HBeAg-negative, anti-HBe antibody positive, detectable serum HBV DNA – treat as per above,
  - – HBeAg-negative, anti-HBe antibody positive, undetectable serum, HBV DNA – monthly monitoring of ALT and HBV DNA, with NA for resection.
  - – Anti-HBe positive patients receiving bone marrow or stem cell transplantation – NA prophylaxis
  - – HbsAg negative recipient of liver graft from anti-HBe-positive donor – indefinite lamivudine prophylaxis
  - – Polyarteritis nodosa (PAN) – think of HBV/HCV infection

- o **Steroid withdrawal**

- • Give the reason why ALF may occur during steroid withdrawal for treatment of polyartritis nodosa (PAN) in HBV, but not in HCV.

  - o Hepatic damage in HBV (but not in HCV) is immune-mediated, and would cause aggressive necrosis upon immune reconstitution resulting from withdrawal of steroids for treatment of PAN.

Please see: Peltekian KM, Hirsch G. Chapter 59. In: Therapeutic Choices. Grey J, Ed. 6th Edition, Canadian Pharmacists Association: Ottawa, ON, 2011, page 789.

137

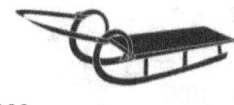

- o **Immune Rebound**

A short course of glucocorticosteroids ("steroids") is no longer used to increase virologic response rates, because of the immune rebound when steroids are stopped.

- Give the explanation for this immune rebound which ccurs when the patient with HBV infection is placed on corticosteroids which are then stopped.
    - o When steroids are stopped, there is ↑ activation of T lymphocytes that promote the Th1 cytokine responses.
    - o The ↑ Th1 cytokine response occurs at the time when there is ↑ expression of HBV.
    - o The combination of ↑ HBV antigen plus ↑ Th1 cytokine response causes hepatic decompensation.
    - o Precore mutant HBV (aka HBe Ag-negative HBV) flares due to a change in the ratio of precore HBV / wild-type HBV.
    - o Mutations in basal core promoter region (with or without precore mutants)
        - ↑ HbeAg
        - ↑ HBV replication
        - ↑ necroinflammation
    - o HBe Ag-negative HBV plus both precore and core mutations
        - ↑ risk of flare with chemotherapy

## HBV Infection and Hepatocellular Cancer (HCC)

- Give clinical and serological characteristics of healthy HBV carriers (no cirrhosis) who are candidates for HCC screening.
    - o Clinical
        - Race
            - African males/females > 20 years
            - Asian male > 40 years
            - Asian female > 50 years
            - Caucasian
                - Inactive or active disease with cirrhosis*
                    - Caucasians with inactive disease and no cirrhosis have a low risk of HCC development, and HCC screening is generally not recommended, but may be considered if there is a family history of HCC, or co-infection with HCV.
        - Family history of HCC
        - Co-infection with HCV, HIV

Adapted from: Sherman M. *Best Practice & Research Clinical Gastroenterology* 2005;19(1): 105.

138

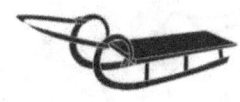

- Give serological factors which are associated with ↑ risk of HCC in HBV infection.
  - HbsAg-positive
  - HBeAg-positive
  - Reversion of anti-HBe to HBeAg$^+$
  - HBV DNA > $10^5$
  - Cirrhosis

---

Clinical Alert !  HBV and HCC
  - HBV and risk of HCC and cirrhosis
    - The level of HBV DNA correlates with the relative risk of HCC and cirrhosis
    - Lowering of HBV DNA is associated with ↓ risk of HCC and cirrhosis
    - Even HBV DNA of 200 IU/mL or 10,000 copies/mL may be associated with ↑ risk of HCC and cirrhosis
    - An argument can be made to use maintenance HBV therapy to suppress HBV and ↓ risk of long-term complications
    - Even HBsAg clearance, … is not on absolute safeguard against the future development of HCC in persons who already have cirrhosis" (Feldman M., et al. Sleisenger and Fordtran's Gastrointestinal and Liver Disease. 9$^{th}$ Edition. Saunders/Elsevier, Philadelphia, 2010, page 1289).
    - Because of vaccine escape mutants in the "a" determinant of the HBsAg, about 2% of vaccinated persons do not mount a protective response.
  - A normal ALT is not a good marker for disease activity
    - ~25% of HBV carriers with normal ALT an serum HBV DNA > $10^4$ copies per mL have stage 2 or greater inflammatory or fibrosis on liver biopsy
  - HCC may develop in HBV
    - In the absence of cirrhosis
    - Even after seroconversion (HBeAg$^+$ → HBeAg$^-$, anti-HBe-positive)
    - Even after loss of HBsAg

---

For more detail regarding treatment of chronic hepatitis B: definitions of response to antiviral therapy, please see Sleisenger and Fordtran's Gastrointestinal and Liver Disease. 10$^{th}$ Edition. Saunders/Elsevier, Philadelphia, 2016, Table 79-4, page 1323; Table 79-5, page 1324; Table 79-6, page 1328.

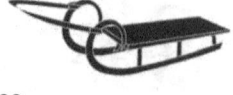

**Hepatitis C Virus** (HCV) **Infection**

- ➤ Demography
  - ○ Perinatal exposure
    - – Transmission rate
      - ▪ HCV ~ 5%
      - ▪ HCV + HIV ~ 15%
    - – Breastfeeding dangerous when HCV > $10^8$ copies/mL
  - ○ Percutaneous
    - – Blood products ($1/2 \times 10^6$)
    - – IV drug use (60% to 90% HCV infected)
    - – Nucleotide accidents
    - – Hemodialysis
  - ○ Non-percutaneous
    - – Sexual contact
    - – Intercourse
      - ▪ Per rectum
      - ▪ During menstruation

- ➤ Pathogenesis
  - ○ About 75% of persons with acute HBV develop chronic HCV because the HBV escapes the immune response to clear the infection.
  - ○ 75% of persons with acute HCV progress to chronic HCV infection because of ineffective immune against the HCV
  - ○ HCV-enters hepatocytes by attachment and transport, using proteins
    - – E1 and E2          envelop proteins
    - – CD81          tetraspan superfamily
    - – SR-B1          scavenger receptor class B type 1
    - – LDL-R          LDL receptor

140

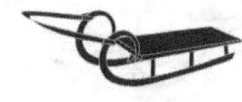

➤ Progression of HCV Infection

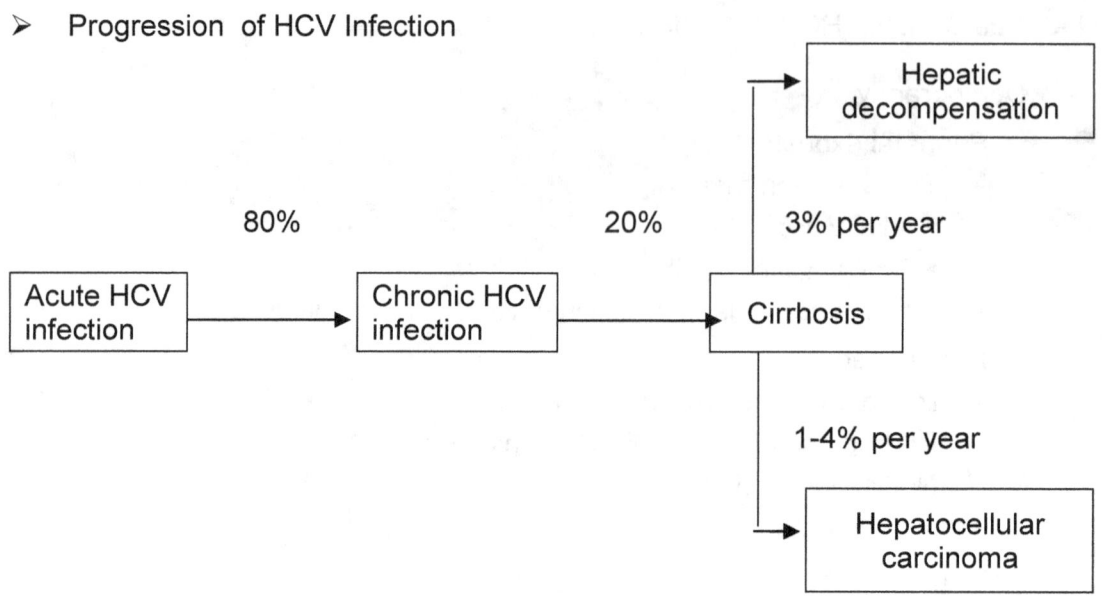

➤ Risk factors

• Give groups of persons at risk for hepatitis C virus (HCV) infection, and give the estimated prevalence of these persons, in these groups in industrialized countries.

| Groups at Risk | Estimated prevalence (range %) |
| --- | --- |
| o A blood transfusion received before 1990/91 | - 5-10 |
| o Children born from HCV positive mothers | - 3-10 |
| o Health care workers | - Related to country of origin |
| o Hemodialysis patients | |
| o Hemophiliac treated before 1990/91 | - 50-90 |
| o HIV infected persons | - 25-35 |
| o Incarcerated persons | - 30-80 |
| o Injection drug users | - 35-90 |
| o Migrants coming from endemic regions | - Related to country of origin |
| o Persons with unexplained persistently elevated ALT | - 15 |
| o Thalassemics | - 42-83 |

Abbreviation: ALT, alanine aminotransferase

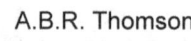

*MASTERING THE BOARDS*
*Hepatology & Pancreaticobiliary Disease*

A.B.R. Thomson

- ➢ Screening

- • Give groups/types of persons who should be screened for HCV.
  - o Concurrent disease
    - – Hemodialysis
    - – Transplantion
    - – Immunosuppressed patients
    - – Hemophylics
    - – Blood transfusion before approximately 1990 (depends on country)
  - o At risk occupations
    - – Needle stick injury
      - ▪ The person pricked with an HCV-contaminated needle should be tested for HCV RNA within 4 weeks, then tested for anti-HCV and ALT at 12 and 24 weeks.

    - – Inmates
  - o At risk behavious
    - – IV drug users
    - – HIV-positive patients
    - – Men who have sex with men (MSM)
    - – Sex trade workers (STWs)
    - – Those with > 50 lifetime sexual partners
    - – Sexually transmitted disease (STD)
    - – Those with a history of STD
  - o Regular folks
    - – Those with unexplained elevated ALT
    - – New Canadians (recent immigrants)

Printed with permission: Van Herck, et al. *Best Practice Res Clin Gastroenterol* 2008;22:6:1009-1029.

- o Family members and sexual contents of HCV-infected persons need to be tested for anti-HCV.

- o Test the children of HCV-infected mothers for HCV RNA when 1 month old.

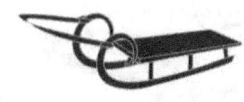

142

- ➤ Clinical
- • Give **extrahepatic manifestations** in patients with HCV infections.
  - o Vitiligo
  - o Lichen planus
  - o PCT (porphyria cutanea tarda)
    - – Sporatic or autosomal dominant heredity
    - – sun exposed areas, especially dorsal aspect of hands
  - o Mixed cryoglobulinemia
  - o Leukocytoclastic vasculitis (palpable purpura in legs)
  - o Reactions
    - – At sites of injection of IFN (interferon)
    - – Localize cellulitis/necrosis
    - – Erythema multiforme major (Steven Johnson Syndrome)
    - – Exfoliative dermatitis
    - – Vesiculobullous reaction
    - – Ribavirin (histamine like reaction)
      - ▪ Localized/confluent lashes
      - ▪ Vesicular lesions
  - o Lung
    - – Idiopathic pulmonary fibrosis
  - o Endocrine
    - – Diabetes mellitus
    - – Autoimmune thyroiditis
    - – Thyroid cancer

- • Give the likely diagnosis of a patient who presents with abdominal pain, leucocytoclastic vasculitis, palpable purpura, and ↓ complement.

  - o Hematology
    - – B cell non Hodgkin's lymphoma
    - – Mixed cryoglobulinemia
    - – Monoclonal gammopathies
    - – Henoch-Schonlein purpura; usually in young adults
    - – Mixed cryoglobulinemia (e.g., associated with HCV)

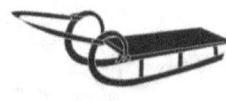

- o Musculoskeletal disorders (MSK)
  - – Chronic polyarthritis
  - – Sicca syndrome
- o Kidney
  - – Cryoglobulinemic nephropathy
  - – Non-cryoglobulinemic nephropathies
  - – Renal cell carcinoma
  - – Membranous nephropathy
  - – MPEN (membranoproliferative) nephropathy
  - – Glomerulonephritis

Adapted from: *Sleisenger and Fordtran's Gastrointestinal and Liver Disease: Pathophysiology/ Diagnosis/ Management.* 10th edition, 2016, Box 80-1, page 1339,

- • Give clinical findings in the patient with HCV which suggests associated cryoglobulinemia.

  - o Skin — Purpuric leucotoclastic vasculitis
  - o CNS/PNS — Peripheral neuropathy
  - o GI — Vasculitis → abdominal pain
  - o Kidney — Acute/chronic renal failure
    - – Nephrotic syndrome
    - – Glomerulonephritis (membranoproliferative)
  - o Laboratory — RF (rheumatoid factor) positive
    - – ↓ complement

- ➤ Laboratory
  - o In acute HCV infection, HCV RNA appears before anti-HCV antibodies.
  - o The presence of HCV RNA plus anti-HCV antibiotics may arise from acute HCV infection or a flare (exacerbation) of chronic hepatitis C.
  - o If hepatitis in the immunosuppressed patient, HCV RNA must be measured to make the diagnosis of anti-HCV antibiotics.

144

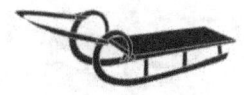

- Give the recommended laboratory assessment prior to therapy of HCV.
  - Anti-HCV
  - HCV RNA (qualitative +/- quantitative)
  - HCV genotyping
  - ALT, ALP, bilirubin, albumin, PT INR, HBsAg, HIV
  - CBC, glucose, TSH, ANA, smooth muscle antibody (SMA), quantitative immunoglobulins, creatinine, B-HCG
  - Abdominal Ultrasound, ECG (if age >50, cardiac disease history)
  - Liver biopsy recommended but not mandatory

- Give the interpretation of anti HCV results.

| Anti HCV by ELISA | Anti HCV by RIBA | Interpretation |
|---|---|---|
| o Positive | – Negative | False positive ELISA; patient does not have true antibody |
| o Positive | – Positive | Patient has antibody[a] |
| o Positive | – Indeterminate | Uncertain antibody status |

Abbreviations: ELISA, enzyme linked immunosorbent assay; HCV, hepatitis C virus; RIBA, recombinant immunoblot assay

[a]Anti- HCV does not necessarily indicate current hepatitis C infection

- Give the reasons why the ALT or AST are not useful markers for the progress of HCV.
  - The transaminases
    - Fluctuate widely in HCV
    - A normal level may occur even though chronic HCV infection is present
    - Women with low levels of HCV RNA may more commonly have low ALT, less inflammation and less fibrosis.

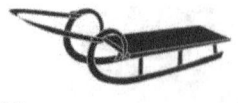

- Give non-biopsy tests to predict the presence of fibrosis in HCV.
  - Blood tests
    - ↑ AST and ↑ ALT, ALT > AST, AST-to-platelet index
    - A2-macroglobulin
      - Haptoglobulin
      - Apolipoproteins A-1
      - GGT
      - Bilirubin
    - FibroSure ®
      - Composite score of blood tests
  - Transient elastography (Fibroscan®)
    - AUC (area-under-the-curve) for predicting cirrhosis, 0.94
    - Note
      - These tests do not accurately categorize
        - Lower grades of cirrhosis
        - Amount of inflammation

- Pathology
  - Liver biopsy grading of HCV is made by a scoring system (e.g., Knodell, Ishak or METAVIR)

---

SO YOU WANT TO BE A HEPATOLOGIST!

Scoring systems have been used in HCV for the estimation of the extent of fibrosis and the presence of cirrhosis.

- Give reasons relating to the performance characteristics of one grading system (such as the METAVIR scoring system), which would shed light on possible limitations of liver biopsy as the test for standard of care.

  - Concordance (intra- and interobserver variation in reporting degree of fibrosis), 85% to 90%

  - Sampling error

  - False negative rate (for correct staging of cirrhosis), 15% difference in reported fibrosis
    - 1 stage, 33%
    - 2 stage, 2%

---

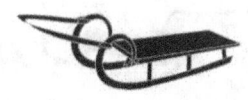

- Give the basis for the simple **METAVIR** scoring system.
  - Inflammation
    - None, mild, moderate, severe
  - Fibrosis
    - None (0)
    - Portal (1)
    - Portal fibrosis with septa (2)
    - Bridging fibrosis (3)
      - Focal
      - Diffuse
      - Marked
      - Cirrhosis

Sleisenger and Fordtran's Gastrointestinal and Liver Disease. 9th Edition. Saunders/Elsevier, Philadelphia, 2010, Figure 79.5, page 1323.

- Give the **METAVIR** system for staging/grading chronic hepatitis C infection on liver biopsy.

| | Piecemeal and Lobular Necrosis *(A) | Fibrosis (F) |
|---|---|---|
| 0 | None | None |
| 1 | Mild activity | Portal fibrosis without septa |
| 2 | Moderate activity | Portal fibrosis with septa |
| 3 | Severe activity | Numerous septa (bridging fibrosis), without cirrhosis |
| 4 | | Cirrhosis |

- Give reasons for biopsying the liver of persons with HCV, genotype 1, without obvious cirrhosis.
  - There is no correlation between ALT or viral load, and stage of fibrosis.
  - Surrogates for the presence of advanced fibrosis such as reversal of ALT/AST ratio, platelet count, pro time-INR are not sensitive.
  - Markers of fibrosis such as hydroxyl proline are not sufficiently specific.
  - Given the variable natural history and the complexity and cost of treatment, informed decision can only be made based on histology.

147

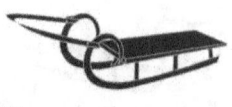

- Over half of persons with acute HCV progress to chronic HCV, and about 1% of persons per year after infection will progress to do compensated cirrhosis.

$$\text{Acute} \xrightarrow{\text{50\%}} \text{Chronic} \xrightarrow{\text{1\% / year}} \text{Cirrhosis}$$

- Patients who do not respond need further advice on what is next and histology may be essential in these persons.

- Liver biopsy may be safer than treatment when you consider alternatives such as treating everyone.

- Post-liver transplantation

- Give the pros and cons of performing a percutaneous liver biopsy in a patient with HCV.

| Issues | Argument in Favor of Biopsy with Acceptable Risk | Reasons for Not Performing a Biopsy |
|---|---|---|
| o Prognosis | – Extent of fibrosis and inflammation are best predictors of disease progression | ▪ Non-invasive markers may accurately stage and grade disease |
| o Decision to treat | – Genotype 1: Identify those most in need of therapy (therapy longer in duration and less likely to succeed) | ▪ Genotypes 2 and 3: Patients motivated for therapy may forgo biopsy (therapy shorter in duration and more likely to succeed) |
| o Treatment-related side effects | – Severity of liver disease helps in deciding of whether to endure or stop therapy | ▪ Commitment to therapy should be independent of disease severity |
| o Previously treated | – Lower success with retreatment. Identify those most in need of therapy (advanced fibrosis) | ▪ Motivated patients who are genotype 2 or 3, were previously treated with interferon monotherapy, are candidates for re-treatment regardless of disease severity |

Printed with permission: Reddy K R. *2006 AGA Institute Postgraduate Course Syllabus:* pg. 81.

148

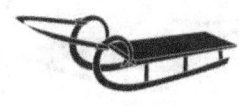

## SO YOU WANT TO BE A HEPATOLOGIST!

- Give the circumstances when liver biopsy needs to be considered in HCV.

  o Genotype 1, 4 – perform liver biopsy when results will change treatment of HCV

  o Genotype 2,3 – perform liver biopsy when treatment of HCV may be postponed

  o Liver biopsy not necessary if clinical, laboratory or diagnostic imaging suggests that cirrhosis is already present

---

Clinical Alert!

o HCV and autoimmune conditions

  – Because autoantibodies are common in HCV, and may not be associated with disease, so be **cautious** making the diagnosis of an autoimmune condition in a person with HCV based just on seropositivity for autoantibodies.

o False-negative HCV serology

  – Even though the EIAs (enzyme immunoassays) for HCV have excellent performance characteristics (sensitivity and specificity of ~ 99%), anti-HCV may be negative in some persons who have HCV replication in the liver.

   ▪ This false-negative HCV serology is seen with
     –Hemodialysis
     –Immune suppression

   ▪ If the person is not at high risk for a false negative HCV (e.g., hemodialysis, immune suppression), a negative anti-HCV on an EIA excludes HCV infection.

   ▪ Anti-HCV positive is diagnostic of HCV infection if there is ↑ serum ALT

  – Early diagnosis of HCV depends on the time after exposure when the test becomes positive:

   ▪ HCV RNA      1 to 3 weeks
   ▪ Anti-HCV      7 to 8 weeks

149

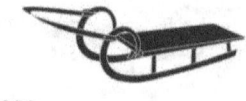

*MASTERING THE BOARDS*
*Hepatology & Pancreaticobiliary Disease*

A.B.R. Thomson

- Give modifiable as well as non-modifiable factors which are associated with the **histological progression** of HCV infection.

There are numerous factors which are established or are possible contributors to the progression of hepatic fibrosis in patients with HCV infection (please see S/F, Table 79.4, page 1325 for extensive details)

- o Patient
  - Age (> 40 yrs)
  - Males
  - Caucasian

- o Lifestyle
  - Obesity
  - Alcohol (> 50 g/day)
  - Smoking
  - Cannabis use (marijuana)

- o Co-morbidities
  - Steatosis
  - Insulin resistance
  - Diabetes (genotypes 1 and 4)
  - Iron overload
  - Co-infection
    - HBV
    - HIV
  - Immunosuppression
  - Schistosomiasis

- o Virus
  - Progression of HCV is not associated with HCV load or genotype

- o Laboratory/ pathology
  - Elevated serum ALT levels (elevated)
  - Histology - Moderate to marked necroinflammation

Adapted from: Berenguer M, and Wright TL. *Sleisenger & Fordtran's gastrointestinal and liver disease: Pathophysiology/Diagnosis/Management* 2006: pg. 1696.; and 2010: pg. 1325.

- Give the clinical feature of acute HCV infection which suggests that the patient will be in the lucky group and clear their HCV without treatment.

  - o Persons with acute HCV associated with jaundice have an increased chance of clearing in HCV.

150

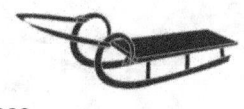

- Give the name of the high mortality-associated subtype variant of HCV infection (> 3 x $10^6$ copies/mL) seen in HCV infected persons who are immune suppressed for organ transplantation.
  - Fibrosing cholestatic variant of HCV-associated hepatitis.

➤ Natural history

| | | |
|---|---|---|
| o Acute → Chronic HCV | | 55% to 89% |
| o Chronic HCV after infection → Compensated cirrhosis | | ~1% per year |
| o Compensated cirrhosis → HCC | | ~2% per year |
| → Decompensation | | ~3% per year |

➤ Treatment

- Give the **management principles** of persons with HCV infection.

  - Prevention, screening, vaccination (none), prophylaxis on exposure
  - General management strategy
  - Assessment of factors predictive of viral response
  - Specific treatments
  - Select optimal agent
  - Reassess therapy
  - Screen for HCC
  - Patients with chronic hepatitis C should be
    - Vaccinated against HAV and HBV
    - Tested for HIV
    - Consider to have possible (treat appropriately)
      - Alcohol abuse and /or
      - Fatty liver

  - Give the objectives of therapy.
    - Eradicate HCV
    - SVR (sustained viral response)
    - Absent serum HCV RNA 6 months after

Adapted from: Berenguer M, and Wright TL. Hepatitis C. *Sleisenger & Fordtran's Gastrointestinal and Liver Disease: Pathophysiology/ Diagnosis/ Management* 2006. pg. 1681-1712.

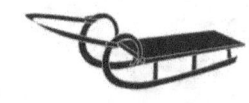

❖ Terminology

o The amazing success of newly introduced protease inhibitors and the possibility of interferon- and ribavirin-free treatment regimens being standard of care in the very near future, some of the following terms may become used much less.

o In the patient with HCV, define the terms RVR, EVR, pEVR, cEVR, PVR, NR, ETR and SVR, as well as the definition and clinical implication of each of the 4 types of responses.

o RVR
– Rapid virologic response
– Undetectable HCV on a serum after 4 weeks of anti-HCV therapy
– Higher chance of SVR; may respond as well with only 24 weeks of treatment

o EVR
– Early virologic response
– 2-log (100-fold) drop in HCV RNA load after 12 weeks of anti-HCV therapy
– Failure to achieve EVR associated with almost no chance of SVR and treatment can usually be stopped

o pEVR
– Partial EVR
– > 2-log (100-fold) decrease in HBV DNA after 12 weeks of anti-HBV therapy (residual HBV RNA still present)

o cEVR
– Complete EVR
– No HCV RNA in serum after 12 weeks of anti-HCV therapy
– On treatment response. Observe for SVR

o PVR
– Partial viral response
– HCV RNA present in serum at 12 weeks, but not at 24 weeks

o NR
– No response, aka will response
– Failure to achieve EVR

o ETR
– HCV RNA undetectable at end of treatment wk 48 – 1 genotype, wk 24 – 2,3

o SVR
– Sustained viral response
– Surrogate marker for eradication of SVR
– No detectable HCV RNA in serum after 24 weeks of anti-HCV therapy

Printed with permission: Sleisenger and Fordtran's Gastrointestinal and Liver Disease. 9th Edition. Saunders/Elsevier, Philadelphia, 2010, Figure 79.7, page 1329.

152

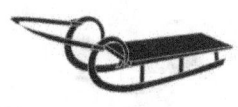

- Give the HCV-RNA levels at week 4,12 and 24 in persons with rapid virologic response (RVR), early virologic response (EVR), slow virologic response (SVR) and no virologic response (NVR).

| | HCV-RNA | | |
|---|---|---|---|
| | Week 4 | Week 12 | Week 24 |
| o Rapid virologic response (RVR) | Undetectable (<50 IU/ml) [a] | Undetectable | Undetectable |
| o Early virologic response (EVR) | >50 IU/ml | Undetectable | Undetectable |
| o Slow virologic response (SVR) | >50 IU/ml | >50 IU/ml, but >log 2 drop | Undetectable |
| o No virologic response (NVR) | >50 IU/ml | >50 IU/ml, but < log 2 drop | Detectable |

[a] Level of detection (LOD) changes with more sensitive test. The currently available new tests have a LOD <15 IU/ml , no prospective studies using these tests have been performed.

Abbreviations: EVR, early virologic response; NVR, no virologic response; RVR, rapid virologic response; SVR, slow virologic response

Printed with permission:  Ferenci P. *Best Practise Res Clin Gastroenterol* 2008;22:1109-1122.

- Lifestyle recommendations
  - Persons with HCV infection should be counselled
    - To avoid sharing toothbrushes and dental or shaving equipment, and be cautioned
    - To cover any bleeding wound to prevent the possibility of others coming into contact with their blood
  - Persons should be counselled to stop using illicit drugs and enter substance abuse treatment.
  - Those who continue to inject drugs should be counselled
    - To avoid reusing or sharing syringes, needles, water, cotton, and other drug preparation equipment
    - To use new sterile syringes and filters and disinfected cookers
    - To clean the injection site with a new alcohol swab; and dispose of syringe and needles after one use in a safe, puncture-proof container
  - Persons with HCV infection should be advised
  - Not to donate blood
  - To discuss HCV serostatus prior to donatation of body organs, other tissue, or semen

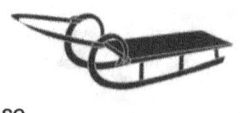

- Pharmaceutical therapy
- Give factors which **predict a poor treatment response** in HCV.
  - Patient
    - Older (age (> 40)
    - Male
    - African racial origin
    - Latino ethnicity
    - Weight: lighter patients (<75kg) more likely to respond (odds ratio 1.91) (fixed dose)
    - Alcoholim
  - Lifestyle
    - Poor adherence to anti-HCV treatment
    - HIV coinfection
  - The virus itself
    - Genotypes1, 4
      - Viral genotype: Genotype 1&4 (42-46%), Genotype 2, 3 (76-82%)
    - When all other factors are taken into account, being in prison improves the clinical outcomes, because all treatment is given (forced high compliance rate)
    - High HCV load
    - No IL-28 B CT, TTgenotype
    - Non-I
    - Lower viral levels: >2 x 10$^6$ (42-53%), <2 x 10$^6$ (62-78%)
    - Early virologic response: negative EVR (defined as 2-log decrease in HCV RNA in first 12 weeks of treatment) is predictive negative SVR (97%)
    - Overall sustained virologic response (SVR) (undetectable HCV RNA 24 weeks after cessation of therapy) to inferon monotherapy: 5-15%, to combined interferon and ribavirin: 30-40%, to combined pegylated interferon and ribavirin: 54-56%.
  - Liver
    - Coinfection with HBV
    - Fibrosis score
    - Decompensated cirrhosis
    - Inadequate drug dose
    - Anemia/thrombocytopenia adverse effects

154

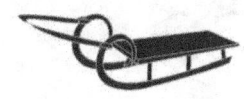

- o Co-morbidities
  - – Insulin resistance / Diabetes
  - – ↓ social support
  - – Renal disease
    - ▪ Ribavirin contraindicated with ↑ GFR
  - – Poor psychiatric comorbidity
  - – Advanced hepatic fibrosis (high fibrosis score)
  - – Steatosis
  - – Decompensated cirrhosis

- o Types of response to anti-HCV therapy
  - – NR > pEVR > cEVR > RVR

- o Absolute or relative contraindications
  - – Pregnancy or attempting conception
  - – Active autoimmune diseases
  - – Significant cardiopulmonary disease
  - – Uncontrolled psychiatric disease
  - – Uncontrolled seizures
  - – Severe cytopenias, including transfusion-dependent anemia

---

MCQ Trick

- Give the effect of incarceration on the response to HCV treatment.
  - o You might think response rate might be lower, but
    - – Treatment-associated SVR depends on HCV genotype and therapy used, for example
      - ▪ I/R (interferon plus ribavirin)
        - – Genotype I 40% to 50%
        - – Genotype II 70% to 80%

---

- Give when mothers with chronic hepatitis C are allowed to breast-feed their children.
  - o As long as they are negative for HIV
  - o Do not use intravenous drugs
  - o Nipples are not cracked

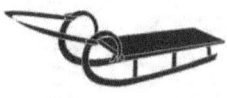

**Ribavirin** (RBV)

- Give possible contraindications to the use of Ribavirin.

  o Pregnancy

  o Inadequate contraception (contraception to prevent conception for 6 mon after RBV stopped

  o Known allergy to ribavirin

  o End-stage renal disease (ESRD)

  o Anemia (cannot give adequate dose, since ribavirin may cause anemia and thus require dose reduction)

  o Angina pectoris (possible)

  o Old age (possible)

- Give the common **adverse effects** (AEs)of Ribavirin (RIB) in the treatment of HCV, and give the management of these AEs.

Clinical: "flu-like symptoms", fatigue, anorexia, nausea, nasal congestion, irritability, cognitive impairment, insomnia

| Laboratory | Level | | Other clinical considerations |
|---|---|---|---|
| o Hemoglobin | 10 gm/dL | - ↓ ribavirin by 200 mg/day | • Consider starting erythropoietin; if Hgb responds poorly to dose reduction, check iron studies and consider reducing peginterferon |
| | 8.5 gm/dL | - Stop ribavirin | • Hold ribavirin and consider stopping; transfuse as necessary |
| o White blood cells | 1500/µL | - ↓ pegIFN by 50% | • Monitor more closely |
| | 1000/µL | - Stop treatment | • Monitor more closely; consider G-CSF |
| o Absolute neutrophils | 750/µL | - ↓ pegIFN by 50% | • Monitor more closely |
| | 500/µL | - Stop pegIFN | • Monitor more closely |
| o Platelets | 50,000/µL | - ↓ pegIFN by 50% | • Individualize dose adjustment |
| | 25,000/µL | - Stop IFN | • Consider platelet transfusion or platelet stimulating factor |

Printed with permission: Davis GL. *2007 AGA Institute Postgraduate Course*: pg. 58.

156

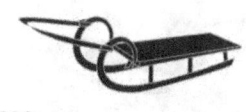

➢ Overall dose reduction of ribavirin in19% of Ribavirin-treated persons, with discontinuation of Ribavarin in 10%

• Give the standard therapy for chronic HCV according to viral genotype.

| Genotype | Interferon Dose (per week) | Ribavirin Dose (mg/day) | Duration (weeks) | SVR |
|---|---|---|---|---|
| 1 | 180 µg PEG alfa-2a or 1.5 µg/kg PEG alfa-2b | 800-1400 mg/day weight-based | 48 | 41-42% |
| 2 | 180 µg PEG alfa-2a or 1.5 µg/kg PEG alfa-2b | 800 mg/day | 24 | 66-75% |
| 3 | 180 µg PEG alfa-2a or 1.5 µg/kg PEG alfa-2b | 800 mg/day | 24 | 66-75% |
| 4 | 180 µg PEG alfa-2a or 1.5 µg/kg PEG alfa-2b | 1000-1200 mg/day | 48 | 55% |
| 5 | 180 µg PEG alfa-2a or 1.5 µg/kg PEG alfa-2b | 1000-1200 mg/day | 48 | 64% |
| 6 | 180 µg PEG alfa-2a or 1.5 µg/kg PEG alfa-2b | 1000-1200 mg/day | 48 | 63% |

Abbreviation: SVR, sustained viral response

Printed with permission: Davis GL. *2007 AGA Institute Postgraduate Course*: pg. 56.

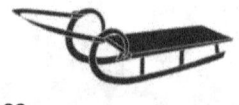

157

- Give the week of assessment of HCV for EVR or SVR in genotype1/4 HCV and genotype 2/3 HCV patients, and the management implications.

| Assessment | Week of assessment | Interpretation | Management implications |
|---|---|---|---|
| ○ Genotype 1, 4 | 4 | HCV RNA <50 IU/ml predicts 90% SVR | Duration of treatment of 24 weeks can be considered |
| – RVR | 12 | HCV RNA <50 IU/ml predicts SVR in 70% | Duration of treatment can be 48 weeks |
| – Complete EVR | 12 | HCV-RNA decline of >2-log but >50 IU/ml is associated with higher relapse (30%) than complete EVR (15%) | Duration of treatment should be extended to 72 weeks to reduce relapse and increase SVR |
| – Partial EVR | 12 | HCV-RNA decline <2 log is associated with SVR in 2% with 48 weeks treatment | Treatment should be stopped |
| – Non-EVR | 24 | HCV RNA >50 IU/ml (detectable) is associated with non-SVR | Treatment should be stopped |
| 24-week Response | | | |
| ○ Genotype 2/3 | 4 | HCV RNA <50IU/ml predicts 90% SVR | Duration of treatment of 12-16 weeks can be considered |
| – RVR | 4 | HCV RNA >50 IU/ml predicts SVR < 50% | Consideration of treatment for duration longer than 24 weeks |
| – Non-EVR | | | |

Abbreviations: EVR, early virologic response; RVR, rapid virologic response

Printed with permission: Terrault N. *2008 ACG Annual Postgraduate course book*: pg. 170-171.

158

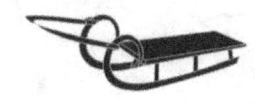

- Give the clinical significance in HCV infection of CC, CT and TT genotypes of the IL-28 gene on chromosome 19.
  - CC genotypes
    - Codes for IFN-λ-3 ("lambda"), with ↑ production of intrinsic IFN
    - ↑ efficacy of PEG-IFN + ribavirin (@x > rate of RVR, complete EVR, and SVR
    - More common in European and Asian ancestry
  - CT and TT genotypes
    - No ↑ lambda IFN1, so lower rates of RVR, EVR, SVR
    - More common in Latino and African ancestry
    - DADs (direct acting anti-viral agents), aka STAT-C (specifically targeted anti-viral therapy) for HCV
    - Telaprevir and baceprevir are linear PIs (protease inhibitors) against the NS 3/4a proteases.
    - PEG-IFN-alpha + RBV (ribavirin) + PI for genotype 1 HCV

## Protease Inhibitors

  - In the past 35 years, three Nobel prizes have been won in the area of gastroenterology/hepatology: the H2-receptor and its antagonists (Black), the LDL receptor, and the rediscovery of Helicobacter pylori and the establishment of its importance in ulcer disease.
  - With the identification of the hepatitis C virus (HCV) by Heyden and the recent "game changing" development of protease inhibitors, the hope for the sustained eradication of HCV has gone from dismall to greater than 95%.
  - This will have a major impact on liver transplantation rates for HCV, and more importantly to the quality of life of sufferers.
  - Unfortunately, with the very high cost of these new anti-HCV medications, this revolutional therapy may not be available to all persons with HCV infection.
  - The rates of regional governmental approval will vary widely in making the drugs available even for the persons of wealth.
  - Most national professional groups have not yet formulated guidelines.
  - Nonetheless, the candidate coming forward for examination will be required to be aware of these existing new development.
  - Therefore, included here are the summarized 2014 AASLD (American Association for Study of Liver Disease) and IDSA (infectious Diseases Society of America) Recommendations.
    These AASLD/IDSA recommendations are available online at

http://www.aasld.org/PRACTICEGUIDELINES/Pages/default.aspx
http://www.idsociety.org/IDSA_Practice_Guidelines/

159

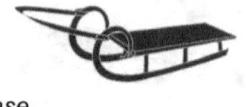

# Interferon (IFN) eligibility

❖ Genotype 1

| Eligible to Receive IFN | **Not** Eligible for IFN |
|---|---|
| o *Recommended regimen for treatmen naïve patients with HCV genotype 1 who are eligible to receive IFN.*<br>  – Daily SOF 400 mgvod and weight-based RBV (1000 mg [75 kg] to 1200 mg [≥ 75 kg]) plus weekly PEG for 12 weeks is recommended for IFN-eligible persons with HCV genotype 1 infection, regardless of subtype. | o *Recommended regimen for treatment-naïve patients with HCV genotype 1 who are not eligible to receive IFN.*<br>  – Daily SOF 400 mg plus SIM 150 mg, with or without weight-based RBV (1000 mg [< 75 kg] to 1200 mg [≥ 75 kg] for 12 weeks is recommended for IFN-ineligible patients with HCV genotype 1 infection, regadless of subtype |
| o *Alternative regimen for treatment-naïve patients with HCV genotype 1 who are eligible to receive IFN.*<br>  – Daily SIM 150 mg for 12 weeks and weight-based RBV (1000 mg [< 75 kg] to 1200 mg [≥ 75 kg]) plus weekly PEG for 24 weeks is an acceptable regimen for IFN-eligible persons with either<br>    ▪ HCV genotype 1b or<br>    ▪ HCV genotype 1a infection in whom the Q80K polymorphism is not detected prior to treatment. | o *Alternative regimens for treatment-naïve patients with HCV genotype 1 who are eligible to receive IFN.*<br>  – Daily SOF 400 mg and weight-based RBV (1000 mg [75 kg] to 1200 mg [≥ 75 kg]) for 24 weeks<br><br>o This regimen may be less effective than daily SOF 400 mg plus SIM 150 mg, particularly among patients with cirrhosis. |

For genotype 1a, baseline resistance testing for Q80K should be performed and alternative treatments considered if this mutation is present.

The following regimens are **not** recommended for treatment-naïve patients with HCV genotype 1.

  o PEG/RBV with or without telaprevir (TEL) or boceprevir (BOC) for 24 to 48 weeks

  o Monotherapy with PEG, RBV, or a DAA

160

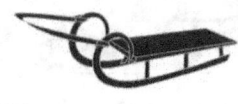

- ❖ **Genotype 2** – Regardless of interferon eligibility
  - o Recommended regimen for treatment-naïve patients with HCV genotype 2, regardless of eligibility of IFN therapy:
    - – Daily SOF 400 mg and weight-based RBV (1000 mg [< 75 kg] to 1200 mg [≥ 75 kg]) for 12 weeks.

The regimens **not** recommended for treatment-naïve patients with HCV genotype 2.

  - o PEG/RBV for 24 weeks
  - o Monotherapy with PEG, RBV, or a DAA
  - o TEL, BOC, or SIM-based regimen

- ❖ **Genotype 3**– Regardless of interferon eligibility
  - o *Recommended regimen for treatment-naïve patients with HCV genotype 3, regardless of eligibility for IFN therapy:*
    - – *Daily SOF 400 mg and weight-based RBV (1000 mg [< 75 kg] to 1200 mg [≥ 75 kg]) for 24 weeks is recommended for treatment-naïve patients with HCV genotype 3 infection.*
    - – *Alternative regimen for treatment-naïve patients with genotype 3 who are eligible to receive IFN.*
      - ▪ Daily sofosbuvir (400 mg) and weight-based RBV (1000 mg [< 75 kg] to 1200 mg [≥ 75 kg]) plus weekly PEG for 12 weeks is an acceptable regimen for IFN-eligible persons with HCV genotype 3.
  - o Regimens **not** recommended for treatment-naïve genotype 3.
    - – PEG/RBV for 24 to 48 weeks
    - – Monotherapy with PEG, RBV, or a DAA
    - – TEL, BOC, or SIM-based regimen should not be used for patients with genotype 3 HCV infection.

- ❖ **Genotype 4**– Interferon eligibility

| Eligible | Not Eligible |
| --- | --- |
| o *Recommended regimen for treatment-naïve patients with HCV genotype 4 who are eligible to receive IFN.*<br>  – Daily SOF 400 mg and weight-based RBV (1000 mg [< 75 kg] to 1200 mg [≥ 75 | o *Recommended regimen for treatment-naïve patients with genotype 4 who are not eligible to receive IFN.*<br>  – Daily SOF 400 mg weight-based RBV (1000 mg [75 kg] to 1200 mg [≥ 75 kg]) for 24 weeks. |

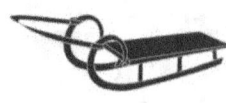

kg]) plus weekly PEG for 12
weeks.

| Eligible | Not Eligible |
|---|---|

- o Alternative regimens for treatment-naïve patients with HCV genotype 4 who are eligible to receive IFN.
  - – Daily SIM 10 mg for 12 weeks and weight-based RBV (1000 mg [< 75 kg] to 1200 mg [≥ 75 kg]) plus weekly PEG for 24 to 48 weeks.

- o Regimens are **not** recommended for treatment-naïve genotype 4.
  - – PEG/RBV for 48 weeks
  - – Monotherapy with PEG, RBV, or a DAA
  - – Telaprevir-, boceprevir-based regimen

❖ **Genotype 5, 6**– Regardless of interferon eligibility

- o *Recommended regimen for treatment-naïve patients with HCV genotype 5 or 6.*
  - – Daily SOF 400 mg and weight-based RBV (1000 mg [< 75 kg] to 1200 mg [≥ 75 kg]) plus weekly PEG for 12 weeks.
  - – *Alternative regimen for treatment-naïve patients with genotype 5 or 6*
    - ▪ Daily weight-based RBV (1000 mg [< 75 kg] to 1200 mg [≥ 75 kg]) plus weekly PEG for 48 weeks is an acceptable regimen for persons infected with HCV genotype 5 or 6.

- o Regimens are NOT recommended for treatment-naïve genotype 5 or 6 HCV.
  - – Monotherapy with PEG, RBV, or a DAA
  - – TEL, BOC-based regimen

Abbreviations: BOC, boceprevir; DAA, direct activity agent; PEG, pegylated interferon; RBV, ribavirin; SIM, simeprevir; SOF, sofosbuvir; TEL, Telaprevir

162

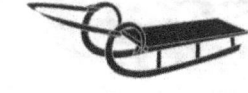

## *Retreatment*

| Genotype | Recommended | Alternative | Not Recommended |
|---|---|---|---|
| Patients in whom previous PEG/RBV has failed (Failure (non response) is defined as partial or null response to treatment with PEG/RBV. Relapse to prior therapy should be treated the same as treatment-naïve) | | | |
| 1 | o SOF + SMV ± RBV x 12 weeks | - SOF x 12 weeks + PEG/RBV x 12 – 24 weeks<br>- SOF + RBV x 24 weeks<br>- SMV x 12 weeks + PEG/RBV x 48 weeks* | - PEG/RBV ± telaprevir or boceprevir<br>- Monotherapy with PEG, RBV, or a DAA<br>- Do not treat decompensated cirrhosis with PEG or SMV |

\* For genotype 1a, baseline resistance testing for Q80K should be performed ans alternative treatments considered if this mutation is present

| Genotype | Recommended | Alternative | Not Recommended |
|---|---|---|---|
| 2 | o SOF + RBV x 12 weeks | - SOF + PEG/RBV x 12 weeks | - PEG/RBV ± telaprevir or boceprevir<br>- Monotherapy with PEG, or direct-acting anti-viral agent<br>- Do not treat decompensated cirrhosis with PEG |
| 3 | o SOF + RBV x 24 weeks | - SOF + PEG/RBV x 12 weeks | - PEG/RBV ± any current protease inhibitor<br>- Monotherapy with PEG, RBV, or a DAA<br>- Do not treat decompensated cirrhosis with PEG |
| 4 | o SOF + PEG/RBV x 12 weeks | - SOF + RBV x 24 weeks | - PEG/RBV ± any current HCV protease inhibitor<br>- Monotherapy with PEG, RBV, or a DAA<br>- Do not treat decompensated cirrhosis with PEG |

| Genotype | Recommended | Alternative | Not Recommended |
| --- | --- | --- | --- |
| 5-6 | ○ SOF x 12 weeks + PEG/RBV 12 weeks | | - PEG/RBV + any current HCV protease inhibitor<br>- Monotherapy with PEG, RBV, or a DAA<br>- Do not treat decompensated cirrhosis with PEG |

Patients in whom previous PEG/RBV plus either telaprevir or boceprevir** has failed†† †††

| Genotype | Recommended | Alternative | Not Recommended |
| --- | --- | --- | --- |
| 1 | ○ SOF x 12 weeks + PEG/RBV x 12-24 weeks | - SOF + RBV x 24 weeks‡<br>- SOF†<br>- PEG/RBV x 24 weeks ‡‡ | - PEG/RBV ± telaprevir or boceprevir or SMV<br>- Monotherapy with PEG, RBV, or a DAA<br>- Do not treat decompensated cirrhosis with PEG or SMV |
| | ○ Note: stop anti HVC therapy | – pEVR in genotype 1, 4 (the use of serum HBV RNA level at week 12) to indicate an EVR, does not apply to genotype 2 or 3 infection<br>– HBV RNA still present at 24 weeks for each of interferon and ribavirin, 30% of HCV patients have to stop therapy because of AEs (adverse effects) | |

***Failure (non-response) is defined as partial or null response to treatment with PEG/RBV plus telaprevir or boceprevir. Relapse to prior therapy should be treated the same as treatment naïve

† Consideration should be given to postponing treatment, pending release of new drugs for patients with limited (F 0-2) hepatic fibrosis

†† A recommendation for simeprevir use for patient with previous telaprevir or boceprevir exposure not provided due to potential risk of preexistant resistance to protease inhibitor treatment.

††† Given the lack of prior approval of protease inhibitor therapy for genotypes 2, 3, 4, 5, 6 and the lack of sufficient data, no recommendations are given for these genotypes at this time

‡ IFN ineligible

‡‡ IFN eligible

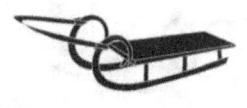

❖ Genotype 1

| Eligible for IFX | Not Eligible for IFX |
|---|---|

- *Recommended regimen for HCV genotype 1 PEG/RBV (without an HCV protease inhibitor) non-responder patients:*
    - Daily SOF 400 mg plus SIM 150 mg, with or without weight-based RBV (1000 mg [< 75 kg] to 1200 mg [≥ 75 kg]) for 12 weeks.

- *Alternative regimen for PEG/RBV (with or without an HCV protease inhibitor) non-responder patients with HCV genotype 1.*
    - Daily SOF 400 mg for 12 weeks and weight-based RBV (1000 mg [75 kg] to 1200 mg [≥ 75 kg]) plus weekly PEG for 12 to 24 weeks.

- *Alternative regimen for PEG/RBV (without an HCV protease inhibitor) non-responder patients with HCV genotype 1 who are eligible to receive IFN.*
    - Daily SIM 150 mg for 12 weeks plus weight-based RBV (1000 mg [< 75 kg] tto 1200 mg [≥ 75 kg]) and weekly PEG for 48 weeks.

- *Recommended regimen for HCV genotype 1 PEG/RBV (with an HCV protease inhibitor) non-responder patients:*
    - Daily SOF 400 m) for 12 weeks plus weight-based RBV (1000 mg [< 75 kg] to 1200 mg [≥ 75 kg]) and weekly.

- Daily SOF 400 mg for 24 weeks and weight-based RBV (1000 mg [< 75 kg] to 1200 mg [≥ 75 kg]) for 24 weeks.

- *The following regimens are NOT recommended for PEG/RBV (with or without an HCV protease inhibitor) non-responder patients with HCV genotype 1:*
    - PEG/RBV with or without telaprevir or boceprevir
    - Monotherapy with PEG, RBV, or a DAA
    - History of decompensated cirrhosis (moderate or severe hepatic impairment; CTP class B or C), treatment is not indicated because of the risks of PEG, BOC and TEL in this population.

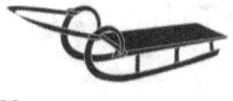

- ❖ Genotype 2– Non-reponder; regardless of interferon eligibility
  - ○ *Recommended regimen for genotype 2 PEG/RBV non-responders.*
    - – Daily SOF 400 mg and weight-based RBV (1000 mg [< 75 kg] to 1200 mg [≥ 75 kg]) for 12 weeks
      - ▪ Patient with cirrhosis may benefit by extension of treatment to 16 weeks.)
  - ○ *Alternative regimen for PEG/RBV non-responder patients with HCV genotype 2 infection who are eligible to receive IFN.*
    - – Retreatment with daily SOF 400 mg and weight-based RBV (1000 mg [< 75 kg] to 1200 mg [≥ 75 kg]) plus weekly PEG for 12 weeks.
  - ○ *Regimens are NOT recommended for non-responder patients with HCV genotype 2:*
    - – PEG/RBV with or without telaprevir, boceprevir or simeprevir
    - – Monotherapy with PEG, RBV, or a DAA

- ❖ Genotype 3
  - ○ *Recommended regimen for HCV genotype 3 PEG/RBV non-responders.*
    - – Daily SOF 400 mg and weight-based RBV (1000 mg [< 75 kg] to 1200 mg [≥ 75 kg]) for 24 weeks.
  - ○ *Alternative regimen for HCV genotype 3 PEG/RBV non-responder patients who are eligible to receive IFN.*
    - – Retreatment with daily SOF 400 mg and weight-based RBV (1000 mg [< 75 kg] to 1200 mg [≥ 75 kg]) plus weekly PEG for 12 weeks.
  - ○ *Regimens are NOT recommended for non-responder patients with HCV genotype 3 infection:*
    - – PEG/RBV with or without telaprevir, boceprevir or simeprevir
    - – Monotherapy with PEG, RBV, or a DAA

- ❖ Genotype 4
  - ○ *Recommended regimen for HCV genotype 4, PEG/RBV non-responder patients.*
    - – Daily sofosbuvir (400 mg) for 12 weeks and daily weight-based RBV (1000 mg [< 75 kg] to 1200 mg [≥ 75 kg]) plus weekly PEG for 12 weeks.
  - ○ *Alternative regimen for HCV genotype 4, PEG/RBV non-responder patients.*
    - – Daily SOF 400 mg and weight-based RBV (1000 mg [< 75 kg] to 1200 mg [≥ 75 kg]) for 24 weeks.

166

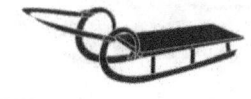

- o *Regimens are NOT recommended for non-responder patients with genotype 4 HCV infection:*
  - – PEG/RBV with or without telaprevir or boceprevir
  - – Monotherapy with PEG, RBV, or a DAA

- ❖ Genotype 5, 6

  - o *Recommended regimen for HCV genotype 5 or 6, PEG/RBV non-responder patients.*
    - – Daily SOF 400 mg for 12 weeks and daily weight-based RBV (1000 mg [< 75 kg] to 1200 mg [≥ 75 kg]) plus weekly PEG for 12 weeks.

  - o Alternate regimen for PEG/RBV non-responder patients with HCV genotype 5 or 6.
    - – None

  - o *Regimens are **not** recommended for non-responder patients with HCV genotype 5 or 6.*
    - – PEG/RBV with or without TEL or BOC
    - – Monotherapy with PEG, RBV, or a DAA

**Renal Impairment**

Dose adjustments are needed for patients with renal impairment

| Renal Impairment | eGFR/CrCl Level (mL/min/ 1.73 m²) | Interferon (IFX) | Ribavirin (RIB) | Sofosbuvir (SOF) | Simeprevir (SIM) |
|---|---|---|---|---|---|
| o Mild | 50-80 | 180 µg PEG (2a) PEG (2b) 1.5 µg/kg | Standard | Standard | Standard |
| o Moderate | 30-50 | 180 µg PEG (2a) PEG alfa-2b 1 µg/kg or 25% reduction | Alternating doses 200 and 400 mg every other day | Standard | Standard |
| o Severe | < 30 | 135 µg PEG (2a) PEG alfa-2b 1 µg/kg or 50% reduction | 200 mg/d | Data not available | Standard |

167

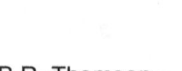

| Renal Impairment | eGFR/CrCl Level (mL/min/ 1.73 m$^2$) | Interferon (IFX) | Ribavirin (RIB) | Sofosbuvir (SOF) | Simeprevir (SIM) |
|---|---|---|---|---|---|
| o ESRD / HD | | PEG (2a) 135 µg/wk or PEG (2b) 1 µg/kg/wk or standard IFN 3 mU 3x/wk | 200 mg/d | Data not available | Data not available |

Abbreviations: ESRD, end stage renal disease; HD, hemodialysis

❖ HIV/HCV coinfection

| Genotype | Recommended | Alternative | NOT Recommended | Allowable anti-retroviral Therapy |
|---|---|---|---|---|
| 1 | o Treatment-naïve and prior PEG / RBV relapsers<br><br>– **IFN eligible:** SOF + PEG / RBV x 12 weeks<br><br>– IFN ineligible: SOF + RBV x 24 weeks<br><br>– SOF + SMV ± RBV x 12 weeks<br><br>o **Treatment experienced (prior PEG/RBV non-responders) regardless of IFN eligibility:** SOF + SMV ± RBV x 12 weeks | Treatment naïve and prior PEG / RBV relapsers<br><br>**IFN eligible:** SMV x 12 weeks + PEG/RBV x 24 weeks*<br><br>Treatment experienced (prior PEG/RBV non-responders)<br><br>**IFN eligibility:** SOF + PEG / RBV x 12 weeks<br><br>**IFN ineligibility:** SOF + RBV x 24 weeks | TVR + PEG / RBV x 24 or 48 weeks (RGT)<br><br>BOC + PEG / RBV x 28 or 48 weeks (RGT)<br><br>PEG/RBV x 48 weeks | For SOF use: ALL except didanosine, zidovudine, or tipranavir<br><br>For SMV use: LIMITEd to raltegravir, rilpivirine, maraviroc, enfuvirtide, tenofovir, emtricitabine, lamivudine, abacavir |

| Genotype | Recommended | Alternative | NOT Recommended | Allowable anti-retroviral Therapy |
|---|---|---|---|---|
| 2 | ○ SOF + RBV x 12 weeks regardless of treatment history | Treatment naïve and prior PEG / RBV relapsers: None<br><br>Treatment experienced (prior PEG/RBV non-responders)<br><br>IFN ineligibility: SOF + PEG / RBV x 12 weeks<br><br>**IFN ineligibility:** Non | PEG/RBV x 24 48 weeks<br><br>Any regimen with TVR, BOC, or SMV | All except didanosine, zidovudine, or tipranavir |

- Give effects of HIV co-infection on the clinical course of HCV.

    - ○ ↓ HCV clearance rate

    - ○ ↑ risk of chronic HCV

    - ○ ↑ risk of progression to fibrosis

    - ○ Use of interferon-based regimen is **contraindicated**, since interferon **accelerates** HIV infection

    - ○ In the setting of HIV plus HCV in the transplantation setting, there is ↑ graft rejection and loss

- Give factors which enhance the risk of accelerated fibrosis in the setting of HCV co-infection with HIV.

    - ○ Patient
        - – Older (> 33 years)
        - – Females

    - ○ HIV
        - – CD4+ < 100 mm3 while on HAART
        - – HIV viral load still detectable while on HAART thei

    - ○ HCV
        - – Untreated

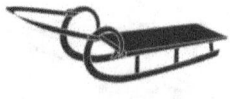

- Give mechanisms for the acceleration of hepatic fibrosis in the patient with HCV and co-infection with HIV.

  - TGF-B1
    - HIV → ↑ TGF-B1
    - ↑ TGFB1 → ↑ HCV replication

  - TJ permeability
    - HIV → ↓ CD4+
    - ↓ CD41 → ↑ TJ permeability
    - ↑ TJ permeability → ↑ bacterial translocation

  - Stellate cells
    - HIV → activate hepatic stellate cells
    - ↑ activated stellate cells → ↑ production of collager

Abbreviation: TJ, tight junctions

| Genotype | Recommended | Alternative | NOT Recommended | Allowable anti-retroviral Therapy |
|---|---|---|---|---|
| 3 | o SOF + RBV x 24 weeks regardless of treatment history | Treatment naïve and PEG/RBV relapsers: None<br><br>Treatment experienced (prior PEG RBV non-responders)<br><br>**IFN eligible:** SOF + PEG / RBV x 12 weeks<br><br>**IFN ineligibile:** None | PEG/RBV x 24-48 weeks<br><br>Any regimen with TVR, BOC, or SMV | All except didanosine, zidovudine, or tipranavir |
| 4 | o Regardless of treatment history:<br><br>– **IFN eligible:** SOF + PEG / RBV x 12 weeks<br>-**IFN ineligible:** SOF + RBV x 24 weeks | None | PEG/RBV x 48 weeks<br><br>Any regimen with TVR, BOC, or SMV | ALL except didanosine, zidovudine, or tipranavir |

### ❖ HCV and Liver Transplantion

- Give hepatic complications following liver transplantation (LT) for HCV.
  - Recurrence of HCV (~100%) post-LT
  - ↑ risk of cirrhosis
    - 20% to 40% in 5 years
  - Rapid progression to cirrhosis
  - High risk of cirrhosis becoming decompensated
    - In 1 year, about half of decompensated HCV cirrhotics will die
  - Fibrosing cholestatic hepatitis

- Give a comparison of the **histologic features** of recurrent hepatitis C virus infection versus acute cellular rejection after liver transplantation.

| Histological Features | HCV Recurrence | Rejection |
|---|---|---|
| o Portal inflammation | – Bland, uniform | ▪ Activated |
| o Lymphocytes, lymphoid aggregates or follicles | – Common (~50%) | ▪ Uncommon |
| o Eosinophils | – Uncommon | ▪ Common |
| o Steatosis | – Common | ▪ Never |
| o Acidophilic bodies | – Common | ▪ Uncommon |
| o Atypical features | – Cholestasis, ballooning degeneration without significant inflammation | ▪ Prominent periportal and lobular necroinflammatory activity w/o sub-endothelial venular inflammation |

Adapted from: *Sleisenger and Fordtran's Gastrointestinal and Liver Disease: Pathophysiology/ Diagnosis/ Management.* Ninth edition, 2010, page 1609.

---

SO YOU WANT TO BE A HEPATOLOGIST!

- Give scientific reasons why the development of a **vaccine** for HCV has been challenging.
  - Requires the production of both
    - Cellular immune response
    - Neutralizing antibodies
  - Anti-HCV does not lead to protective immunity (escape from antibody recognition)
  - High mutational rate of HCV
  - Heterogeneity of HCV envelop proteins

---

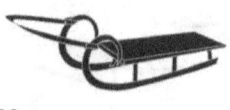

### ❖ HCV and HBV/HCV Coinfection

- Give the risk of cirrhosis, hepatocellular carcinoma (HCC) and mortality in hepatitis B and hepatitis C virus (HBV/HCV) monoinfected and coinfected patients.

| Feature | Cirrhosis | HCC | Mortality (SMR) |
|---|---|---|---|
| ○ HBV monoinfection | 22% | OR 16-23 | 1.4-5.3 |
| ○ HCV monoinfection | 30% | OR 8-17 | 2.4-3.1 |
| ○ HBV/HCV coinfection | 50% | OR 36-165 | 5.6-49 |

Abbreviations: HBV, hepatitis B; HCC, hepatocellular carcinoma; HCV, hepatitis C; OR, odds ratio; SMR, standard mortality ratio

Printed with permission: Wursthorn, et al. *Best Practice Res Clin Gastroenterol* 2008;22:1063-1079. (Studies: Amin et al, 2006; Di Marco et al, 1999; Donato et al, 1998 ; Shi et al, 2005; Zarski et al, 1998)

"There are two ways of spreading light: to be the candle or the mirror that reflects it".

Edith Wharton

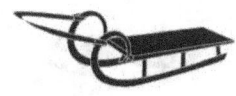

# OTHER HEPATOTROPIC VIRUSES

## Cytomegalovirus (CMV)

- Give types of hepatobiliary disorders associated with CMV infection.
    - Transminitis
    - Hepatitis
        - Acute
        - Granulomatous
        - Cholestatic
    - Fulminant hepatic failure
    - Post liver transplantation
        - Fibrosing cholestatic hepatitis
    - Graft rejection-like picture
    - Typical pathological changes on liver biopsy
        - Multinucleated giant cells
        - Owl's eye nuclear inclusions
        - Mononuclear portal and parenchymal inflammatory infiltration

## Epstein-Barr Virus (EBV)

- Mononucleosis-like illness (IgM anti-EBV)
- Worse clinical course in persons > 30 years
- May cause
    - Chronic hepatitis
    - Granulomatous hepatitis
    - PTLT (post-transplantation lymphoproliferative disease)

## Hepatitis D Virus (HDV)

➢ Virology

- Nuclear antigen in hepatocytes of persons infected with HBV.
- 3 genotypes HDV RNA encodes HDag
- HBsAg protects the complex of HDV-RVA-HDag hepatocyte injury is likely immune-mediated
- Serological markers

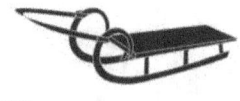

- Clinical
  - HDV infection may occur associated with severe HBV
    - Severe chronic HBV (decompensation)
    - Fulminant HBV
    - HBV carriers (especially IV drug users [IVDU])
    - HBV: HBV DNA, HBsAg
      - Previously HBsAg⁻, now anti-HBC⁺
      - More common in IVDUs chronic HDV in ~ 5%
      - Usually HDV resolves as HBV resolves
    - After HBV (coprimary infection)
    - After HBV (superimposed HDV infection)
      - Development of chronic HDV in ~70%
      - Previously HBsAg⁺, non IgM anti-HBC⁻
      - Progress to cirrhosis
    - HDV replication inhibits HBV replication
    - HBV DNA and HBsAg must be present for HDV replication

---

SO YOU WANT TO BE A HEPATOLOGIST!

- The patient tests positive for
  - HBV DNA⁺
  - HBsAg⁺
  - IgM anti-HDV⁺

- On the basis of their IgM anti-Hbc, determine if the HDV infection represents a coinfection of HBV, or if the person previously had HBV and the HDV was acquired (superinfection) afterwards.

| Type of infection | Previous HBsAg | ALT | IgM anti-HBc+ | Clinical course |
|---|---|---|---|---|
| o Coinfection | Negative | Double peak* | Positive | Usually resolves as HBV improves |
| o Superinfection | Positive | ↑ from baseline** | Negative | Progresses to cirrhosis |

*first with HBV infection, then later with HDV
**baseline may be increased because of initial HBV infection

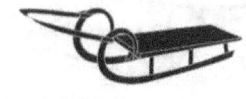

**Hepatitis E Virus** (HEV)

➤ Demography

  o More common in adults and males

  o High attack and mortality rates in pregnant women (each trimester)

  o Increased spontaneous abortions
    – Stillbirths
    – Neonatal deaths

• Give the "PRIM" countries where HEV is endemic.

  o Pakistan

  o Russia

  o India

  o Mexico

➤ Virology

  o RNA virus

  o Transplacental transmission (mother-to-new-born)

  o Fecal-oral transmission (water contaminated with HEV)

➤ Clinical

  o Presentations
    – Acute icteric or non-icteric hepatitis
    – Fulminant hepatic failure (22%)

**Herpes Simplex Virus** (HSV)

➤ Clinical

  o Acute HSV hepatitis from an infection with HSV-1 or HSV-2 may occur in immunocompetent as well as immunocompromised persons.

  o Microcutaneous and genital HSV lesions

  o Pregnant women
    – 3rd trimester
    – Fulminant hepatic failure

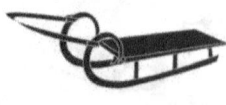

> Laboratory

   o Transaminitis
      - Immune suppressed persons

• Give laboratory features and which should alert the physician about the
  possibility of HSV hepatitis and the need to begin empiric therapy with acyclovir.

   o ↑↑ ALT, AST (> 1000)
   o ↓ WBC
   o Fever / abdominal pain
   o Associated HSV
      - Pneumonitis
      - Encephalopathy

> Histopathology

• Give the typical pathological changes of HSV on liver biopsy.

   o Focal or extensive
      - Hemorrhage
      - Necrosis

   o Hepatocytes
      - Cowdry A type inclusions in hepatocytes near the necrosis
      - Hepatocytes in periportal area
         ▪ Multinucleated
         ▪ Ground glass

Please see: Peltekian KM, Hirsch G. Chapter 59. In: Therapeutic Choices.
Grey J, Ed. 6th Edition, Canadian Pharmacists Association: Ottawa, ON,
2011, Table 7: Drug used in viral hepatitis, page 799-800.

The liver biopsy of the patient with acute viral hepatitis shows inclusions in the
nuclei of the hepatocytes.

• The histopathological features which help to differentiate between CMV- vs
  HSV- associated hepatitis.

   o CMV hepatitis   - Hepatocytes contain intra-nuclear inclusion with a
                       surrounding halo
                     - This halo is aka "owl's eye" inclusion
                     - Positive CMV immunohistochemistry

   o HSV hepatitis   - Hepatocytes with "glassy" nuclear inclusions (no
                       halo)
                     - Multi-nucleated giant cells

– Extensive necrosis

**Leptospirosis** (aka Weil Syndrome)

➤ Microbiology

   o Leptospira interrogans

➤ Clinical

   o General
- – Fever
- – Rigors

   o Clinical
- – Eyes
  - ▪ Conjunctivitis jaundice
- – Heart
  - ▪ Temperature-pulse dissociation
- – Lung
  - ▪ Cough, no sputum
- – MSK
  - ▪ Myalgias
- – Kidney
  - ▪ $\downarrow Na^+$, $\downarrow K^+$
  - ▪ Renal insufficiency
- – Hematology
  - ▪ lymphadenopathy
- – Liver
  - ▪ ALF (rare)
  - ▪ Hepatitis

➤ Laboratory

   o $\uparrow$ AST, $\uparrow$ bilirubin

> Clinical Gem
> - Give infectious causes of liver disease which cause fever and temperature-pulse dissociation.
>   - o Amebiasis
>   - o Leptospirosis

"There is no achievement without goals."
Robert J. McKaine

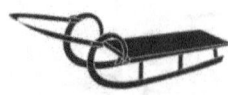

## OTHER INFECTIONS

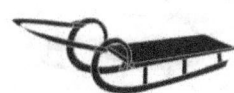

*MASTERING THE BOARDS*
*Hepatology & Pancreaticobiliary Disease*

A.B.R. Thomson

## SO YOU WANT TO BE A HEPATOLOGIST!

- Give mechanisms responsible for the common finding of cholestasis on liver biopsy from a person with sepsis.

Sepsis releases

- Exotoxins and endotoxins
  - Inhibits transport across hepatocyte sinusoidal and canalicular membrane
- TNF-α
  - Same effect as exo- / endotoxins

- In the context of the right upper abdominal pain and a urogenital infection, give the definition of **Fitz-Hugh-Curtis Syndrome**. Also, give its most common causes.

The Fitz-High-Curtis is perihepatitis, usually caused by salpingo-oophoritis from

- Chlamydia trachomatis
- Gonococcus

## Amebic Liver Disease

➢ Clinical
  - When to suspect amebic liver abscess
    - ↑ AP, leukocytes without eosinophilia
    - Temperature-pulse dissociation

➢ Diagnosis
  - Serology positive (in 95% after only 1 week of infection)

- Give reasons why percutaneous biopsy/aspiration of a suspected amebic liver abscess is generally **contraindicated**.
  - Right Lobe
    - Subcapsular peritonitis
  - Left lobe
    - Extension to
      - Peritoneum
      - Pleural space
      - Pericardium

179

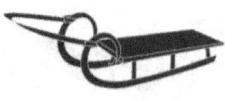

> Diagnostic imaging
  o CT scan
    – Elevated R. hemidiaphragm (50%)
    – Solitary
    – Large, round lesion
    – Usually right lobe of liver
    – Low attention (dark)
    – Enhancing rim of hepatic tissue

- Give reasons why it is sometimes necessary to accept the above potential complications, and to aspirate or drain "anchovy paste" (mixture of blood and liver tissue) from a solitary hepatic amebic abscess.
  o No clinical improvement after 3-5 days of metronidazole
  o Negative for amebic serology (occurs in 5% of patients)
  o Left lobe abscess
  o Rim of tissue < 1 cm large abscess

Source: Spiegel BM, Karsan AA. Acing the hepatology questions on the GI board exam. Slack Incorporated 2012, Table 38.1, page 106.

Curiosity: stool cultures are usually negative for Entamoeba cysts or trophozoites in persons with an amebic abscess

> Prognosis
  o When to suspect poor prognosis
    – ↑ bilirubin
    – ↓ albumin


## Echinococcal ("hydratid") Cyst of the Liver

> Epidemiology
  o Sheepherder (also think of fasciolosis)

> Cinical
  o Cough
  o Hepatomegaly (especially right lobe of liver)

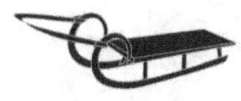

- Complications of
  - Enlarging cyst
    - Obstruction of biliary tree
    - Cholangitis
    - Pancreatitis
  - Compression on blood vessels
    - PV (portal hypertension)
    - HV (Budd-Chiari syndrome)
    - IVC (leg edema)
- ↑↑ AP

➤ Diagnostic imaging
  - US/CT scan
    - Round, smooth cyst
    - Daughter cyst
    - Internal septations
    - Ring-like calcification, especially "eggshell" calcification

➤ Treatment
  - Albendazole
  - When cysts are not active and not under pressure → aspirate (caution: may cause anaphylaxis)
  - Surgical resection for cyst ≥ 10 cm

"Always do your best. What you plant now, you will harvest later."

Og Mandino

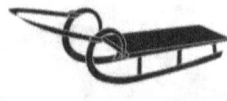

# INHERITED METABOLIC DISORDERS OF LIVER

| ➢ Terminology | Meaning |
| --- | --- |
| o Cosmopolitan SNPs | – Present in all ethnic groups |
| o Haplotype | – Group of variants or SNPs that occur together on a single chromosome |
| o Insertions and deletions | – One or more base pairs are inserted or deleted into the genome (rare) |
| o Linkage disequilibrium | – Variants that are linked to one another |
| o Missense mutation (non-synonymous) | – Base pair substitution that results in an amino acid change |
| o Polymorphism | – Variation in DNA sequence present in an allele with a frequency of 1% or greater in a population |
| o Population-specific SNPs | – Occur in specific ethnic groups |
| o Recombination | – Cross-over events that occur during meiosis that result in unlinking of genes or variants |
| o Sense mutation (synonymous) | – Base pair substitution that does not alter the coded amino acid |
| o Single nucleotide polymorphism (SNP) | – Most common form of DNA sequence variation |

Printed with permission Wright TL. *2007 AGA Institute Postgraduate Course*. pg. 45.

"Be aware of the big picture in the patients' life, not just blinkers on the obvious medical problem."

Dr. Joel Huurwitz

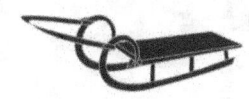

*MASTERING THE BOARDS*
*Hepatology & Pancreaticobiliary Disease*

A.B.R. Thomson

# IRON OVERALOAD DISORDERS

## Hereditary Hemochromatosis (HH)

➤ Pathophysiology

- Give the role of hepcidin in iron hemostasis in iron deficiency, inflammation and hereditary hemochromatosis.
  - ○ HFE binds to TFR1 and TFR2
  - ○ The HFE-TFR1 complex on the surface of the hepatocyte senses transferrin saturation (TS)
  - ○ When TS↑, diferric transferrin displaces HFE from the HFE-TFR1 complex
  - ○ HFE now binds to TFR2
  - ○ HFE-TFR2 complex causes the hepatocytes to sense ↓ TS (and ↓ BIS), so expression of hepcidin falls, and iron absorption increases
  - ○ As BIS increase → ↑ BMP6 binding to hepatocyte receptors → ↑ SMAD4
  - ○ In HH, the mutation in HFE provides abnormal "sensing" of the body iron stores the intestinal crypts "sense" that the body iron stores (BIS) are low, despite these BIS actually being high in HH.
  - ○ The sensing of ↓ BIS leads to ↓ hepcidin, ↑ active ferroportin, and ↑ iron absorption
  - ○ The ↑ iron absorption continues, unresponsive to the ↑ BIS because of the mutation of HFE
  - ○ Hepcidin decreases iron "release" from enterocytes (↓ transport of FE across the enterocyte BLM), and hepcidin also decreases iron release from macrophages.
  - ○ The ↓ hepcidin in HH causes ↑ iron release from macrophages

➤ Genetics

- Give the interpretation of the following genetic test results in persons suspected as having hereditary hemochromatosis (HH).
  - ○ C282Y homozygote
    - – Seen in >90% of genetic Hemochromatosis (HH). Wide range of clinical iron overload from no disease to total body iron overload and organ failure. Siblings of a homozygote should be screened with genetic tests, transferring saturation and serum ferritin, since they have a 1 in 4 chance of also being homozygous. Children of a homozygote are obligate heterozygotes but will only be homozygous if the other parent is at least a heterozygote. Testing of the second parent can identify the risk to the children with further testing of the children only recommended if the second parent is at least heterozygous for C282Y mutation.

183

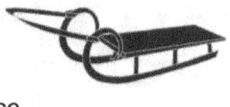

- False genetic results may occur but are rare.
- Approximately 50% of homozygotes do not have clinical iron overload (normal serum ferritin and transferring saturation). Such individuals are considered to be non-expressing homozygotes and may never develop disease. They should probably be followed with repeat serum ferritin and transferring saturation every 5 years.

o C282Y/H63D compound heterozygote
- Patients can carry one major mutation and one minor mutation. Typically iron studies are normal, although mild to moderate iron overload may occur. Severe iron overload is typically only seen in the setting of other causes of liver disease.

o C282Y heterozygote
- Occurs in approximately 10 per cent of the Caucasian population in which individuals carry one copy of a major mutation. Typically associated with normal iron studies. In rare circumstances that biochemical iron studies suggest significant iron overload (e.g., serum ferritin >1000µg/l) liver biopsy for hepatic iron index may be helpful in distinguishing between the genetic disorder and other causes of liver disease. It is recommended that siblings of a C282Y heterozygote be tested for this mutation.

o H63D homozygote
- Patients carry two copies of a minor mutation. Iron studies are typically normal, although mild to moderate iron overload is occasionally seen. In patients with biochemical evidence of iron overload, liver biopsy may be helpful to quantitate hepatic iron and determine need for treatment with phlebotomy.

o H63D heterozygote
- Occurs in approximately 20 per cent of the Caucasian population in which individuals carry one copy of a minor mutation. If biochemical iron studies are abnormal, these changes are more likely due to other non-genetic causes of iron overload.

o No HFE mutations
- If iron overload is present without any HFE mutations, non-genetic causes of iron overload are likely. Rarely patients may have mutations of other iron-related proteins such as transferring receptor-2, but these variants cannot be readily detected by genetic tests.

Printed with permission: Wright TL. *2007 AGA Institute Postgraduate Course*. pg. 47.

184

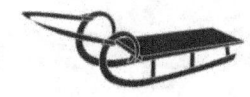

➢ Clinical

- Give the **physical findings** in patients with HH.
    - o Skin
        - – Increased pigmentation in sun-exposed areas
            - ▪ Melanocyte stimulation of ↑ melanin in skin
            - ▪ Iron in basal layers of skin
        - – Porphyria cutanea tarda (PCT)
    - o Liver
        - – Hepatomegaly
        - – Cutaneous stigmata of chronic liver disease
        - – Splenomegaly
        - – Signs of PHT (ascites, encephalopathy, jaundice, coagulopathy)
    - o Joints
        - – Arthritis
        - – Joint swelling
        - – Chondrocalcinosis
    - o Heart
        - – Dilated cardiomyopathy
        - – Congestive heart failure (CHF)
        - – Arrhythmias
    - o Endocrine
        - – Testicular atrophy
        - – Hypogonadism
        - – Hypothyroidism

Abbreviations: Hereditary hemochromatosis (HH); PHT, portal hypertension

Adapted from: Bacon BR, et al. Hepatology. 2011;54(1):328-43.

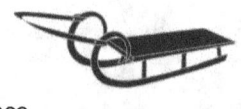

- ➤ Laboratory
  - o Transferrin concentration (TS) > 45%
  - o Ferritin saturation
  - o ALT, AST
  - o Genotyping C282Y, H63D
  - o TS (transferrin saturation) is more sensitive and specific for HH than is serum ferritin concentration.
  - o Serum ferritin concentration may be normal, even when TS > 45%
  - o Serum iron studies but not hepatic iron levels may be abnormal in PCT (porphyria cutanea tarda), NASH, chronic HCV, and alcoholic liver disease.
  - o About 40% of PCT patients have a mutation in C282Y, and NASH patients have a higher prevalence of C282Y mutations.
  - o The prevalence of HFE mutations is not increased in chronic HCV, but
    - – 22-62% of these persons have elevated serum ferritin concentrations, and
    - – 18-32% have elevated transferring saturation levels. There is no enrichment of HFE mutations in persons with alcoholic liver disease and elevated iron studies.

- • Give the clues that the patient with hereditary hemochromatosis does not have cirrhosis.
  - o < 40 years
  - o No hepatomegaly
  - o Ferritin < 1000 mg/mL
  - o AST normal

- • Give the role of ↑ Fe in hepatocytes and development of fibrosis.
  - o ↑ hepatocyte Fe → lipid peroxidation of hepatocytes
  - o Injured hepatocytes release profibrogenic cytokines
  - o Profibrogenic cytokines activate stellate cells
  - o Activated stellate cells lead to hepatic fibrosis

186

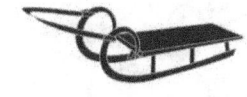

> ➤ Diagnostic algorithm

- Give a suggested **algorithm** to investigate HH-based on serum transferrin saturation, serum ferritin concentration, and HFE genotype.

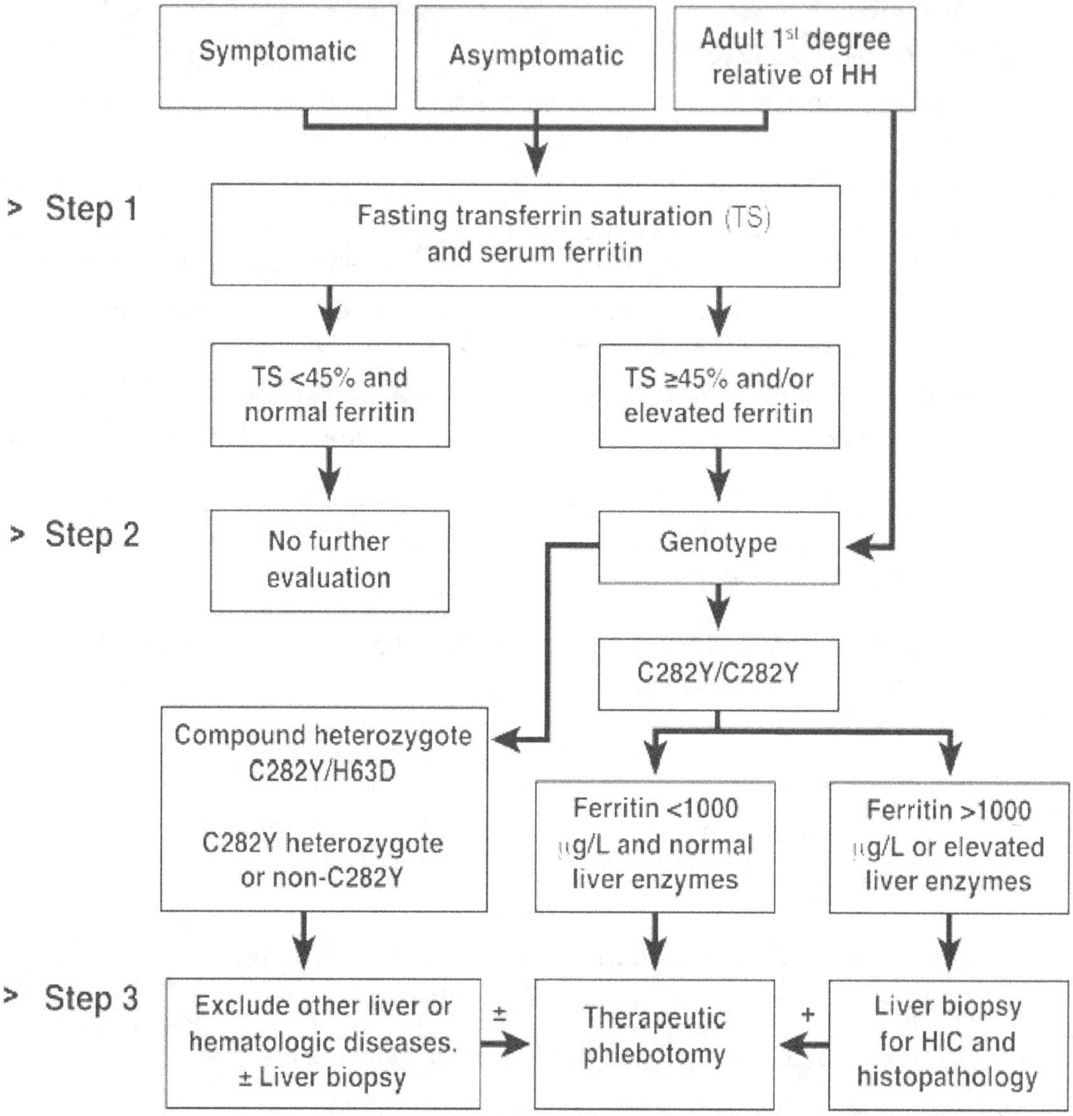

```
┌──────────────┐  ┌──────────────┐  ┌──────────────────┐
│  Symptomatic │  │ Asymptomatic │  │ Adult 1ˢᵗ degree │
│              │  │              │  │  relative of HH  │
└──────────────┘  └──────────────┘  └──────────────────┘
```

> **Step 1**

Fasting transferrin saturation (TS) and serum ferritin

| TS <45% and normal ferritin | TS ≥45% and/or elevated ferritin |

> **Step 2**

No further evaluation

Genotype

C282Y/C282Y

Compound heterozygote
C282Y/H63D

C282Y heterozygote
or non-C282Y

Ferritin <1000
µg/L and normal
liver enzymes

Ferritin >1000
µg/L or elevated
liver enzymes

> **Step 3**

Exclude other liver or
hematologic diseases.
± Liver biopsy    ±→

Therapeutic
phlebotomy    ←+

Liver biopsy
for HIC and
histopathology

Algorithm for an approach to a patient with elevated transferrin saturation and/or serum ferritin.

Printed with permission: Adams PC. Evaluation of cirrhosis with an elevated ferritin. Clin Gastroenterol Hepatol. 2012;10(4):368-70.

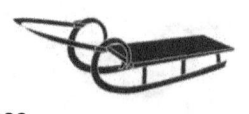

187

- ➢ Indications
  - o Liver biopsy in the person with HH is not necessary if
    - – They are young (< 40 years)
    - – Liver enzymes are normal, and if serum ferritin concentration is < 1000 mg/ml.
    - – Otherwise, fibrosis or cirrhosis might be suspected, and liver biopsy would be indicated
  - o Perl Prussian blue stain shows excess iron in the hepatocytes in HH, with fibrosis around the portal area, especially when the hepatic iron concentration is > 16, 000 µg/g liver dry weight
  - o Cirrhosis
  - o ↑ risk of HCC, even without cirrhosis

- ➢ Diagnostic imaging

- • Give the typical MRI findings in early HH, without cirrhosis or HCC.
  - o ↓ Signal intensity (darker) of liver as compared with spleen, on T-2 weighted image

- • Give the radiological features of the arthropathy of HFE-related HH.
  - o Second and third metacarpophalangeal joints, or knees
  - o Joint space – narrow
  - o Joint swelling
  - o Chondrocalcinosis
  - o Subchondral cysts
  - o Osteopenia

- ➢ Histopathology

A liver biopsy is performed in a C282Y/C282Y homozygote because of ↑ transaminases or serum ferritin > 1000 ng/mL:

- • Give the tests related to iron which can be performed on the liver biopsy tissue.
  - o Pearl pressure blue stain
    - – Location of iron
      - ▪ Hepatocytes
      - ▪ Kupffer cells
    - – Semi-quantitative grading of amount of iron

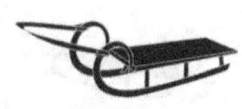

- HIC (hepatic iron concentration)
  - Normal, < 1500 µg/gm liver, dry weight
  - HH with symptoms, > 10,000 µg/gm
  - HIC level when fibrosis/cirrhosis occurs, > 20,000 µg/gm
  - Note: if patient has HH and for example HCV or NASH, fibrosis/cirrhosis will develop at HIC < 20,000 µg/gm liver, dry weight
- HII (hepatic iron index) = HIC / age of patient (years)
  - > 1.9, HH
  - < 1.9, likely secondary iron overload

➢ Differential diagnosis

• Give a classification of iron overload syndromes affecting the liver.

➢ Hereditary Hemochromatosis

- *HFE*-related
  - C282Y/C282Y
  - C282Y/H63D
  - Other *HFE* mutations (TFR gene)

- Non–*HFE*-related
  - Neonatal hemochromatosis
  - Juvenile hemochromatosis
  - Hemojuvelin (HJV)
  - Hepcidin (HAMP)Transferrin receptor-2 (TfR-2)
  - Atransferrinemia
  - Ferroportin (SLC40A1)

➢ Secondary Iron Overload

- Iron-loading anemias
  - Thalassemia major
  - Sideroblastic
  - Chronic hemolytic anemia
  - Aplastic anemia
  - Ineffective erythropoiesis
  - Pyruvate kinase deficiency
  - Pyridoxine-responsive anemia

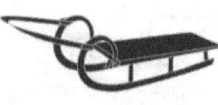

- ↑ iron intake
  - ↑ oral intake chronic
  - African iron overload
  - Parenteral iron overload
  - Hemojuvelin BMP (bone morphogenetic protein) binding to its receptor on the hepatocyte surface.
  - Loss-of-function mutation or gain-of-function
    - Multiple red blood cell transfusions
    - Iron–dextran injections
    - Long-term hemodialysis
- Chronic liver disease
  - Alcoholic liver disease (ALD)
  - Hepatitis B
  - Hepatitis C
  - Nonalcoholic fatty liver disease (NAFLD/NASH)
  - Porphyria cutanea tarda (PCT)
- Dysmetabolic iron overload syndrome
- Miscellaneous
  - Neonatal iron overload
  - Aceruloplasminemia
  - Congenital atransferrinemia

Printed with permission: Bacon BR, et al. Hepatology. 2011;54(1):328-43.

- Give the mechanism of iron overload which occurs with inflammation.
  - Iron metabolism is altered in inflammatory disorders (e.g., anemia of chronic disease)
  - In inflammatory disorders the ↑ proinflammatory IL-6 increases STAT3 signaling
  - ↑ STAT3 signaling increases hepcidin
  - This inflammation-associated ↑ hepcidin causes
    - Retention of iron in duodenocytes → ↓ iron absorption
    - Retention of iron in macrophages → loading of iron in RES (reticuloendothelial system), with less iron being available for synthesis of heme, and thus the development of anemia

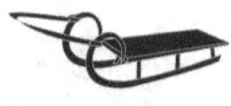

- Give the mechanisms of Fe overload in ALD and HCV.
  - In ALD (alcoholic liver disease) and HCV, ↑ ROS (reactive oxygen species) are formed
  - ↑ ROS
    - Acts on a C/EBP (CCAAT / enhancer binding protein) → ↓ hepcidin expression
  - ↓ hepcidin → ↑ iron absorption and release of iron from macrophages → iron overload

- ➢ Treatment
  - Phlebotomy of one unit (500 mL) of blood (250 mL of packed red blood cells) removes about 250 mg of iron: the serum ferritin falls by about 25 ng/mL
  - Phlebotomy is performed weekly until the serum ferritin is< 50 mg/ml (removal of 1 unit of blood lowers serum ferritin concentration by about 30 mg/ml) and transferrin saturation is < 50%
  - It is important to treat the patient with HH, to prevent the 20x ↑ risk of HCC. Even when the HH cirrhosis patient has a liver transplant, they remain at ↑ risk of cardiac disease.
  - With phlebotomy in HH, serum ferritin falls slowly and progressively, while TS remains abnormally increased until just before body iron stores are normal, and treatment frequency for phlebotomy may be switched from a treatment to a maintenance program.
  - Liver transplantation corrects the defect in HFE (inHH, but the 5 year survival rate is less than in non-HFE Fe-overload:
    - Normal iron stores (in HH), 75%
    - Non-HFE Fe overload, 63%
    - HFE, Fe overload, 34%
  - Although HCC risk is increased in HH even without the presence of cirrhosis, there are no accepted guidelines for HCC screening in HH without cirrhosis.

- Give the effect of phlebotomy on the following complications of HH.
  - Development of HCC
  - Regression of cirrhosis
  - Arthropathy
  - Hypogonadism
  - Little, if any

192

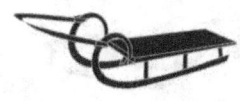

- Give the expected response to phlebotomy treatment in patients with HH, in addition to the fall in serum transferrin saturation and ferritin concentration.
  - ↑ sense of well-being, energy level
  - ↓ in abdominal pain
  - ↑ survival if diagnosis and treatment before development of cirrhosis and diabetes
  - Liver
    - ↓ tissue iron stores in hepatocytes
    - No reversal of established cirrhosis
    - No (or minimal) improvement in arthropathy
    - No reversal of testicular atrophy
    - Normalization of elevated liver enzymes
    - Reversal of hepatic fibrosis (in approximately 30% of cases)
    - Decline in hepatic iron concentration (HIC) and hepatic iron idex (HII)
    - Eliminate of risk of HH-related HCC if iron removal is achieved before development of cirrhosis
    - ↓ portal hypertension in patients wih cirrhosis
  - Extrahepatic
    - Improved cardiac function
    - Improved control of diabetes
    - Reduction in skin pigmentation

Adapted from: Bacon BR, et al. Hepatology. 2011;54(1):328-43.

➢ Prognosis

- Give the common causes of death after liver transplantation (LT) for HH.
  - HCC (Hepatocellular cancer)
  - Infections (↑ risk of infection in iron-loaded patients)
  - Cardiac and ventricular dysrhythmias
  - HF (heart failure)

- A 30-year-old man's biological father died of cryptogenic cirrhosis, and the young man requests genetic testing for hemochromatosis. He is found to be a C282Y homozygote (C282Y +/+). What are the next steps for him and his family?*
  - Normal iron studies → repeat iron studies every 5 years.
  - Abnormal iron studies → liver biopsy and liver iron index, >40years, ferritin >1000, ↑ AST; exclude HCV, alcohol, NAFLD/NASH
  - Assess liver enzymes and function – blood, ultrasound
  - Education

193

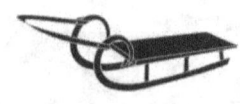

❖ Assess and treat
  o Extraintestinal manifestations (diabetes, heart, arthritis)
  o Avoid liver toxins, including alcohol
  o Screen for HCV, HCC
  o Preventative care: vaccinate against HAV, HBV
  o Phlebotomy if ↑ liver iron index

❖ Screen
  o Siblings – screen
  o Spouse - screen to determine if their children should be screened
  o Avoid high intake of Fe, vitamin C

*Remember, there is non-expression of the phenotypic abnormality in approximately 50% of the hereditary hemochromatosis genotype

---

**SO YOU WANT TO BE A HEPATOLOGIST!**

- Give the reason why the prevalence of HH associated with celiac disease may be underestimated.

  o Risk of CD (celiac disease) in HH (hereditary hemochromatosis), OR (odd ratio) ~ 2.2

  o The clinical expression of HH may have been reduced by CD, due to malabsorption of iron.

  o So the OR of CD + HH may be even higher

---

- Give the interventions which may be used to treat 4 different liver diseases, in which the treatment may lead to the reversal of hepatic fibrosis.

| Liver Disease | Intervention |
|---|---|
| o Hemochromatosis (HH) | – Phlebotomy |
| o Secondary iron overload | – Desforoximine |
| o Hepatitis B infection | – Anti-HBV therapy |
| o Hepatitis C infection | – Anti-HCV therapy |
| o Non-alcoholic steatohepatitis | – Weight reduction |
| | – Management of associated metabolic syndrome |

Source: Adams P. Gastroenterology 2011; 1142-1143

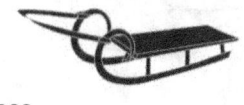

# WILSON DISEASE

➤ Definition

    o Wilson disease (WD) is an autosomal recessive condition caused by a mutation in ATP1B WD gene on chromosome 13, resulting in reduced secretion of copper from the liver into the bile, and accumulation of excessive copper in numerous tissues such as CNS, eye, liver, red blood cells, kidney.

• Give the copper metabolism in the hepatocyte.

Portal Venous Blood

Cu

Sinusoidal Membrane

CFTR

CCS      COX17      ATP7B

SOD    Mitochondrial cytochrome oxidase

Copper chaperones
ATOX1, CCS, COX17
Targets
ATP7B, SOM

Trans golgi network

Apo CER

Metallothionein copper storage protein

CER    COMD

Canalicular Membrane

Hepatic Bile

Abbreviations: ATOX, antioxidant 1 copper chaperone; ATP7B, cytochrome oxidase; CCS, copper chaperone for superoxide diastase; CER, ceruloplasmin; COMD1, copper excretion protein; COX17, cytochrome C oxidase 17; Cu, copper; SCO1, synthesis of cytochrome C oxidase 1; SOD, superoxide dismutase

Adapted from: Sleisenger and Fordtran's Gastrointestinal and Liver Disease. 10th Edition. Saunders/Elsevier, Philadelphia, 2016, Figure 72-2, page 1271.

195

➤ Pathophysiology

• Give the pathophysiology of Wilson disease.

  o In health

    - Copper (Cu) from albumin and other carriers in the blood is taken up into the hepatocyte by the copper transporter CTR1.
    - Copper (Cu) enters the liver and binds to Cu chaperones CTR1, COX17, and ATOX1.
    - Copper in the liver binds to apoceruloplasmin, forming ceruloplasmin (α2-glycoprotein).
    - Under basal conditions, the Wilson ATPase is located in the trans-Golgi network (TGN), where it receives Cu from the Cu chaperone ATOX1.
    - Cu transfer to the transmembrane domain is accompanied by ATP hydrolysis and formation of transiently phosphorylated intermediates of the Wilson ATPase ('phosphorylation').
    - The Wilson ATPase participates in the mechanism for incorporating Cu into apo-ceruloplasmin to generate holo-ceruloplasmin.

196

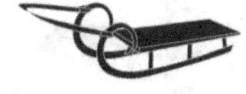

- In Wilson disease, there is
  - Misfolding of Wilson ATPase
  - Retention of WD ATPase in the endoplasmic reticulum
  - Failure to bind to ATOX1
  - Abnormal trafficking of WD ATPase
  - Abnormal phosphorylation and copper transfer
  - ↓ biliary excretion of Cu
  - Copper accumulation and toxicity in hepatocytes and other tissues (e.g., eye, kidney)

Abbreviations: BC, bile canaliculus; Mt, metallothionein; RER, rough endoplasmic reticulum; SER, smooth endoplasmic reticulum; TGN, trans-Golgi network.

Printed with permission: Ferenci P, et al. Defining Wilson disease phenotypes: from the patient to the bench and back again. Gastroenterology 2012;142(4):692-6.

➢ Clinical

- Give clinical features that suggest the diagnosis of WD.
  - Hepatic
    - Acute liver failure
    - Acute hepatitis
    - Chronic hepatitis
    - Autoimmune-like hepatitis
    - Asymptomatic hepatomegaly
    - Isolated splenomegaly
    - Persistently elevated serum aminotransferase activity (AST, ALT)
    - Fatty liver
    - Cirrhosis: compensated or decompensated
  - Neuropsychiatric symptoms
    - Depression
    - Neurotic impulsive behavior
    - Basal ganglia involvement
      - Disorder of gait
      - Rigidity

197

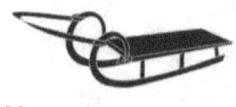

- o Neurological
  - – Movement disorders (tremor, involuntary movements)
  - – Drooling, dysarthria
  - – Rigid dystonia
  - – Pseudobulbar palsy
  - – Dysautonomia
  - – Migraine headaches
  - – Insomnia
  - – Seizures
  - – Depression
  - – Neurotic behaviours
  - – Personality changes
  - – Psychosis
- o Eyes
  - – Sunflower cataracts
  - – Kayser-Fleisher rings
- o Hemolytic anemia
- o Hyperphonia (soft voice)
- o Kidney
  - – Aminoaciduria
  - – Nephrolithiasis
  - – Fanconi syndrome
  - – Nephrolithiasis
- o Gallbladder
  - – Cholelithiasis
- o Pancreas
  - – Pancreatitis
- o MSK
  - – Arthritis of larger joints
  - – Osteoporosis
  - – Osteochondritis
  - – Rickets
  - – Rhabdomyolysis

198

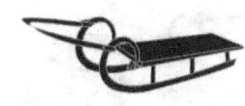

- Heart
  - Cardiomyopathy
  - Arrhythmias
  - SCD (sudden cardiac death)
- Endocrine
  - Hypoparathyroidism
  - Amenorrhea
  - Infertility
  - Spontaneous abortion
  - Menstrual irregularities
  - Repeated miscarriages
- Skin
  - Lunulae ceruleae

Modified in part from: Roberts EA, Schilsky ML; American Association for Study of Liver Diseases (AASLD). Diagnosis and treatment of Wilson disease: an update. Hepatology. 2008 ;47(6):2089-111.

---

Clinical Gems and Pearls

- A young person with liver disease in WD who develops neurological symptoms usually has cirrhosis.
- Hemolytic anemia in WD occurs in
  - Acute hepatitis
  - ALF (acute liver failure)
- Basal ganglia symptoms / signs
  - Plus KF rings = WD
  - No KF rings ≠ WD

---

➢ Histopathology

- Give the histopathological changes in the liver in WD.
  - Lysosomal deposits of Cu-metallothionon (orcein stains), especially in Kupffer cells
  - Inflammation, including interstitial hepatitis
  - Mallory bodies
  - Patchy involvement of cystic dilation of mitochondrial cristae

199

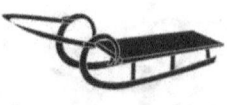

- ➤ Laboratory
- Give laboratory features that suggest the diagnosis of WD.
  - o Transaminases < 1500 U/L (may be normal)
  - o AST/ALT > 2.2
  - o ↓ AP (alkaline phosphatase)
  - o ↑↑ bilirubin (B) (from liver disease plus RBC hemolysis)
  - o AP/B < 4
  - o ↓ serum ceruloplasmin
  - o ↓ serum copper (ceruloplasmin-bound)
  - o ↑ non-ceruloplasmin-bound copper
  - o ↑ copper in the urine (reflects ↑ non-ceruloplasmin-bound copper)
  - o ↑ liver copper (> 250 µg per g dry weight of liver)

- ➤ Tests for **diagnosis** of Wilson disease
  - o The gold standard for diagnosis of WD
    - – Hepatic copper > 250 µg/g dry tissue – Yes
    - – ↓ serum ceruloplasmin
    - – ↑ free copper, ↑ urine copper – No (seen in heterozygotes, and other chronic cholestatic conditions)

| | Test | Typical Finding | False Negative | False Positive |
|---|---|---|---|---|
| o | Serum ceruloplasmin | Decreased by 50% of lower normal value | Normal levels in patients with marked hepatic inflammation<br><br>Overestimation by immunologic assay<br><br>Pregnancy, estrogen therapy | Low levels in:<br>- Malabsorption<br>- Acerulo-plasminemia<br>- Heterozygotes |
| o | 24-hour urinary copper | > 1.6 µmol / 24 hr<br><br>> 0.64 µmol / 24 hr in children | Normal<br>- Incorrect collection<br>- Children without liver disease | Increased<br>- Hepatocellular necrosis<br>- Cholestasis<br>- Contamination |
| o | Serum "free" copper | > 1.6 µmol/L | Normal if ceruloplasmin overestimated by immunologic assay | |

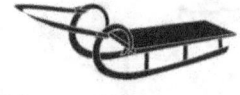

| Test | Typical Finding | False Negative | False Positive |
|------|-----------------|----------------|----------------|
| Hepatic copper | > 4 µmol/g dry weight | Due to regional variation<br>- In patients with active liver disease<br>- In patients with regenerative nodules | Cholestatic syndrome |
| Kayser-Fleischer rings by slit lamp examination | Present | Absent<br>- In up to 50% of patients with hepatic Wilson<br>- In most asymptomatic siblings | Primary biliary cholangitis |

Printed with permission: European Association for Study of Liver. EASL Clinical Practice Guidelines: Wilson disease. J Hepatol. 2012;56(3):671-85.

SO YOU WANT TO BE A HEPATOLOGIST!

The serum concentration of ceruloplasmin is decreased in WD, but the reduction is not diagnostic for the condition.

- Give a classification of the other causes of reduced ceruloplasmin levels.
  - Chronic liver disease
  - Malnutrition
  - Malabsorption
  - Nephrotic syndrome
  - Hereditary aceruloplasmin

- Give the reasons why measurement of liver copper may be normal or non-diagnostic in early WD.
  - In early WD the lysosomal Cu may be distributed unevenly in the liver, so there is a possible sampling error.

- Give the mechanism for the iron deficiency which may occur in WD.
  - $Fe^{2+}$ stored in ferritin must be oxidized in order for the $Fe^{2+}$ to become $Fe^{3+}$ and to be then bound to transferrin and be transported to bone marrow for production of RBC.
  - Ceruloplasmin is a feroxidase (oxidase activity).
  - ↓↓ ceruloplasmin, as occurs in WD, results in less oxidation of $Fe^{2+}$ in ferritin, so ↓ $Fe^{3+}$ is bound to transferrin and transported to the bone marrow to produce RBC, thereby leading to anemia.

201

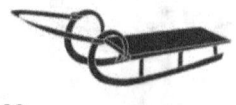

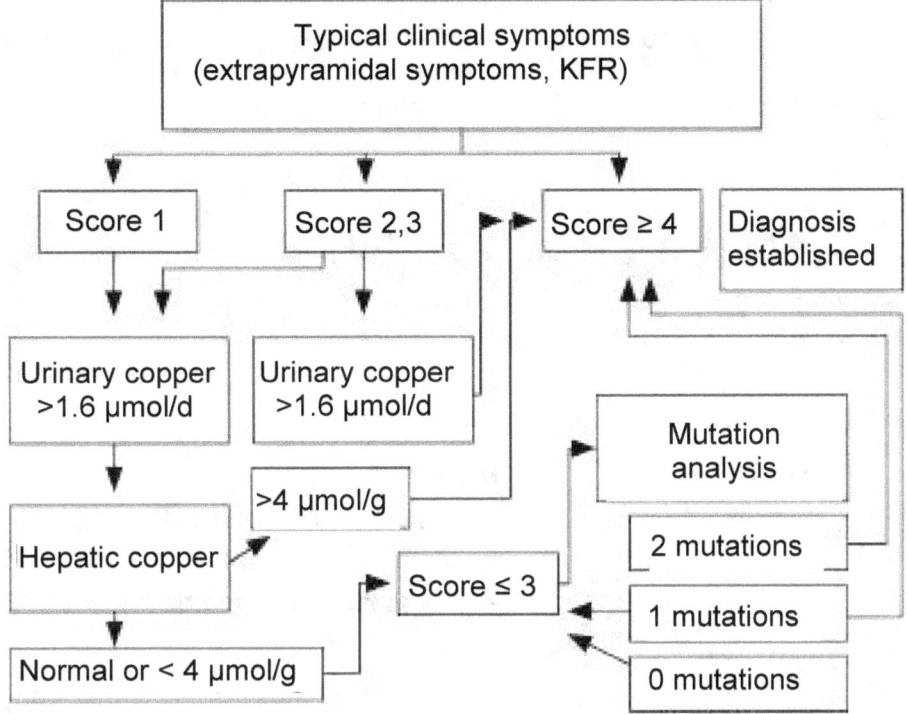

Printed with permission: European Association for Study of Liver. EASL Clinical
Practice Guidelines: Wilson disease. J Hepatol. 2012;56(3):671-85, Figure 1.
Approach to diagnosis of Wilson disease (WD) in a patient with unexplained liver
disease.

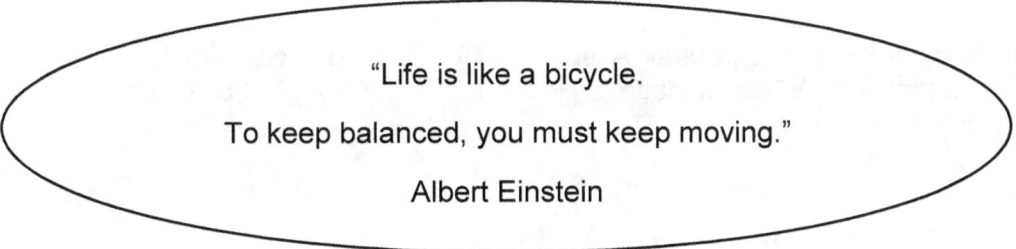

"Life is like a bicycle.

To keep balanced, you must keep moving."

Albert Einstein

MASTERING THE BOARDS                                    A.B.R. Thomson
Hepatology & Pancreaticobiliary Disease

❖ **Scoring system** (Leipzig) developed at the 8th International Meeting on Wilson disease.

| Findings | Score | Findings | Score |
|---|---|---|---|
| **KF rings** | | **Liver copper** | |
| - Present | 2 | - > 5x ULN (>4 µmol/g) | 2 |
| - Absent | 0 | - 0.8-4 µmol/kg | 1 |
| | | - Normal (< 0.8 µmol/g) | -1 |
| **Neurologic symptoms** | | - Rhodamine-positive granules | 1 |
| - Severe | 2 | | |
| - Mild | 1 | **Urinary copper (in the absence)** | |
| - Absent | 0 | - Normal | 0 |
| | | - 1.2x ULN | 1 |
| | | - > 2x ULN | 2 |
| **Serum ceruloplasmin** | | - Normal but > 5x ULN | 3 |
| - Normal (> 2 g/L) | 0 | | |
| - 0.1- 0.2 g/L | 1 | | |
| - < 0.1 g/L | 2 | | |
| **Coombs-negative hemolytic anemia** | | **Mutation analysis** | |
| - Present | 1 | - On both chromosome detected | 4 |
| - Absent | 0 | - On 1 chromosome detected | 1 |
| | | - No mutations detected | 0 |

| TOTAL SCORE | Evaluation |
|---|---|
| ≥ 4 | Diagnosis of WD established |
| 3 | Diagnosis possible, more tests needed |
| ≤ 2 | Diagnosis very unlikely |

Printed with permission: European Association for Study of Liver. EASL Clinical Practice Guidelines: Wilson disease. J Hepatol. 2012;56(3):671-85, Table 5.

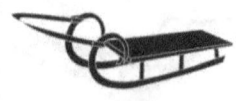

➢ Treatment

- • Give why it is important to appreciate that it takes ~ 6 months for D-penicillamine and trientine to improve neurological symptoms and liver enzymes in WD.
    - o So that therapy is not considered to be unsuccessful and incorrectly stopped prematurely.
    - o Plan pregnancy
        - – Switch from chelators to oral zinc ~ 3 mon before conception
    - o If pregnancy not planned and patient still on chelator → reduce to lower dose

- • Give the **adverse effects** of therapy of WD (Wilson disease).

- ❖ D-penicillamine

| | | |
|---|---|---|
| o CNS | – ↑ neurological symptoms | |
| o Hypersensitivity reaction | – Fever | |
| | – Rash | |
| | – Lymphadenopathy | |
| | – Neutropenia (↓ PMV) | |
| | – Thrombocytopenia | |
| o Endocrine | – Hypothyroid | |
| o Skin lesions | – Pemphigoid lesions | |
| | – Lichen planus | |

204

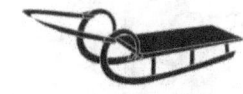

- o Hematology
  - ↓ RBC
  - ↓ WBC
  - ↓ platelets
  - Lymphadenopathy
- o MSK
  - Lupus-like syndrome
  - Arthralgias
- o Lung
  - Goodpasture syndrome
- o Kidney
  - Proteinuria
- o Pregnancy
  - Teratogenic
  - Iron deficiency
  - Suppression of bone marrow

❖ Trientine
  - o Gastritis
  - o Iron deficiency
  - o Bone marrow suppression

❖ Ammonium tetrathiomolybdate
  - o Suppression of bone marrow
  - o Hepatotoxicity

Please see: Swan MG. Chapter 58. In: Therapeutic Choices. Grey J, Ed. 6th Edition, Canadian Pharmacists Association: Ottawa, ON, 2011, Table 7: Wilson disease, page 780.

---

➤ Clinical Alert in Treatment of WD: Stopping Rules

  - o **Do not** suddenly stop chelating treatment in WD

  - o Suddenly stopping chelating therapy may
    - ↑ neurological defects
    - ↑ risk of acute liver failure (ALF); requires liver transplantation
    - ↑ risk of being refractory to treatment when Cu-chelating therapy is reintroduced

---

➤ Screening

  - o WD is caused by autosomal recessive ↓/absent function of the gene ATP7B; who needs to be screened for WD in the patient's family.
    - First-degree relatives

  - o Suggested algorithm for Wilson disease, based on the Leipzig Score

205

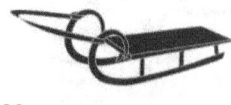

# α1- TRYPSIN (α1-AT) **DEFICIENCY**

- ➤ Genetics
  - o Autosomal recessive disorder associated autosomal co-dominant mutation in α1AT (serine protease inhibitors) on chromosome 14
    - – Leads to chronic disease of lungs (emphysemia) and liver (cirrhosis)
  - o Mutation in codon 342 of the 1-AT gene, changing a single amino acid from lysine to glutamate

- ➤ Pathophysiology

- • Give the pathogenesis of α1-AT deficiency.
  - o Replacement of glutamine with lysine from a mutation at position 342 of the α1-AT (SERPINA 1) gene leads to degradation of the serine proteases in the serum and tissues
  - o Loss of serum α1-AT activity results in
    - – Loss of normal inhibition of the activity of the elastase protease
    - – ↑ neutrophil elastase activity
    - – ↑ proinflammatory effect of ATZ polymers on neutrophils
  - o The AT protein is misfiled and polymerized and malprocessed.
  - o This abnormal structure of the AT2 protein lead to its retention in the ER, and ↓ intracellular degeneration (abnormal "quality control" of the protein)
  - o Loss of normal inhibition of the activity of the elastase protease
  - o The gain-in-function alter intracellular signaling pathways, with the changes in processes include
    - – ↑ autophagy
    - – Mitochondrial injury
    - – ↑ apoptosis

- ➤ Histopathology

- • Give the histopathology of α1-AT deficiency.
  - o ↓ bile ducts
  - o Intracellular cholestasis
  - o Inflammation
  - o Steatosis
  - o PAS (periodic acid-Schiff) – positive, diastase-resistant globular inclusions of polymers of α1-ATZ protein in periportal hepatocytes and Kupffer cells

206

- IHC (immunohistochemistry)
  - Staining with monoclonal antibody to α1-ATZ confirms α1-ATZ proteins in the globular inclusions.

- Clinical
  - Pulmonary emphysema
  - Hepatic cirrhosis
  - Panniculitis, ulcerative, neutrophilic
  - Aneurysm of aorta, cervical artery

Note; recombinant plasma A1AT replacement therapy useful for lung but not liver A1AT changes

- Treatment
  - Liver transplantation (LTx) corrects the metabolic disorder
  - 5-year survival rate after LTx for α1-AT
    - Children, 83%
    - Adults, 90%
  - Curiosity!
    - "Liver transplantation with grafts from donors with unrecognized α1-AT deficiency appear to have a comparable outcome to transplants using grafts without unrecognized liver disease" (*Sleisenger and Fordtran's Gastrointestinal and Liver Disease*. 10th Edition. Saunders/Elsevier, Philadelphia, 2016, page 1282).

"When we are no longer able to change a situation, we are challenged to change ourselves."

Viktor Frankl

207

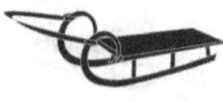

## AUTOSOMAL DOMINANT POLYCYSTIC KIDNEY DISEASE (ADPKD)

➢ Clinical

The patient with ADPKD (autosomal dominant polycystic kidney disease) develops esophageal varice but no ascites. There are no signs of portal hypertension /cirrhosis.

- Give the explanation for the **non-cirrhotic portal hypertension**, and the lack of ascites.
  - In the high liver (massive hepatomegaly), the cysts may compress veins and lead to non-cirrhotic portal hypertension.
    - Hepatic function is normal
  - Depending upon which vein(s) is obstructed determines which hepatic complications are present

| Compression | Sign |
|---|---|
| – PV (portal vein) | ▪ Esophageal varices (EV) |
| – HV (hepatic vein) / IVC (inferior vena cava) | ▪ Ascites |

Clinical Pearl

- Portal hypertension can occur in ADPKA the absence of obstruction of PV, HV or IVC, due to the association of ADPKD with CHF (congenital hepatic fibrosis)
- Large hepatic cysts may cause gastric outlet obstruction

  - The patient with massive hepatic cysts from APPKD may have no cirrhosis, normal hepatic function, and a low MELD score, but liver transplantation is justified for their non-cirrhotic portal hypertension, esophageal varices and ascites.
    - A MELD exception may be requested to make the ADPKD patient with massive hepatic cysts and non-cirrhotic PHT eligible for liver transportation.

- Give the most common causes of abdominal pain in the patient with ADPKD.

  - Renal      – Cyst
    - Hemorrhage
    - Infection
    - Perforation

  - Abdominal wall    – Hernia
  - Colon      – Diffuse diverticulitis

208

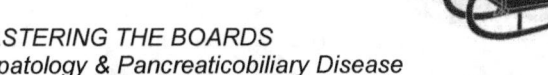

# CYSTIC FIBROSIS (CF)

- Give the hepatobiliary lesions which are specific to CF itself, and those secondary to extrahepatic disease.

  - Specific    – FBC (focal biliary cirrhosis)
    - Obstruction of small bile ducts
    - Inflammatory
    - Steatosis
    - Proliferation of bile ducts
    - Portal fibrosis
    - Multilobular biliary cirrhosis (MBC)
      - 10% of FBC progress to MBC and portal hypertension

  - Secondary    – Cardiopulmonary disease
    - Centrilobular necrosis
    - Drug hepatotoxicity
      - Cirrhosis

  - Specific and/or secondary
    - Muscocele
    - Mucous hyperplasia
    - Microgallbladder
    - Biliary sludge
    - Cholelithiasis
    - Cholangiocarcinoma
    - Bile duct compression/stricture from pancreatic fibrosis

➢ Suspecting and Diagnosing Liver Disease in CF

  - "Liver biochemical test levels may remain relatively normal despite histological evidence of cirrhosis" (Feldman M., et al. Sleisenger and Fordtran's Gastrointestinal and Liver Disease. 9th Edition. Saunders/Elsevier, Philadelphia, 2010, page 1277).

  - Hepatic lesions may be focal biliary cirrhosis (FBC), so there is considerable sampling error, and liver biopsy may underestimate the severity of the associated liver disease.

  - A normal abdominal ultrasound does not exclude clinically important hepatic fibrosis.

209

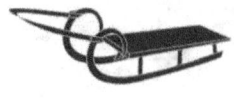

## Sickle Cell Disease

- Give hepatobiliary complications of sickle cell disease.

  o Liver diseases
    - Acute sickle hepatic crisis
    - Hepatic sequestration
    - Sickle cell intra-hepatic cholestasis
    - Hepatic infarction
    - Hepatic iron overload
    - Viral hepatitis

  o Biliary system
    - Cholelithiasis and choledochalithiasis
    - Acute cholecystitis and cholangitis
    - Ischemic cholangiopathy

Printed with permission:  Ahmed S, et al. *Best Practice & Research Clinical Gastroenterology* 2005;19(2): 299.


## Mitochodrial Cytopathies

- Give the causes and features of mitochondrial cytopathies.

  o Causes
    - Acute fatty liver of pregnancy
    - Reye syndrome
    - Genetic defects in mitochondrial function
    - Drug-related liver injury (DILI)

  o Features
    - Clinical
      - Vomiting and apathy
    - Laboratory
      - Lactic acidosis
      - Hypoglycemia
      - Hyperammonemia
    - Histopathology
      - Microvesicular fat in organs

Adapted from: Sleisenger and Fordtran's Gastrointestinal and Liver Disease. 10th Edition. Saunders/Elsevier, Philadelphia, 2016, page 1300-1301.

210

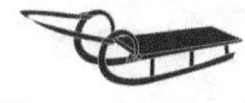

## Miscellaneous Other Inherited Disorders

- Give other inherited disorders, which affect the liver.

  - Alagille syndrome
  - Benign intrahepatic cholestasis
  - Cholesterol ester storage disease
  - Dubin-Johnson syndrome
  - Gilbert syndrome
  - Lysosomal lipase deficiency
  - Progressive familial intrahepatic cholestasis
  - Wolman disease
  - Zellweger syndrome

Printed with permission: Wright TL. *2007 AGA Institute Postgraduate Course*. pg. 44.

- Give the dietary therapy of **hereditary liver diseases** (in addition to always avoiding alcohol).

| Disorder | Dietary intervention |
|---|---|
| o Hemochromatosis | – Avoidance of excess dietary iron, selection of foods containing phytates or tannins to reduce iron absorption (together with appropriate phlebotomy treatment) |
| o Wilson disease | – Low-copper diet, zinc supplementation (together with chelating agent); green tea |
| o Cystic fibrosis | – High-fat diet, pancreatic enzyme supplements, fat-soluble vitamin supplements, medium chain triglycerides (MCT) |
| o Hereditary fructose intolerance | – Low fructose, low sucrose diet |
| o Galactosemia | – Galactose-free diet |
| o Tyrosinemia | – Low phenylaline and tyrosine diet |
| o Glycogen storage disease | – Continuous glucose feeding |
| o Cerebrotendinous xanthomatosis | – Deoxycholic acid supplementation |

Adapted from: Thapa BR. *Indian J Pediatr.* 1999; 66(1 Suppl): S110-9.

211

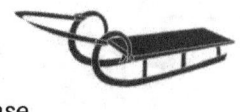

# DRUG- INDUCED LIVER INJURY (DILI)

➢ Methods and metabolism

SO YOU WANT TO BE A HEPATOLOGIST!

- Give the meaning of Phase I, II and III reactions involved in hepatic drug **metabolism**.

  o Phase I reactions
    – Microsomal drug oxidases and the CYP gene superfamily
      ▪ Involves the hemoprotein f the CYP gene
      ▪ Drugs are converted to a toxic metabolite (e.g., acetaminophen → NAPQI)

  o Phase II
    – Conjugation
      ▪ Through glucuronic acid or inorganic sulfate by formation of ester links with the drug

  o Phase III
    – Secretion of drugs or their metabolites by transporters
      ▪ ATP-binding cassette (ABC) protein
      ▪ MDR1 (multidrug resistance protein C1)
      ▪ MRP1 (multidrug resistance-associated proteins)
        – MRP-3   sinusoidal membrane of hepatocytes
        – MRP2   canalicular membrane (CM) of hepatocytes

- Give the reason why DILI resulting from drugs metabolized by phase I reactions (e.g., acetaminophen) is localized in zone 3 (around the terminal hepatic venules [THV]).

  o Phase 1 reactions are catalyzed by microsomal drug oxidase, the key component of when is a hemoprotein of the CYP gene superfamily.

  o CYP2E1 is located in hepatocytes which form a 1 to 2 hepatocyte thick rim around the THV.

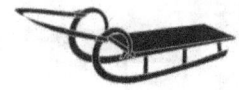

212

➤ Pathophysiology

• Give major **mechanisms** of drug-induced liver injury, leading to hepatocyte apoptosis and necrosis.
  o Direct hepatotoxicity
    – Injury to
      ▪ Mitochondria
      ▪ Plasma membrane
  o ROS (reactive oxygen species)
    – "the liver is exposed to oxidative stress by the propensity of hepatocytes to reduce oxygen...."
    – Some drugs (e.g., acetaminophen) may be converted by CYP into pre-oxidant reactive metabolites
    – CYP-mediated metabolism → formation of reactive metabolites → ↓ glutathione → injury to mitochondria → 1) release of cytochrome C and 2) operation of MPT (mitochondrial permeability transition) → activation of caspase → apoptosis
    – Formed from injured hepatocytes and kupffer cells
    – Reactive metabolites undergo covalent binding to proteins
    – Protein-drug adducts
      ▪ Inactive important enzymes
      ▪ May be acted upon by immunodestructive processes
  o Glutathione system
    – Pro-oxidants signal Nrf (the redox-sensitive transcription factor)
    – Nrf → ↑ CYP 2E1 expression → ↑ hepatic glutathione synthesis (from cysteine) → ↑ antioxidant effects
    – Cystolic glutathione
      ▪ In the reduced state, resulting from the effect of NADPH and glutathione reductase
      ▪ Glutathione deficiency injures mitochondria, releases cytochrome C and MPT (mitochondrial membrane permeability transition), leading to activation of caspases and apoptosis
  o Biochemical pathways of cellular damage
    – Covalent binding of drug to cellular proteins
    – Oxidation of proteins
    – Post-translational modification of proteins
    – Lipid peroxidation
    – Cleavage of DNA
    – ↑ $Ca_i^{2+}$ (intracellular concentration of $Ca^{2+}$)

213

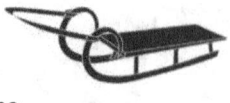

- o Hepatic non-hepatocyte cells
  - – Kupffer cells
    - ▪ Act as macrophages and antigen-presenting cells
    - ▪ Activated Kupffer cell may release TNF, ROS and as-L, which may lead to hepatocyte apoptosis/necrosis
  - – Endothelial cells
    - ▪ Their low glutathione context make then susceptibility to vascular injury
  - – Stellate cells
    - ▪ When activated, will deposit matrix and lead to fibrosis
- o Immunologic mechanisms
  - – Formation of ligands with death receptors
  - – Porin-mediated introduction of granzyme
  - – "altered antigen" drug metabolite interacts with cellular proteins to form drug-protein adducts (haptens)
  - – Drug-induced autoimmunity

➢ Clinical

- Give drugs that have been reported to have an increased risk of hepatotoxicity in patients with chronic liver disease.

| Drug | Underlying liver disease as a risk factor |
|------|-------------------------------------------|
| o Methotrexate | – Alcoholic liver disease, NAFLD |
| o Vitamin A (high doses) | – Alcoholic liver disease |
| o Rifampin | – Primary biliary cholangitis |
| o Methimazole | – Chronic hepatitis B |
| o Ibuprofen (NSAIDs) | – Hepatitis C |
| o Antiretrovirals ( e.g., zalcitabine, saquinavir) | – Hepatitis B, C |
| o Antiandrogens | – Chronic viral hepatitis B, C |
| o Oral contraceptives | – Women with liver tumours, or history of jaundice of pregnancy |

Adapted from: Gupta NK, and Lewis JH. *Aliment Pharmacol Ther* 2008; 28(9): 1021-41.

- In the context of DILI, give the meaning of the Hy law.

  - o In DILI, the finding of clinical jaundice plus increased ALT or AST has a mortality rate of ~ 10%.

214

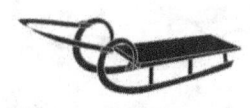

- Give drugs which are **relatively contraindicated** and must be used cautiously in persons with liver disease.

  o  Clonazepam

  o  Conjugated estrogen/medroxyprogesterone

  o  Dantrolene

  o  Felbarnate

  o  Gemfibrozil

  o  Lovastatin and other HMG-CoA reductase inhibitors (statins)

  o  Metformin

  o  Methotrexate

  o  Naltrexone

  o  Niacin

  o  Pemoline

  o  Phenelzine

  o  Tacrine (in persons with prior jaundice)

  o  Ticlopidine

  o  Tolcapone

  o  Valproic acid

  o  Zalcitabine

Suggestion from the author: you have better things to do tthan to memorize this list. In the patient with liver disease, look up this list, or look up the dugs to be used

Adapted from: Gupta NK, and Lewis JH. *Aliment Pharmacol Ther* 2008; 28(9): 1021-41.

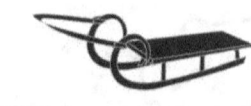

*MASTERING THE BOARDS*
*Hepatology & Pancreaticobiliary Disease*

A.B.R. Thomson

- Give drugs for which lower doses are recommended in patients with cirrhosis ("hepatic dosing").
  - o Acetaminophen
  - o Benzodiazepines
  - o Beta blockers
  - o Cetirazine
  - o Fluoxetine
  - o Indinavir
  - o Lamotrigine
  - o Losartan
  - o Moricizine
  - o Narcotics
  - o PPIs
  - o Repaglinide
  - o Risperidone
  - o Sertraline
  - o Topiramate
  - o Tramadol
  - o Valproic acid
  - o Venlafazine
  - o Verapamil

Adapted from: Gupta NK, and Lewis JH. *Aliment Pharmacol Ther* 2008; 28(9): 1021-41.

➢ Causes/associations

- Give **risk factors** of the development of DILI (drug-induced liver injury).
  - o Older age
  - o Female gender
  - o Polypharmacy
  - o Past history of adverse drug reaction
  - o Alcohol
    - – ↓ dose threshold and ↑ severity of hepatotoxicity of some drugs, e.g., acetaminophen, isoniazid, niacin, methrotrexate
  - o Nutritional status
    - – Obesity
      - ▪ Halothane
    - – Malnutrition
      - ▪ Methotrexate
      - ▪ Tamoxifen

216

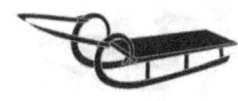

- o Pre-existing liver disease
  - – Methotrexate (treatment for psoriasis)
  - – HBV, HCV, HIV/AIDs
    - ▪ Anti-TB drugs
    - ▪ HAART therapy
    - ▪ Anti-cancer drugs
    - ▪ Ibuprofen
    - ▪ Myeloablation
    - ▪ Anti-androgens
    - ▪ Sulfonamides
  - – HCV sinusoidal obstruction syndrome

- ➢ Histopathology

- • Give types of histopathological changes in the liver seen in DILI.
  - o Acute hepatitis
  - o Fulminant hepatic failure
  - o Chronic granulomatous hepatitis
  - o Chronic hepatitis
  - o Autoimmune hepatitis
  - o Cholestasis with/without hepatitis
  - o Steatohepatitis with/without fibrosis
  - o Vascular toxicity
    - – SOS (sinusoidal obstruction syndrome; aka veno-occlusive disease)
    - – Sinusoidal dilation
    - – Cavernous hemangioma
    - – NRH (nodular regenerative hypertension
    - – Peliosis hepatitis
  - o Tumour
    - – FNH
    - – Hepatic adenoma
    - – HCC
    - – Cavernous hemangioma

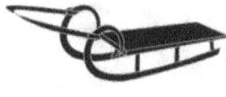

# Methotrexate

- Give risk factors for methotrexate induced hepatic fibrosis, their clinical importance, and their implications for prevention.

| Risk Factors | Importance | Implications for Prevention |
|---|---|---|
| o Age | – ↑ risk > 60 yr, possibly related to renal clearance and/or biological effect on fibrogenesis | ▪ Care in use of methotrexate in older persons |
| o Dose | – Incremental dose<br>– Dose frequency<br>– Duration of therapy<br>– Cumulative (total) dose | ▪ 5-15 mg/wk is safe<br>▪ Weekly bolus (pulse) safer than daily schedules<br>▪ Consider liver biopsy every 2 years<br>▪ Consider liver biopsy after each 2 g methotrexate |
| o Alcohol consumption | – ↑ risk with daily levels > 15 g (1-2 drinks) | ▪ Avoid methotrexate use if alcohol intake not curbed. Consider pre-treatment liver biopsy with relevant history of alcohol use. |
| o Obesity | – ↑ risk | ▪ Consider pre-treatment and interval liver biopsies |
| o Diabetes mellitus | – ↑ risk in obese persons (type 2 diabetes mellitus) | ▪ Consider pre-treatment and interval liver biopsies |
| o Pre-existing liver disease | – ↑↑ risk, particularly related to alcohol, obesity, and diabetes (NASH) | ▪ Pretreatment liver biopsy mandatory<br>▪ Avoid methotrexate, or used scheduled interval biopsies according to severity of hepatic fibrosis, total dose, and duration of methotrexate therapy |

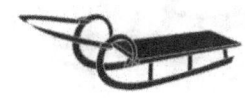

| Risk Factors | Importance | Implications for Prevention |
|---|---|---|
| o Systemic disease | – Possibly risk greater with psoriasis than rheumatoid arthritis (may depend on preexisting liver disease, alcohol intake) | ▪ None |
| o ↓ renal function | – ↑ risk because of reduced clearance of methotrexate | ▪ Reduced dose, greater caution with use |
| o Other drugs | – NSAIDS, vitamin A, and arsenic may increase risk | ▪ Greater caution with use<br>▪ Monitor liver biochemical tests |

- o Other diseases
  - – Rheumatoid arthritis
    - ▪ Salicylates
    - ▪ Sulfasalazine
  - – Diabetes, obesity
    - ▪ Methotrexate
  - – Chronic renal disease
    - ▪ Methotrexate → fibrosis
    - ▪ Renal transplantation → azathioprine-associated hepatic vascular damage

Abbreviations: Nash, non-alcoholic steatohepatitis; NSAIDS, nonsteroidal anti-inflammatory drugs

Printed with permission: *Sleisenger and Fordtran's Gastrointestinal and Liver Disease: Pathophysiology/ Diagnosis/ Management*. Ninth edition, 2010, Table 86.7, pg 1443.

---

CLINICAL CHALLENGE

Jaw clenching and teeth grinding (bruxism) are uncommon extrahepatic manifestations of liver disease. In the patient with these signs plus tender hepatomegaly, sweating, fever and transaminases > 1000, give the likely diagnosis.

- o Acute hepatitis with sweating, fever, jaw clenching and teeth grinding would be suggestive of drug induced liver injury, for example from "ecstasy".

- • For an extra mark, give the chemical name for ecstasy (clue: MDMA).
  - o Ecstasy is **methylenedioxymethamphetamine**.

---

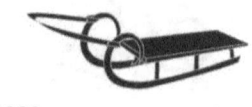

*MASTERING THE BOARDS*
*Hepatology & Pancreaticobiliary Disease*

A.B.R. Thomson

## Oral Contraceptive Agents (OCA)

- Give hepatobiliary complications of the use of oral contraceptive agents (OCAs).

  o Gallstones

  o Cholestasis

  o Unmasking PBC, and other cholestatic diseases such as familial intrahepatic cholestasis

  o Unmasking porphyria

  o Tumours
    - Adenomas
    - ↑ size of FNH (focal nodular hyperplasia)
    - Hepatocellular carcinoma (rare)

  o Increased risk of NASH (non-alcoholic steatohepatitis)

  o Vascular
    - Budd-Chiari syndrome
    - Peliosis hepatic (sinusoidal dilation)

## Mushroom Poisoning

- Give the pharmacological treatment of mushroom poisoning (Amanita phalloides) and DILI (drug-induced liver injury).

  o NAC, in IV or po doses as per acetaminophen toxicity, plus

  o Penicillin G IV 1 million units/kg BW/day, plus

  o Silibinin (silymarin, milk thistle) IV/po 30-40 mg/kg BW/day for 3-4 days.

Abbreviation: BW, body weight

---

**SO YOU WANT TO BE A HEPATOLOGIST!**

- Give the mechanism of hepatotoxicity caused by Amanita phalloides.

  o Alpha-amatoxin
    - ↓ mRNA
    - ↓ protein synthesis

  o Phalloidin
    - Interferes with polymerization of actin
    - Disrupts cell membranes

---

## Dress Syndrome

- o Glucocorticosteroids, only for Drug-induced liver injury (DILI) associated DRESS syndrome
    - Drug rash
    - Eosinophilia ⎤ plus DILI → corticosteroids
    - Systemic symptoms ⎦

## Acetaminophen Poisoning

- Give the management of the patient with acetaminophen (ACM) overdose.

  - o Initial measures
    - Suspect acetaminophen overdose if the transaminases are > 1000 IU/mL, and if the serum bilirubin concentrations are normal (in the absence of possible ischemic hepatitis, i.e., hypotension or CV collapse).
    - ABC`s
    - Determine likelihood of hepatotoxicity from nomogram (except in non-intentional cases)
    - Immediately give activated charcoal (1gm/kg body weight [BW] po in a slurry (does not reduce the effect of NAC [N-acetylcysteine]) if presenting within 12 hours
    - Rule out other co-ingestions
    - Serum acetaminophen (ACM) level, urine toxicology screen, LFT's, LEs, INR, arterial lactate
    - Stratify risk for possible need for liver transplantation
    - Contact liver transplantation centre

CLINICAL PEARL: DILI

The dose of acetaminophen which places the ordinary patient at risk for acute liver failure (ALF) is 8 gm, but the dose level may be lower, especially for the smaller person. It is better to remember the threshold as < 150 mg/kg, rather than 6-8 gm.

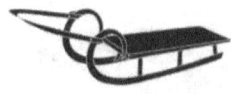

## Acetaminophen Toxicity **Nomogram**

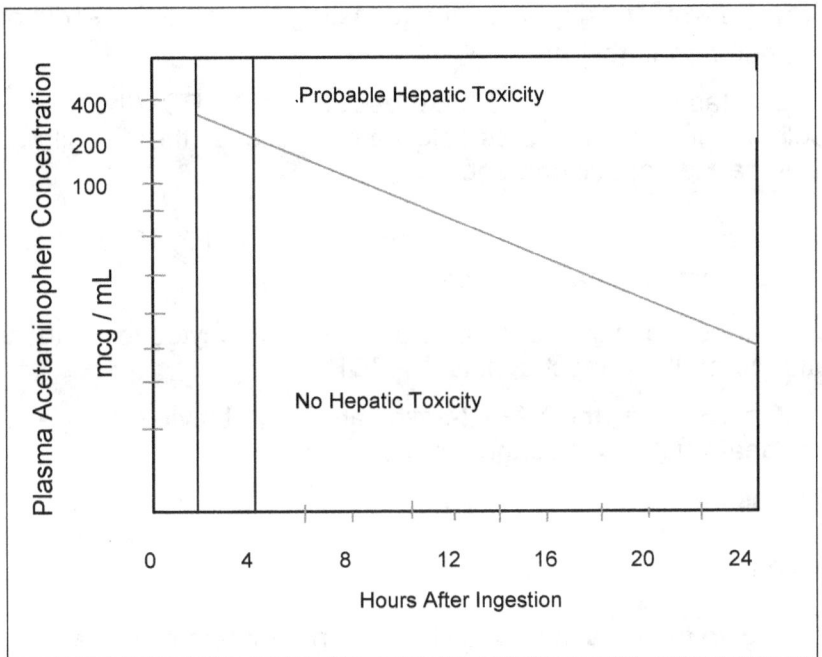

Printed with permission: Spiegel BM, Karsan AA. Acing the hepatology questions on the GI board exam. Slack Incorporated 2012, Figure 27-1, page 83.

SO YOU WANT TO BE A HEPATOLOGIST!

A toxic nomogram is available to predict how long after ingestion NAC remains effective. Because of the relative safety of the use of NAC, and that it may be efficacious even 48 hours after overdose, or in persons with non-acetaminophen ALF, the nomogram is **not always strictly followed**. In addition, the nomogram may have limitations.

- Give examples of when the standard acetaminophen toxicity nomogram may not correctly reflect possible severe liver disease.
    - Multiple doses of acetaminophen taken, rather than > 4 g taken at once
    - Unknown time of overdose ingestion
    - Alcoholic patient
    - Fasting patient

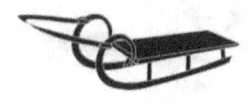

## SO YOU WANT TO BE A HEPATOLOGIST!

- Give the reason why drinking alcohol and fasting lower the threshold of acetaminophen hepatotoxicity.
  - Alcohol and fasting →↑ CYP2E1 expression → ↑ NAPQI (the toxic metabolite) ↓ glutathione stores below a critical level, thereby allowing NAPQI to cause hepatic damage

- Give the reason why NAC has to be given PO or IV within 12 to 16 hours of an acetaminophen overdose.

  - NAC provides the cysteine to stimulate the hepatocytes to synthesize glutathione and to protect against NAPQI

  - After 12 to 16 hours, the NAPQI-associated hepatocyte damage and the cell death pathways cannot be reversed.

  - Further, as the hepatocytes are destroyed, there are not enough metabolically healthy cells to convert the cysteine from NAC to glutathione.

- If this is true, give the reason why is NAC given for acetaminophen toxicity even 36 hours after poisoning.

  - NAC will stabilize vascular reactivity in persons with liver failure, so it may have some benefit beyond the mechanisms of glutathione and NADPQI.

- **N-acetylcysteine** (NAC)**, and other measures**
  - Oral N-Acetylcysteine (NAC)
    - Loading dose: 140 mg/kg po/NG x 1
    - 70 mg/kg q 4 hours x 17 doses
    - Stopping rules after 72 hours, or when liver chemistry improves
    - Compazine/raglan for nausea prn
    - Cimetidine (P450 inducer)
  - IV N-Acetylcysteine (NAC)
    - Dose 1. Loading dose: 140 mg/kg NAC in 200 ml D5W over 1 hour
    - Dose 2. 50 mg/kg NAC in 500 ml D5W over 4 hours.
    - Dose 3. 125 mg/kg NAC in 1000 ml D5W over 19 hours.
    - Dose 4. 150 mg/kg NAC in 1000 ml D5W over 24 hours.
    - Dose 5. 150 mg/kg NAC in 1000 ml D5W over 24 hours.

223

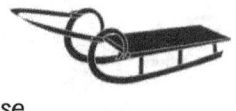

- o Caution regarding use of NAC
  - − NAC should be given within 4 hours of overdose, but may still be of value 48 or more hours after ingestion.
  - − Do not administer NAC to patients with known sulfa allergy
  - − Administer IV formulation of oral NAC through a leukopore filter in a monitored setting after consent obtained from patient/family.
  - − IV infusion of NAC leads to anaphylactoid/hypersensitivity reactions in 3 to 5% most commonly during loading dose.
  - − Hold and reduce infusion rate by 50% if rash/nausea occurs. Administer fluids, IV benadryl, IV steroids as needed.
  - − For causes of ALF other than acetaminophen, and in patients with stages I or II encephalopathy, NAC may improve outcomes.

- Give the use of NAC (N-acetylcysteine) in non-acetaminophen associated acute liver failure (ALF).

| End Point | NAC | No-NAC |
|-----------|-----|--------|

- ❖ Adults
  - o Liver transplantation-free survival

| | NAC | No-NAC |
|---|---|---|
| − All patients | 40% | 27% |
| − Stages ½ at entry | 52% | 31% |

  - o MOFS
    - − ↑ tissue oxygenation
- ❖ Children
  - o ↓ LOS (length of hospital stay)
  - o ↑ rate of spontaneous recovery
  - o Manage coma (stages III-IV in ALF)
    - − Intubation
    - − Epidural monitoring of intracerebral pressure (ICP) of < 25 mmHg, and cerebral perfusion pressure of 50-80 mmHg
    - − 30° elevation of the head of the bed
    - − Factor VII or FFP to get INR < 1.8
    - − Mannitol infusion
    - − Hypothermia, or indomethacin
    - − Cultures
    - − Antifungal coverage
    - − Vasopressors (norepinephrin)
    - − To maintain cerebral perfusion pressure > 50 mmHg, enteral nutrition
  - o Psychological assessment of overdose
  - o Treat complications if ALF present

Adapted from: Chun LJ, et al. *J Clin Gastroenterol* 2009;43(4):342-9.

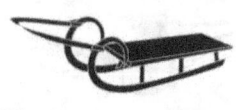

## VASCULAR DISEASES

- Classify, and give examples of vascular diseases of the liver.

    o Disorders of portal venous inflow
    - Acute mesenteric/portal venous thrombosis (PVT)
    - Chronic mesenteric/PVT

    o Disorders of hepatic arterial (HA) inflow
    - HA thrombosis
    - Hepatic arteriovenous fistula
    - Ischemic hepatitis

    o Disorders of hepatic venous outflow
    - Veno-occlusive disease (VOD)
    - Budd-Chiari syndrome (BCS)

Printed with permission: Kamath PS. *Mayo Clinic Gastroenterology and Hepatology Board Review* 2008: pg. 337.

## Portal Colopathy

➢ Defination

    o Portal colopathy is the "....vascular manifestations of portal hypertension in the colon" (Sleisenger and Fordtran's Gastrointestinal and Liver Disease. 10th Edition. *Saunders/Elsevier*, Philadelphia, 2016, page 628).

➢ Causes

    o Varices

    o Hemorrhoids

    o Telangiectasias (spider—nevi-like lesions)

    o Patchy diffuse redness, colitis-like

---

SO YOU WANT TO BE A GASTROENTEROLOGIST!

- What is the postulated pathogenesis of the hemangioblastomas seen in persons with von Hippel-Lindau disease (vHLD).

    o In vHLD, the vHL protein is lost, there is increased hypoxia-inducible factor, and increased production of VEGF (vascular endothelial growth factor).

Note: Inhibitors of VEGF receptor 2 (eg semaxanib) reduce the elevated VEGF in vHLD, and have been found to be useful to treat the hemangiomas.

---

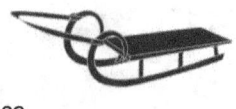

**Budd-Chiari Syndrome** (BCS)

➢ Definition

    o Obstruction of the hepatic venous outflow from the right atrium to the small hepatic venules

➢ Causes/associations

• Give causes of the Budd-Chiari Syndrome (BCS).

    o Hypercoagulable states
       – Inherited
          ▪ Factor V Leiden mutation
          ▪ Prothrombin mutation
          ▪ Antithrombin deficiency
          ▪ Protein C deficiency
          ▪ Protein S deficiency
          ▪ Antiphospholipid syndrome
       – Acquired
          ▪ Myeloproliferative disorders
          ▪ Cancer
          ▪ Pregnancy
          ▪ Oral contraceptive use
          ▪ Paroxysmal nocturnal hemoglobinuria (PNH)
          ▪ Polycythemia rubra vera (PRV)

    o Tumour invasion
       – Hepatocellular carcinoma
       – Renal cell carcinoma
       – Adrenal carcinoma

    o Miscellaneous
       – Aspergillosis
       – Behçet's syndrome
       – Inferior vena cava webs
       – Trauma
       – Inflammatory bowel disease
       – Dacarbazine therapy

    o Idiopathic

    o Commonest causes
       – Africa, Asia
          ▪ MOVC (membranous obstruction of the inferior vena cava)

226

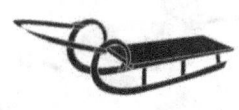

- NA/Europe
  - Thrombosis of hepatic veins, from thrombogenic states, e.g., myeloproliferative disorders ($JAK_2$ mutations of the gene coding for tyrosine kinase Janus kinase 2)

Please see Sleisenger and Fordtran's Gastrointestinal and Liver Disease. 10th Edition. Saunders/Elsevier, Philadelphia, 2016, page 1395 for a more extensive list.

- ➢ Clinical
  - o Abdominal pain
  - o Hepatomegaly
  - o Ascites
  - o Hepatic failure (if acute)
  - o Note: Presentation: BCS "….should be considered in patients presenting with decompensated cirrhosis or refractory ascites out of proportion to the magnitude of liver biochemical test abnormalities (Sleisenger and Fordtran's Gastrointestinal and Liver Disease. 10th Edition. Saunders/Elsevier, Philadelphia, 2016, page 1395).

- ➢ Diagnostic imaging
  - o Doppler ultrasound
  - o MRI (contrast enhanced); multiphasic CT

---

**CLINICAL CHALLENGE**

A young woman presents with a rapid onset of abdominal pain, hepatomegaly and ascites. MRI demonstrates an enlarged caudate lobe.

- Give clinical diagnosis, and explain the changes on diagnostic imaging.
  - o Budd-Chiari syndrome (BCS) is caused by obstruction of blood flow in the hepatic vein, with flow away from the liver.
  - o The damage occurs mostly in zones 3 and 2; because of the ↓ total in the HV, and because the caudate lobe has additional blood flow through the accessory hepatic veins, the caudate lobe may hypertrophy.
  - o If a venogram were peformed, it might show a "spider web" appearance suggestive of BCS (BCS → ↓ HV flow → ↑ accessary HV flow → spider appearance on venography).
  - o Curiosity: a very large candate lobe may compress the IVC (inferior vena cava) and further ↓ HV outflow.

---

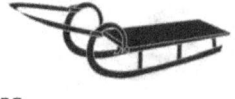

*MASTERING THE BOARDS*
*Hepatology & Pancreaticobiliary Disease*

A.B.R. Thomson

➢ Histopathology

• Give the acute and chronic histopathological changes of Budd-Chiari syndrome.

| o Acute centrilobular | – Congestion |
| | – Sinusoidal distention |
| | – Hemorrhage |
| | – Necrosis |
| | – Little inflammation |

| o Chronic | – Patchy, asymmetrical involvement |
| | – Perivenular sclerosis |
| | – Venular (↑ subendohelium) |
| | – Hepatocellular necrosis |
| | – Regenerative nodules |
| | – Cirrhosis |

➢ Management    o Cause
  – Treat any esophageal varices
  – Anticoagulants, thrombolysis, venesection
  – Cytotoxic drugs

o Surgical
  – Porta-caval shunt
  – TIPS (if incomplete obstruction)
  – Embolectomy (selected cases)
  – Liver transplantation

Abbreviations: HV, hepatic vein; IVC, inferior vena cava; PV, portal vein

Adapted from: Sleisenger and Fordtran's Gastrointestinal and Liver Disease. 10th Edition. Saunders/Elsevier, Philadelphia, 2016, page 1394.

➢ Treatment
  o Acute
    – Supportive care, including
      ▪ Large volume paracentesis of ascites
      ▪ Treating underlying condition
    – Anticoagulation
    – Thrombolysis
    – Angioplasty (obstruction of IVC plus HV → form portocaval shunt)
    – Stent placement
    – TIPS ("bridge" to liver transplantation)

228

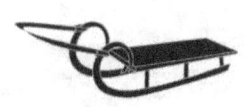

- - Fulminant
    - – Hepatic failure (↑ MELD score)
    - – Liver transplantation (LT)
  - Chronic
    - – If acute care as per above fails and there is decompensated cirrhosis, then
      - ▪ TIPS
      - ▪ Liver transplant
      - ▪ Portosystemic shunt surgery (PSS)
        - – PV becomes the hepatic outflow tract
        - – No IVC stenosis
        - – IVC pressure < 20 mmHg
  - Note: the "uncorrected" MELD score does not take into account the refractory ascites which is common in BCS

- Give the treatment options and indications for the use different modalities in the patient with Budd-Chiari Syndrome (BCS), and also give their advantages and disadvantages.

| Treatment | Indication | Advantages | Disadvantages |
|---|---|---|---|
| ○ Thrombolytic therapy | Acute thrombosis | Reverses hepatic necrosis | Risk of bleeding<br>Limited success |
| ○ Angioplasty with and without stenting | IVC webs<br>IVC stenosis<br>Focal hepatic vein stenosis | No long-term sequelae<br>Averts need for surgery | High rate of restenosis or shunt occlusion |
| ○ TIPS | Possible bridge to transplantation in fulminant BCS<br>Acute BCS (HE) | Low mortality<br>Useful even with compression of IVC by caudate lobe | High rate of shunt stenosis<br>Extended stents may interfere with liver transplantation |
| ○ Surgical shunt | Subacute BCS if portacaval pressure gradient <10 mmHg or occluded IVC | Definitive procedure for many patients<br><br>Low rate of shunt dysfunction with portacaval shunt | Risk of procedure-related death<br>Limited applicability |

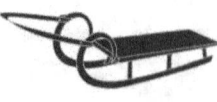

| Treatment | Indication | Advantages | Disadvantages |
|---|---|---|---|
| o  Liver transplantation | Subacute BCS Portacaval pressure gradient >10 mmHg Fulminant BCS Presence of cirrhosis Failure of portosystemic shunt | Reverses liver disease<br><br>May reverse underlying thrombophilia | Risk of procedure-related death<br><br>Need for long-term immunosuppression |

Abbreviations: HE, hepatic encephalopathy; IVC, inferior vena cava; TIPS, transjugular intrahepatic portasystemic shunt

Printed with permission:  Kamath PS. *Mayo Clinic Gastroenterology and Hepatology Board Review* 2008: pg. 344.

---

Therapeutic Trick

- Give what must be excluded in the patient with Budd-Chiari Syndrome before considering liver transplantation.

    o  Associated malignancy, causing a procoagulative state → HV thrombosis → BCS

---

**Sinusoidal Obstruction Syndrome** (SOS, aka Veno-occlusive Disease)

- ➢ Definition
    - o  Diffuse, ideopathic endothelial injury causing non-thrombotic obstruction of central hepatic venules, leading to dilation of sinusoids and hepatic congestion

- ➢ Causes
    - o  Common associations
        - – Bone marrow transplantation (BMT) occurs
            - ▪ Within 2 weeks after BMT
            - ▪ In 50% of BMT
            - ▪ 70% mortality rate
        - – Chemotherapy
        - – Azathioprine
    - o  Hepatic irradiation
    - o  Older age
    - o  HCV
    - o  C282Y (HH, hereditary hemochromatosis)
    - o  Other pre-existing chronic liver diseases
    - o  Recent bacterial/viral infections

230

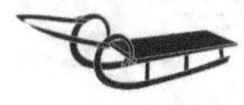

- ➢ Clinical
  - o Clinical associations
    - – BMT (bone marrow transplantation)
    - – Chemotherapy
    - – Jamaican herbal teas
    - – Azathioprine use
  - o Symptoms/signs
    - – Painful hepatomegaly
    - – Rapid weight gain
    - – Ascites

- ➢ Laboratory abnormalities
  - o Conjugated hyperbilirubinemia > 2 mg/dL
  - o Thrombocytopenia

- ➢ Diagnostic imaging
  - o Liver, spleen
    - – Hepatosplenomegaly
  - o Portal vein (PV)
    - – Dilated
    - – Flow in PV slow or reversed
  - o Umbilical vein
    - – Recanalization
  - o Gallbladder
    - – Thick wall

- ➢ Differential
  - o SOS develops after BMT on days 10 to 20
    - – Distinguish from GVHD (graft-versus-host disease) which develops after day 15
      - ▪ Sepsis and drug toxicity do not usually cause painful hepatomegaly or ascites, as does SOS

- ➢ Predictors of severity
  - o Jaundice
  - o Ascites
  - o HVPG (hepatic venous pressure gradient) > 20 mmHg
  - o Multiorgan failure
  - o Mortality rate ~25% from multiorgan failure, and not liver failure

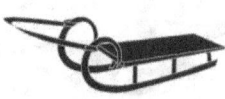

## Stem Cell Transplantation

- Give the timing and method of diagnosis liver and biliary diseases following stem cell transplantation.

| Disease | Timing | Diagnosis |
|---|---|---|
| o Sinusoidal obstruction syndrome (SOS) | – Onset before day 20 | ▪ Typical clinical features plus exclusion of other causes of jaundice and weight gain<br>▪ Imaging (Doppler ultrasound or CT)<br>▪ Transvenous measurement of wedged hepatic venous pressure gradient and liver biopsy<br>▪ Note atypical presentations (acute hepatitis, anasarca) |
| o Cholestasis of infection (cholangitis lenta) | – Following sepsis or neutropenic fever (usually before day 30) | ▪ Exclude other causes of cholestasis<br>▪ Inferential diagnosis in a patient with cholestatic jaundice |
| o Acute GVHD | – Day 15-50 | ▪ Confirm GVHD in skin, gut<br>▪ Exclude other causes of cholestasis<br>▪ Liver biopsy |
| o Acute viral hepatitis | – HSV, day 20-50<br>– Adenovirus, day 30-80<br>– VZV, day 80-250<br>– HBV and HCV, during immune reconstitution | ▪ Pre-transplant blood test (antigen, antibodies, PCR results)<br>▪ Isolation of virus from other sites (stool and urine for adenovirus)<br>▪ PCR of serum for specific viruses |
| o Fungal abscess | – Day 10-60 | ▪ Liver biopsy histology/PCR/immunostains<br>▪ Hepatic pain, fever |
| o Bacterial infection | – Day 10-80 | ▪ Liver imaging (MRI>CT)<br>▪ Serum fungal antigen(s)<br>▪ Hepatic pain, fever<br>▪ Liver imaging<br>▪ Liver biopsy, culture |

232

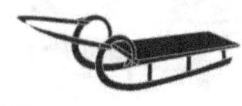

| Disease | Timing | Diagnosis |
|---|---|---|
| o Drug-liver injury | – Day 0-100 | ▪ Clinical evidence linking elevations of serum ALT or alkaline phosphatase to drugs known to cause liver injury |
| o Ischemic liver disease | – Day 0-30<br>– Day 15-60 | ▪ Clinical evidence linking shock to subsequent rises in serum ALT |
| o Biliary obstruction | – Day 10-50 | ▪ History, examination<br>▪ Biliary ultrasound |
| o Idiopathic hyper-ammonemia | – After day 80 | ▪ ERCP>magnetic resonance cholangiography<br>▪ Unexplained confusion, coma<br>▪ Blood ammonia |
| o Chronic hepatitis C | – Pre-transplant<br>– Long-term follow-up after transplant | ▪ HCV RNA in serum<br>▪ ↑ serum ALT after immune reconstitution |
| o Iron overload | – After day 80 | ▪ Transferrin saturation<br>▪ Marrow iron qualification<br>▪ Liver iron quantification (Ferriscan MRI, liver biopsy quantification) |
| o Chronic GVHD | – Years after transplant | ▪ Prior acute GVHD history<br>▪ Chronic GVHD in other organs<br>▪ Consistent ↑ serum ALT, alkaline phosphatase<br>▪ Note hepatitis-like presentation |
| o Nodular regenerative hyperplasia (NRH) | | ▪ Liver biopsy (reticulin stain)<br>▪ Signs of portal hypertension but preserved liver function<br>▪ Laparoscopic appearance of the liver |

Abbreviation: GVHD, graft-versus-host disease

Printed with permission:  McDonald, G.B., and Frieze, D. *Gut* 2008; 57:987-1003, Table 3 pg. 995.

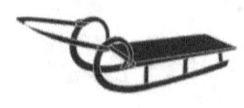

**Portal Vein Thrombosis** (PVT)

- ➢ Causes/associations
  - o Hypercoagulable states
    - – Antiphospholipid syndrome
    - – Antithrombin deficiency
    - – Factor V Leiden mutation
    - – Methylenetetrahydrofolate reductase mutation TT677
    - – Myeloproliferative disorders
    - – Nephrotic syndrome
    - – Oral contraceptives
    - – Paroxysmal nocturnal hemoglobinuria
    - – Polycythemia rubra vera
    - – Pregnancy
    - – Prothrombin mutation G20210A
    - – Protein C deficiency
    - – Protein S deficiency
    - – Sickle cell disease
  - o Impaired portal vein flow
    - – Budd-Chiari syndrome
    - – Cirrhosis
    - – Nodular regenerative hyperplasia
    - – Sinusoidal obstruction syndrome
  - o Inflammatory diseases
    - – Umbilical vein (infants)
    - – Behçet syndrome
    - – Inflammatory bowel disease
    - – Pancreatitis
  - o Infections
    - – Appendicitis
    - – Cholangitis
    - – Cholecystitis
    - – Diverticulitis
    - – Liver abscess
  - o Intraabdominal cancer
    - – Pancreas
    - – Cholangiocarcinoma
    - – HCC
    - – Bladder cancer

234

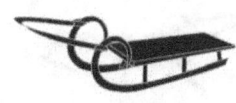

- o Intra-abdominal procedures
  - – Alcohol injection
  - – Abdominal surgery
  - – Colectomy
  - – Fundoplication
  - – Gastric banding
  - – Hepatic chemoembolization
  - – Hepatobiliary surgery
  - – Islet cell injection
  - – Liver transplantation
  - – Peritoneal dialysis
  - – Radiofrequency ablation of hepatic tumour (s)
  - – Sclerotherapy of esophageal varices
  - – Splenectomy
  - – TIPS procedure
  - – Umbilical vein catheterization

Adapted from: Stevens WE. *Sleisenger & Fordtran's gastrointestinal and liver disease: Pathophysiology/Diagnosis/Management* 2006: pg. 1762; and 2010, 1378.

For more details, please see Feldman M., et al. Sleisenger and Fordtran's Gastrointestinal and Liver Disease. 9th Edition. Saunders/Elsevier, Philadelphia, 2010, Table 83.2, page 1378, for "Causes of Portal Vein Thrombosis".

---

Clinical Alert!

"....long-term anti-coagulation does not increase the risk or severity of variceal bleeding and prevents further portal and mesenteric venous thrombotic complications" (Feldman M., et al. Sleisenger and Fordtran's Gastrointestinal and Liver Disease. 9th Edition. Saunders/Elsevier, Philadelphia, 2010, page 1379).

---

235

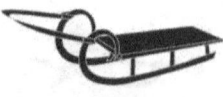

## Portal Vein Stenosis

➤ Clinical

Progression over time of obstruction of PV

- o Thrombus

    ↓

- o Constriction/compression (invasion)

    ↓

Collagenous formation

↓

Cavernous transformation of venous channels

↓

Portal cavernoma

➤ Laboratory

- o Slight increase in LFTs, Portal hypertension, Ascites

➤ Treatment

- o Resection and end-to-end reconstruction

## Hepatic Artery Thrombosis/Stenosis

➤ Clinical

- Give the clinical features and treatment of hepatic artery stenosis and thrombosis, as well as portal vein stenosis or thrombosis.

| Time of Occurrence | Leading Symptoms | Treatment |
|---|---|---|
| ❖ Hepatic artery thrombosis | | |
| o Early | – Fulminant increase in LFTs<br>– Acute liver failure<br>– Hemodynamic instability | ▪ Urgent acute thrombectomy or<br>▪ Urgent retransplantation |
| o Late | – Biliary complications Strictures<br>– Intrahepatic abscesses<br>– Cholangitis and sepsis | ▪ Management of biliary complications using ERC, PTC Rt-PA lysis therapy<br>▪ Elective retransplantation |

236

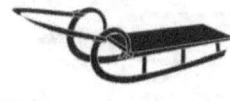

| Time of Occurrence | Leading Symptoms | Treatment |
|---|---|---|
| ❖ Hepatic artery stenosis | – Slight increase in LFTs<br>– Mild or late biliary complications | ▪ Reoperation, with resection of the anastomosis and end-to-end reconstruction |
| ○ Early | – Acute liver failure<br>– Fulminant increase in LFTs<br>– Hemodynamic instability<br>– Ascites<br>– Variceal bleeding | ▪ Urgent thrombectomy<br>▪ Urgent retransplantation |
| ○ Late | – Slight increase in LFTs<br>– Portal hypertension<br>– Ascites<br>– Variceal bleeding | ▪ Endoscopic treatment Rt-PA lysis therapy<br>▪ Elective retransplantation |

Printed with permission: Mueller AR, Platz KP, and Kremer B. *Best Practice & Research Clinical Gastroenterology* 2004;18(5): pg. 884.


## Splenic Vein Thrombosis

- Give the anatomical reasons why thrombosis of the splenic vein (SV) may cause gastric fundal varices, but not esophageal varices.

  ○ Thrombosis of SV (SVT) causes ↑ pressure in short gastric veins.

  ○ Obstruction of SV is distant to the joining of the SV to the SMV (superior mesenteric vein), which form the portal vein and from there the esophageal veins.

  ○ Thus, EV do not form with SVT (but do form with PVT)

---

An MCQ Trick Question

The usual surgical treatment for isolated gastric fundal varices due to splenic vein thrombosis (SVT) is sphenectomy.

- Give the circumstance whe splenectomy would not be curative for SVT.

  ○ A SVT combined with a portal vein thrombosis (PVT) would not be cured by splenectomy.

---

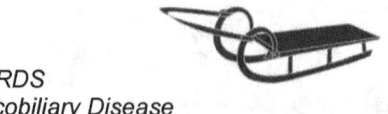

> Treatment

Abdominal ultrasound demonstrates a cystic mass, and CT which confirms a HAA (hepatic artery aneurysm).

- Give the surgical management of HAA.
  - o Extrahepatic
    - – Proximal to gastroduodenal artery
      - ▪ Proximal and distal ligation of HA (collateral blood supply still occurs in gastroduodenal artery)
    - – Distal to gastroduodenal resection artery
  - o Intrahepatic
    - – partial hepatic resection

> Mortality rate of ruptured HAA        o  ~ 30%


## Ischemic Hepatitis

> Definition

- Give reasons why "Ischemic" or "Hypoxic" hepatitis may not be a satisfactory term.
  - o Reduced hepatic blood flow from any cause, such as congestive heart failure, respiratory failure, systemic hypotension, cause the following pathological changes:
    - – Very little inflammatory infiltrate (i.e., no "hepatitis")
    - – Centrilobular necrosis
    - – Loss of hepatocytes
    - – RBC in sinusoids
    - – May progress to centrilobular fibrosis

- In the context of chronic centrilobular vascular congestion, give the meaning of "reverse lobulation".
  - o Reverse lobulation is the formation of bridging necrosis between central veins, (the reverse of bridging necrosis between portal tracts), which is characteristic of cardiac cirrhosis.

Note: Same answer for different question: Give the pathological feature distinguishing portal cirrhosis from cardiac cirrhosis.

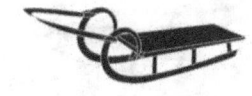

➢ Laboratory

- Give laboratory measurements which suggest ischemic hepatitis.
  - ↑ AST
  - ↑↑ LDH
  - ALT-to-LDH ratio of < 1.5
  - Rapid fall of LDH and AST, usually within 4 days
  - In congestive hepatopathy
    - ↑ SAAG
    - ↑ protein in ascites

**Hepatic Artery Aneurysm** (HAA)

➢ Causes/associations
  - Atherosclerosis (may also cause hepatic infarction)
  - Mycotic infection
  - Vasculitis
  - Pseudoaneurysms
    - Liver biopsy
    - Percutaneous transhepatic cholangiogram
    - Liver transplantation

xxxxxxxxxxxxxxxxxxxxxxxxxxxxxxxxxxxxxxxxxxxxxxxxxxxxxxxxxxxxx

SO YOU WANT TO BE A HEPATOLOGIST!

Atherosclerosis may involve the hepatic artery, and cause a hepatic artery aneurysm (HAA), which may rupture, and is associated with a 30% mortality rate.

- Give another but chronic hepatobiliary complication of artherosclerosis of the hepatic artery.

  - Slow obstruction of the hepatic artery may reduce the blood supply to the bile duct (aka [common bile duct]), leading to
    - Ischemic cholangiopathy
      - CBD strictures
      - Obstruction

xxxxxxxxxxxxxxxxxxxxxxxxxxxxxxxxxxxxxxxxxxxxxxxxxxxxxxxxxxxxx

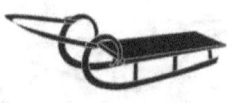

➢ Clinical

- Give the physical finding on the abdominal wall of the person the person with cirrhosis which suggests that the hepatic bruit is from recanalization of the umbilical vein.

    o The presence of a caput medusa suggests ↑.blood flow in the abdominal wall veins, arising from recanalization of the umbilical vein, producing the C-B (Cruveilhier – Baumgarten) murmur.

---

Clinical CUriosity

    o Some patients with ascites despite salt restriction and taking appropriate diuretics lose the ascites when a hepatic bruit develops.

---

SO YOU WANT TO BE A HEPATOLOGIST!

- Give the name of the bruit, and the mechanism of the spontaneous clearance of ascites.

    o C-B (Cruveilhier – Baumgarten) murmur.

    o The development of spontaneous portosystemic shunt as a result of portal hypertension helps to partially bypass the liver blood flow blocked by the cirrhotic nodules; the result is an abdominal bruit, ↓ PHT, and ↓ ascites.

"The real voyage of discovery consists not in seeking new lands but seeing with new eyes."

Marcel Proust

240

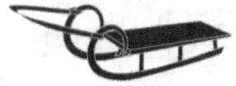

## ACUTE LIVER FAILURE (ALF)

➢ Definitions

  o A sudden (usually < 24 weeks length of illness) loss of hepatic function in a patient without preexisting liver disease, with the development of coagulopathy) INR > 1.5) and hepatic encephalopathy (Ritt DJ, et al. *Medicine (Baltimore)* 1969:151-72.)

  o ALT is defined as "….the rapid development of hepatocellular dysfunction, specifically coagulopathy and mental status changes (encephalopathy) [and often jaundice] in a patient without prior liver disease".

  o Coagulopathy (INR ≥ 1.5) and encephalopathy in patient without previous cirrhosis and with an illness of < 26 weeks duration

  o ALF is "….a clinical syndrome that represents the final common pathway of severe liver injury resulting from numerous infections, immunologic, metabolic, vascular and infiltrative disorders", leading to severe cellular or mitochondrial dysfunction and hepatocellular necrosis".

  o "Hepatic encephalopathy is a defining criteria" for ALF. (Feldman M., et al. Sleisenger and Fordtran's Gastrointestinal and Liver Disease. 9th Edition. *Saunders/Elsevier* 2010, page 1557).

  o The time interval between the onset of illness and the development of ALF is < 8 weeks, although some authors suggest a range of different time intervals:
    – Hyperacute     ≤ 1 week
    – Acute          1 to 4 weeks
    – Subacute       4 to 24 weeks

Note: since these subgroups have no prognostic significance, the use of these terms is no longer wide-spread

➢ Demography

  o < 1 / $10^5$ per year

  o 1-year survival ~ 65%

➢ Types

  o ALF (acute liver failure) syndrome
    – HE (hepatic encephalopathy)
    – Coagulation abnormalities
    – Jaundice
    – No prior liver disease
    – ↑ inflammatory cytokines
    – ↓ immunity
    – ↓ metabolism of albumin-bound toxins

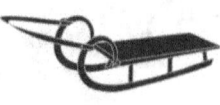

241

- o Acute on chronic liver failure (AoCLF)
  - – ↑ NO (nitric oxide)
  - – ↑ vasodilation
  - – ↓ cardiac output

- Give the pathogenesis of major **complications** of acute liver failure.

| Complication | Pathogenesis |
|---|---|
| o Hypoglycemia | – ↓ hepatic glucose synthesis |
| o Encephalopathy | – Cerebral edema |
| o Infections | – Reduced immune function<br>– Invasive procedures |
| o Gastrointestinal hemorrhage | – Stress ulceration<br>– Esophageal varices (PHT) |
| o Coagulopathy | – ↓ clotting factor synthesis<br>– Thrombocytopenia<br>– Fibrinolysis |
| o Hypotension | – Hypovolemia<br>– Decreased vascular resistance |
| o Respiratory failure | – ARDS (DAD) |
| o Pancreatitis | – Unknown |
| o Renal failure | – Hypovolemia<br>– Hepatorenal syndrome<br>– Acute tubular necrosis<br>– NSAID damage |

Abbreviations: ARDS, Acute respiratory distress syndrome; CT, computed tomography; DAD, diffuse alveolar damage; ICP, intracranial pressure; NSAIDs, nonsteroidal anti-inflammatory drugs; PHT, portal hypertension.

Adapted form: *Sleisenger and Fordtran's Gastrointestinal and Liver Disease: Pathophysiology/ Diagnosis/ Management.* Ninth edition, 2010, Table 93-4: pg. 1561.

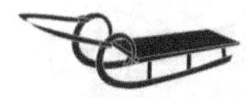

> Causes/associations

- The causes of ALF in America are as follows:
  - Acetaminophen overdose, 46%
  - Indeterminate, 14%
  - Drug-related (other than acetaminophen), 11%
  - HBV, 7%
  - Other causes, 7%
  - Autoimmune, 5%
  - Ischemic, 4%
  - HDV, 3%
  - Wilson disease, 2%

- The commonest causes of ALF worldwide are:
  - Acetaminophen overdose
  - HBV
  - HAV
  - DILI (drug-induced liver injury) from drugs other than acetaminophen.

- Other less common drugs and toxins causing ALF are isoniazid, propylthiouracil, phenytoin, valproic acid

- Don't forget the mushroom! – Amanita phalloides poisoning

- The spontaneous recovery rate is 58-64% for acetaminophen, ischemia and HDV, and 20-25% for all other causes of ALF (Lee WM, et al. *Hepatology* 2008;47:1401-15.)

- Give a classification of the causes of acute hepatic failure (ALF), and give examples.

  - Viral infections
    - Hepatitis A-E
    - With the extent of international travel, it remains mindful for us to recall the countries where HEV is endemic, and therefore should be suspected as cause of ALF, especially in a pregnant woman.
    - Cytomegalovirus (CMV)
    - Epstein-Barr virus (EBV)
    - Herpes simplex (HSV)
    - Parvovirus B19
    - Adenovirus
    - Viral hemorrhagic fever
    - Rarely Herpes zoster, Human herpes virus-6, West Nile virus, coxsackie B virus

243

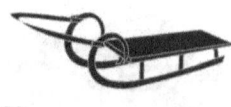

- o Drugs (Iatrogenic)
    - – Acetaminophen, isoniazid, NSAIDs, sulfonamides
    - – Tetracycline, rifampin, valproic acid, phenytoin, halothane
    - – Telithromycin, orlistat, amiodarone
- o Immune reconstitution
    - – In HBV use and then withdrawal of steroids, chemotherapy or anti-TNF drugs (immune suppression, followed by immune reconstitution with withdrawal of these drugs).
- o Primary graft non-function post-liver transplantation
- o Post-liver transplantation
    - – Primary graft non-function
- o The cause of ALF is not always identified
- o Inherited
    - – Wilson disease
    - – Alpha-1 antitrypsin deficiency
    - – Galactosemia
    - – Tyrosinemia, Reye's syndrome, hereditary fructose intolerance
    - – Neonatal iron storage disease
    - – Lecithin-cholesterol acyltransferase deficiency
- o Ischemic
    - – Left heart failure
    - – Shock (cardiogenic/non-cardiogenic)
    - – Venocclusive disease (SOS, sinusoidal obstruction syndrome)
    - – Budd-Chiari syndrome (BCS)
    - – Heat stroke (Inadvertent occlusion if portal vein at surgery)
- o Infiltration
- o Leukemia, lymphoma, metastatic carcinoma
- o Pregnancy
    - – Eclampsia
    - – Preeclampsia
    - – HELLP
    - – AFLP (acute fatty liver of pregnancy)
    - – HEV
- o Massive hepatomegaly

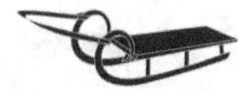

- o History of cancer
  - – Breast
  - – Lung (small cell)
    - ▪ Lymphoma
    - ▪ Melanoma
    - ▪ Myeloma
  - o Syncythial giant cell hepatitis

Adapted from: Khashab M, et al. *Curr Gastroenterol Rep* 2007;9(1):66-73.

- • Give the cause of ALF in which there is a marked increase in both ALT and LDH.
  - o Acute ischemic injury of the liver

- ➢ Laboratory
  - o Blood work
    - – AFP
    - – ALT, AST, AP, GGT
    - – Albumin, INR, bilirubin
    - – 1° /2° electrolytes
    - – Type and screen
    - – Factor V, lactate
    - – Serum copper, ceruloplasmin, 24 hour urine copper
    - – Ferritin, iron, % saturation
    - – Alcohol, drug screen
    - – Autoimmune markers
  - o Serologies
    - – HIV
    - – HAV – IgM
    - – HBV - HBsAg, HBsAb, IgM anticore
    - – HDV (if HBV positive), HEV (if pregnant)
    - – HCV
    - – CMV/HSV/EBV/Toxoplasmosis titers
  - o Cultures/Microbiology
    - – Blood, urine, and peritoneal fluid
    - – PPD and Candida

245

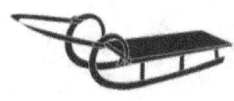

- Give laboratory measures which suggest a poor prognosis in ALF (acute liver failure), including ALF from EHS (exertional heat stroke).

  o AFP < 3.9 ng/mL on the day after the value of ALT reaches a peak.

  o Normal phosphate (yes, a normal phosphate is a sign of poor prognosis in ALF, since the liver is not taking up ↑ $PO_4^-$ to help the liver regenerate).

  o ↓ factor V

---

Trivia

- Give the standard laboratory changes in ALF from acetaminophen which helps to distinguish it from the other common causes of ALF.

  o ALF from acetaminophen has ALT > 2000 , ↑ INR but normal or non-normal serum bilirubin concentration.

- Give the cause of ALF in which there are the following changes in liver enzymes.

  o ↑ ALT, ↑↑ LDH, ALT/LDH < 4

  o EHS (exertional heat stroke)

---

➤ Clinical

Major complications of ALF include HE, coagulopathy, jaundice, GI bleeding, and hypoglycemia.

- Give other major complications of ALF.

  | | | |
  |---|---|---|
  | o Bacterial and fungal infections | – | Bacterial infections in 80% of ALF patients (Staphylococcus and gram-negative aerobes) |
  | | – | Bacteremia in 25% |
  | | – | Fungal infections (Candida albicans, Aspergillus) in ~30% |
  | o MOFS (multiple Organ Failure Syndrome) | – | Hypotension (↓ MAP [mean arterial pressure] from peripheral vasodilation) |
  | | – | Pulmonary edema |
  | | – | Renal failure |
  | o DIC (disseminated intravascular coagulopathy) | | |

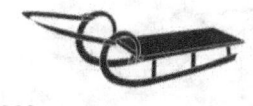

- o Acute pancreatitis
  - – Seen in 44% of patients dying from ALF, especially from acetaminophen overdose
- o Acute respiratory failure
  - – Pulmonary edema
  - – ARDS (acute respiratory distress syndrome); DAD, diffuse alveolar damage)
- o Acute renal failure
  - – Acute renal failure in 50% of ALF, from HRS (hepatorenal syndrome) and ATN (acute tubular necrosis)
  - – Intermittent hemodialysis, continuous hemofiltration, hemoadsorption, MARS (albumin dialysis using the molecular adsorbent recirculating system)

➢ Diagnostic Imaging
- o Liver US with Doppler
- o Chest x-ray
- o CT head
  - – CT of the head in ALF is neither sensitive nor specific to detect early intracerebral hypertension, but can identify the advanced stages of intracerebral hypertension and brainstem herniation (Larsen FS, Wendon J. *Liver Transpl* 2008;14:S90-6.)
- o Cardiopulmonary evaluation
  - – ECG
  - – 2-D surface echo with Doppler
  - – Pulmonary function tests
- o Cancer Surveillance
  - – Pelvic, prostate, breast, colon and HCC, as indicated

Adapted from: Gill RQ, and Sterling RK. *J Clin Gastroenterol* 2001;33:191-8.

➢ Differential
- o The diagnosis of ALF is based on clinical findings, and must be differentiated from conditions with similar clinical findings:

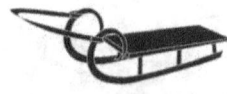

- Give the important hepatic and non-hepatic conditions which may **mimic** the clinical presentation of ALF.
    o Acute decompensation of chronic liver disease
    o Acute HBV
    o Acute flares of chronic HCV
    o Alcoholic hepatitis
    o Sepsis (low factor VIII in sepsis; normal factor VIII in ALF)
    o SLE (systemic lupus erythematosus)
    o TTP (thrombotic thrombocytopenic purpura)

---

**SO YOU WANT TO BE A HEPATOLOGIST!**

The AASLD Position Paper on ALF defines ALF as coagulopathy and encephalopathy

"……. In a patient without pre-existing cirrhosis and with an illness of < 26 weeks duration".

- Give the hepatic conditions in which often unrecognized pre-existing cirrhosis may be present.
    o HBV, vertically-acquired
    o WD (Wilson disease)
    o AIH (autoimmune hepatitis)

---

- Give the **performance characteristics** of scoring systems for ALF.

| System | Sensitivity | Specificity | PPV | NPV |
|---|---|---|---|---|
| KCC ≥ 1 | 26 – 47% | 83 – 92% | 0.63 – 0.70 | 0.65 – 0.69 |
| Apache II | | | | |
| ≥ 12 | 67% | 76% | 0.69 | 0.75 |
| ≥ 20 | 68% | 87% | 0.77 | 0.81 |
| MELD ≥ 35 | 61% | 71% | 0.54 | 0.76 |
| SOFA ≥ 12 | 67% | 80% | 0.74 | 0.74 |

Abbreviations: APACHE, acute physiology and chronic health evaluation; KCC, Kings College Criteria; MELD, Model for End-Stage Liver Disease; NPV, negative predictive value; PPV, positive predictive value; SOFA, sequential organ failure assessment

Adapted from: Feldman M., et al. Sleisenger and Fordtran's Gastrointestinal and Liver Disease. 9th Edition. *Saunders/Elsevier* 2010, Table 93.6, page 1564.

248

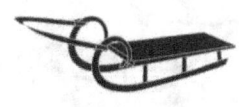

- ➤ Treatment
  - o Treatment of
    - – Liver-related and -nonrelated complication
      - ▪ Assess for possible adrenal insufficiency (present in ~ 2/3 of ALF patients) with a cosyntropic stimulation test, or empirically treat with IV steroids
    - – Prepare for possible liver transplantation
      - ▪ Assess for possible liver transplantation (LT), using MELD or modified MELD scores.
      - ▪ List for LT if no contraindications
        - – Medical/Surgical Candidacy
        - – Transplant hepatology evaluation
        - – Transplant surgery evaluation
        - – Transplant social work/psychosocial/nutritional evaluation
        - – Dental examination
        - – Risk stratification (MELD or modified MELD)

- • Give specific treatments for the causes of ALF.
  - o Acetaminophen-n-acetylcysteine (NAC)
  - o AFLP (acute fatty liver of pregnancy), pre-eclampsia
    - – Delivery of fetus
  - o Amanita phalloides poisoning
    - – NAC IV/po
    - – Penicillin G IV
    - – Silibinin IV
  - o Herpes
    - – Acyclovir
  - o Autoimmune hepatitis
    - – Steroids
  - o HBV
    - – Nucleoside or nucleotide analogues
  - o DILI plus DRESS syndrome
    - – Glucocorticosteroids, NAC

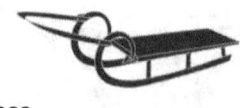

➢ Prognosis

• Give the **King's College Criteria** (KCC) risk stratification criteria for liver transplantation in ALF.

    ○ Acetaminophen

        – INR > 6.5 (PT > 100 sec), serum creatinine > 3.4 mg/dl, stage 3 or 4 encephalopathy

        – Arterial lactate > 3.5 at 4 hours after resuscitation

        – pH < 7.30 or arterial lactate > 3.0 at 12 hours after resuscitation

    ○ Non-acetaminophen

        – INR > 6.5 (PT > 100 sec); or

        – Any 3 of the following:

            ▪ INR > 3.5 (PT > 50 sec)

            ▪ Age < 10 or > 40 years

            ▪ Bilirubin > 17.5 mg/dl

        – Duration of jaundice > 7 days

        – Etiology: drug reaction

Printed with permission: Fontana RJ, and Chung RT. *AGA Institute 2007 Spring Postgraduate Course Syllabus*: 636.

"Motivation is what gets you started,

Habit is what keeps you going."

Jim Rohn

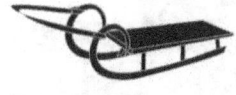

## PORTAL HYPERTENSION (PHT)

- ➢ Definition
  - o Hepatic sinusoidal pressure ≥ 6 mmHg

- ➢ Pathophysiology
  - o After a meal, portal blood flow increases, with no ↑ portal pressure, because the hepatic sinusoids have
    - – High
      - ▪ Compliance
      - ▪ Accommodation
    - – Low
      - ▪ Resistance
  - o Blood supply to the liver is
    - – 70% portal vein (PV, blood from mesenteric circulation)
    - – 30% hepatic artery (HA, from celiac artery)
  - o With the dual blood supply (portal venous inflow) to the liver, when blood flow increases in the PV, it decreases in the AA, and vice versa, through an autoregulatory mechanism
    - – Recall that we are dealing with three distinct vascular beds
      - ▪ Intrahepatic
      - ▪ Splanchnic
      - ▪ Systemic

- • Give components of each of the vasodilating and vasoconstricting systems involved in the disturbed hemodynamics in cirrhosis.

- ❖ Vasodilator systems
  - o Adenosine
  - o Adrenomedullin
  - o Arterial natriuretic peptide (ANP)
  - o Bradykinin
  - o Brain natriuretic peptide (BNP)
  - o Calcitonin gene-related peptide (CGRP)
  - o Carbon monoxide (CO)
  - o Endocannabinoids
  - o Endothelin-3 (ET-3)
  - o Endotoxin
  - o Enkephalins
  - o Glucagon
  - o Histamine
  - o Hydrogen sulphide
  - o Interleukins
  - o Natriuretic peptide of type C (CNP)
  - o Nitric oxide (NO)
  - o Prostacyclin (PGI$_2$)
  - o Substance P
  - o Tumour necrosis factor-α (TNF-α)
  - o Vasoactive intestinal polypeptide (VIP)

251

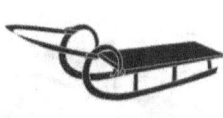

❖ Vasoconstrictor systems

   ○ Adrenaline and noradrenaline

   ○ Angiotensin II

   ○ Endothelin-1 (ET-1)

   ○ Neuropeptide Y

   ○ Renin-angiotensin-aldosterone system (RAAS)/

   ○ Sympathetic nervous system (SNS)

   ○ Vasopressin (ADH)

Printed with permission: Møller S, and Henriksen JH. *GUT* 2008; 58: pg. 271.


- Give the **pathophysiological components** producing the hyperdynamic circulation and cardiovascular dysfunction in persons with cirrhosis.

  ❖ The overall effect is

    ○ ↓ intrahepatic NO and ↓ intrahepatic vasodilation (effect on endothelial cells as well as possibly on HSCs) → ↑ intrahepatic vasoconstriction → ↑↑ intrahepatic resistance (law of Poiseuille)

  ❖ ↑ Portal flow and resistance

    ○ ↑ portal flow

    ○ ↑ resistance

      – Mechanical factors

      – Regenerative nodules

      – Fibrotic bands

      – Defenestration and capillarization of sinusoids

      – Swelling of hepatocytes and Kupffer cells

      – Vascular factors

    ○ ↑ collaterals (↑ angiogenesis)

    ○ ↓ fenestration

    ○ Ohm law

$$\Delta P = F \times R$$

F, flow
$\Delta P$, change in pressure
R, resistance

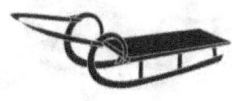

- ❖ Hepatic vasoconstriction and ↑↑ increased intrahepatic resistance
  - ○ ↑ sheer stress on sinusoids
    - – ↑ eNOS → NO (nitric oxide) → intrahepatic vasodilation
    - – ↑ ET-1 (endothelin-1) → binds to
      - ▪ ET-A receptors on HSC → ↑ HSC contraction → intrahepatic vasoconstriction
      - ▪ Also binds to ET-B receptors on endothelial cells → activates eNOS → vasodilation
    - – In cirrhosis, there may be ↑ NO production
    - – In splanchnic endothelial cells from ↑ sheer stress → ↑ cytokines, and ↑ phosphorylation of eNOS → vasodilation in splanchnic and systemic vascular beds (note below that in cirrhosis there is ↓ intrahepatic NO, ↓ intrahepatic vasodilation, ↑ intrahepatic vasoconstriction)
  - ○ In cirrhosis
    - – ↓ activation of eNOS protein in endothelial cells → ↓ production of NO
    - – ↑ caveolin-1 (an eNOS inhibiting protein)
    - – ↓ AKT (protein kinase B)
    - – Phosphorylation of eNOS
    - – ↑ GRK (G protein-coupled receptor kinase, which inhibits eNOS)
    - – ↑ VEGF (vascular endothelial growth factor) from shear stress may ↑ eNOS (VEGF is a NO stimulatory growth factor)
    - – ↑ intestinal endotoxin (LPS) → ↑ TGF-β, ↑ ET-1, with binding to ET-A receptors on HSC → intrahepatic vasoconstriction
  - ○ Law of poiseuille $R = 8\,\eta L / \P r^4$
  - ○ Resistance (R) is affected by the length and radius (r) of the vessel, and by the viscosity of the blood; in cirrhosis, the radius becomes less as a result of the vasoconstriction; because the effect of radius (r) on resistance (R) is to the fourth power ($r^4$), a small fall in r causes a large ↑ R.
  - ○ Give NO in cirrhosis will restore the intrahepatic vasodilation arising from the endothelial cells, but the HSC in cirrhosis contribute to the vasoconstriction and are less responsive to NO. Replacement in cirrhosis, so benefit of restoring ↓ NO levels does not fully restore the vessel diameter to normal

- ❖ Peripheral and splanchnic arterial vasodilatation
  - ○ Baroreceptor-induced increase in heart rate
  - ○ The vasodilation in splanchnic and systemic (peripheral) vascular beds leads to

253

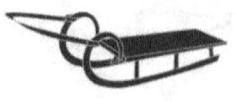

- ↑ cardiac output (hyperdynamic circulation)
- ↓ mean arterial pressure
- ↑ systemic blood flowing into splanchnic circulation

❖ Autonomic dysfunction

  o ↑ sympathetic nervous system (SNS) activity → ↑ intrahepatic vasoconstriction from
  - Norepinephrine
  - Angiotension
  - Leukotrienes
  - Thromboxane

  o Vagal impairment

❖ Alterations in cardiac preload

  o ↑ portosystemic shunting

  o ↑ blood volume

  o Effects of posture

  o ↓ blood viscosity

❖ Alterations in oxygen exchange

  o Anemia

  o Hypoxemia

  o Hepatopulmonary syndrome

  o Portopulmonary hypertension

❖ Collateral Circulation

  o As the portal pressure increases
  - There is ↑ flow of blood into the portal vein-systemic collateral circulation
  - The direction of blood flow reverses, and blood flows abnormally from the portal circulation into the venous component of the systemic system.

Abbreviations: HSC, hepatic stellate cell; LPS, lipopolysaccharide; eNOS, endothelial NO synthase


- In the setting of the portal hypertension (PHT) and hepatic cirrhosis, give the meaning of "**hepatofugal**" **blood flow**.

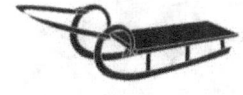

- In PHT, when the HVPG (hepatic venous portal gradient) > 12 mmHg, blood flows backwards up into the esophageal vein, and from there into portal vein.
  - This backward flow is known as "hepatofugal blood flow"
- Give sites of communication of the portal to thesystemic circulation which develop in portal hypertension, and name the involved/connected blood vessels in this abnormal flow.

| Site | Vessel(s) |
|---|---|
| o Rectum | Inferior mesenteric vein → pudendal vein |
| o Umbilicus | Umbilical vein → left portal vein |
| o Retroperitoneum (in women) | Ovarian vessels → iliac veins |
| o Gastroespohageal area | Hepatic venous pressure gradient<br>- > 10 mmHg for collaterals to develop<br>- > 12 mmHg for esophageal varices to bleed<br>- > 16 mmHg for gastric varices to bleed<br><br>Most common site of bleeding, palisade zone, do not drain to periesophageal veins, and from there to the azygous system |

Printed with permission: Møller S, and Henriksen JH. *Gut* 2008; 58:271.

- Give the anatomical site of increased resistance when liver disease is associated with ↑ portal pressure (PP) and HVPG is normal.

  - There will be ↑ PP but normal HVG when the site of ↑ resistance is presinusoidal.

➢ Causes/associations

- Give the causes of portal hypertension based on the site of **increased resistance**.
  - o Prehepatic
  - o Intrahepatic
    - Presinusoidal
    - Sinusoidal
    - Post-sinusoidal
  - o Posthepatic

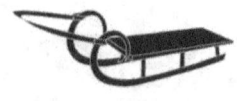

- Give causes of liver disease in which there may be **portal hypertension without cirrhosis**, due to a presinusoidal component of the intrahepatic disease (non-cirrhotic portal hypertension).
  - ALD (alcoholic liver disease: presinusoidal perivenular lesions)
  - AIH (autoimmune hepatitis)
  - PBC (Primary Biliary Cholangitis)
  - ADPKD (autosomal dominant polycystic kidney disease)
  - HH (hereditary hemochromatosis)
  - Schistosomiasis (S. mansoni, S. japonicum)
    - Presinusoidal granulomas
    - Inflammation
    - Periportal fibrosis
  - Sarcoidosis (early disease; later the site of ↑ intrahepatic resistance is postsinusoidal)
  - 1° or 2° liver malignancy

**Hypertensive Gastropathy** (PHG)

➢ Endoscopy

- Give the mucosal changes in the stomach associated with portal hypertensive gastropathy*.
  - Mosaic- like mucosal pattern
    - Small, polygonal areas surrounded by a whitish- yellow depressed border (snake skin appearance) can be categorized as mild (pink mucosa), and moderate (diffuse red mucosa)
  - Red point lesions
    - Small (<1 mm), red, flat, point like marks
  - Cherry red spots
    - Large (> 2 mm), round, red coloured, protruding lesions
  - Black-brown spots
  - Irregularly shaped black and brown flat spots that do not fade upon washing (these changes might represent intramucosal hemorrhage)

  * These changes are characterized endoscopically by the presence of four main findings, as described by the New Italian Endoscopic Club (NIEC).

  Printed with permission: Perini et al. *Nature Clinical Practice Gastroenterology and Hepatology* 2009; 6(3):150-8.

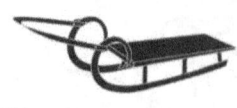

- Compare and contrast portal hypertensive gastropathy (PHG) and gastric antral vascular ectasia (GAVE).

|  | PHG | GAVE |
|---|---|---|
| o Distribution | Proximal stomach | Distal stomach |
| o Mosaic pattern | Present | Absent |
| o Red signs | Present | Present |
| o Biopsy | | |
|   – Thrombi | - | +++ |
|   – Spindle cell proliferation | + | ++ |
|   – Fibrohyalinosis | + | +++ |
| ➢ Treatment | Beta-blockers<br>TIPS | Argon laser<br>Banding<br>Cryotherapy<br>Antrectomy |

Printed with permission: Garcia-Tsao G., and Kamath PS. *2007 AGA Institute Postgraduate Course*: pg. 619.


**Tranjugular Intrahepatic Portosystemic Shunt** (TIPS)

➢ No benefit

   o GAVE

   o No change in overall survival

➢ Proven benefit of TIPS

   o Primary prophylaxis of bleeding from EV or GV  - No

     – Prevent rebleeding from

       ▪ EV, GV, ECTV - Yes

       ▪ PHG failing BB - Yes

       ▪ GAVE - No

     – Refractory cirrhotic ascites, intolerant to LVP

     – Hepatic hydrothorax, resistant to ↓ $Na^+$ & diuretics

     – Budd-Chiari syndrome, moderate disease, failed anti-coagulation

     – HRS

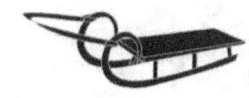

➤ Loss of patency

o In about 10% of TIPS, thrombosis occurs within 24 hrs, and the prophylactic use if anticoagulation is not established.

o Over the longterm, dysfunction of the shunt will occur in ~ half because of pseudointimal hyperplasia in the parenchymal tract or outflow hepatic vein, associated with development of a coating of collagenous matrix covered by endothelial cells.

o Doppler ultrasound may be used to establish the potency of the TIPS.

o There are numerous signs reported on Doppler ultrasound which have been used to predict the presence of dysfunction of the shunt, but these signs have a low sensitivity rate (10% - 2.6%) and an acceptable specificity (88% - 100%).

o Patency of TIPS is best demonstrated with re-catheterization of the TIPS.

Abbreviations: BB, beta blocker; ECTV, ectopic varices; EV, esophageal varices; GAVE , gastric antral vascular hyperplasia; GV, gastric varices; HRS, heptorenal syndrome; LVP, large volume paracentesis; PHG, portal hypertensive gastropathy

- Give **relative contraindications** to TIPS.

o Liver failure
   – Hepatic encephalopathy
   – Jaundice (serum bilirubin > 5 mg/dL)
   – Coagulopathy (INR > 2)

o Progressive renal failure

o Associated acute infection

o Severe cardiopulmonary disease

o MELD > 18

o R-HF

```
Clinical Caution

TIPS make HE worse.
```

Abbreviations: HE, hepatic encephalopathy; R-HF, right heart failure; TIPS, transjugular intrahepatic portosystemic shunts

- Give **complications** of the TIPS (transjugular intrahepatic portosystemic shunt) procedure.
  - Technical complications
    - Neck puncture
    - Indequate access to hepatic vein
    - Creation of parenchymal tract to portal vein
    - May make later liver transplantation technically more difficult
  - Vessels
    - Puncture of pulmonary artery (PA), pulmonary vein (PV), liver capsule
    - Ischemia (hepatic artery thrombosis)
  - Stent
    - Inadequate deployment of stent across parenchymal tract
    - Stent-related complications – thrombosis, stenosis
    - Stent migration into portal vein or inferior vena cava ( IVC)
  - Liver
    - Hepatic encephalopathy (HE) (new, or worse, or chronic)
    - Intraperitoneal bleeding
    - Hepatic infarction
    - Hepatic rupture
    - Fulminant hepatic failure (acute liver failure [ALF])
  - CPS
    - Pulmonary hypertension and right heart failure
  - Unique
    - Unique complications of TIPS – hemolytic anemia, infectious endotipsitis
  - Systemic
    - Sepsis
    - Multiple organ failure syndrome
    - Long-term presence of foreign body

Abbreviation: CPS, cardiopulmonary systems

Adapted from: Sanyal AJ. *2006 AGA Institute Postgraduate Course:* pg. 195.

260

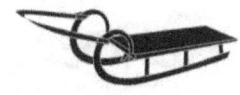

> Practical Tips for Liver Biopsy (LBx)

| Peri-LBx Management | Days to Stop Before LBx | Days to Restart After LBx |
|---|---|---|
| o Drugs | | |
| – Antiplatelet drugs | 10 | 2-3 |
| – Anti-coagulants | 5 | 1 |
| – Heparin | 1 | |
| o Restrictions | | |
| – Food | No | |
| – Exercise | No | |
| – Sedation | No | |
| – Heavy lifting | Probably a good idea | |
| o Post-biopsy | | |
| – Monitoring of vital signs | Yes | |
| – Observation time | 4 hr | |

- o Hemostasis
  - – "the time to spontaneous cessation of surface bleeding (from the liver after biopsy with a 1.8 mm diameter Menghini needle) …… did not correlate with abnormalities in the PT, platelet count, or whole-blood clot time".
  - – In patients with hemophilia, correct bleeding diathesis before LBx
  - – Inpatients on hemodialysis or with chronic renal failure
    - ▪ DDAVP (desmopressin) 0.3 mg/kg BW may be given pre-LBx
    - ▪ Patients on chronic hemodialysis should be dialyzed before LBx.

"Goals in writing are dreams with deadlines."

Brian Tracy

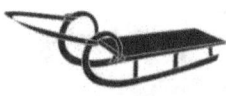

# CIRRHOSIS

➢ Pathophysiology

- Give pathophysiological factors responsible for the development of hepatic fibrosis and cirrhosis.
  - o Extracellular matrix proteins (EMP)
  - o Hepatic stellate cells (HSC)
  - o Activation of HSC to form myofibroblasts
  - o Other mesenchymal cell populations and bone marrow-derived cells
  - o Hepatocyte growth factor (HGF)
  - o TGF-β
  - o Renin-angiotensin system (RAS)
  - o Angiotensin-converting enzyme (ACE)
  - o Angiotensin I and II receptors
  - o Endotoxin, lipopolysaccharide (LPS)
  - o Toll-like receptor (TLR4)
  - o Angiogenesis
    - – Vascular endothelial growth factor (VEGF)
    - – Angioporetin 1, 2

Adapted from: Jiao J, et al. *Curr Opin Gastroenterol* 2009;25(3):223-9.

➢ Causes/associations
  - o Viral hepatitis
    - – HBV, HCV, HDV
  - o Metabolic
    - – Non-alcoholic steatohepatitis (NASH)
    - – Hemochromatosis (HH)
    - – Wilson disease (WD)
    - – 1-antitrypsin deficiency (α1 ATD)
    - – Galactosemia
    - – Tyrosinemia
    - – Sclerosing cholangitis (SC)
    - – Primary biliary cholangitis (PBC)
    - – Autoimmune hepatitis (AIH)
  - o Drugs/toxins
    - – Alcohol

262

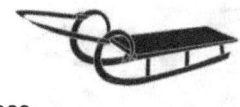

- o Congestive
    - – Cardiac failure
    - – Budd-Chiari syndrome (BCS)
- o Cystic fibrosis (CF)

➢ Diagnostic imaging

- Give hepatic and extrahepatic signs of cirrhosis on CT and/or MRI.

    - o Hepatic
        - – Nodularity
        - – ↑ periportal space
        - – Posterior notch
        - – ↑ caudate and lateral segment
        - – ↑ candate-to-right lobe size
        - – Enlarged gallbladder
    - o Extrahepatic
        - – Splenomegaly
        - – Varices
        - – Ascites

Adapted from: Ito K, et al. *Magn Reson Imaging Clin N Am* 2002;10(1):75-92, vi.

- Give examples of **endocrine complications** affecting patients with PBC-, alcohol – , or hemochromatosis – associated cirrhotic disease.
    - o Alcoholic cirrhosis
        - – Gonadal insufficiency
        - – Hypothalamic dysfunction
        - – Gynecomastia
    - o Hemochromatosis
        - – Gonadal insufficiency
        - – Hypothalamic dysfunction
        - – Diabetes mellitus
    - o Primary biliary cholangitis
        - – Autoimmune thyroid disease
        - – Metabolic bone disease

Adapted from: Sleisenger and Fordtran's Gastrointestinal and Liver Disease. 10th Edition. Saunders/Elsevier, Philadelphia, 2016, page 1588-1589.

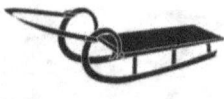

- Give examples of the effect of cirrhosis on the assessment of endocrine function.
  - o Hypothyroidism
    - – ↓ T3
    - – N/↑ thyroxine binding globulin (TGB) level
    - – ↑ ALT/AST (also seen with hyperthyroidism)
  - o Diabetes mellitus (or insulin resistance)
    - – Elevated fasting blood glucose level
  - o Feminization and hypogonadism
    - – ↑ estrogen level
    - – ↑ sex hormone-binding globulin level
    - – ↓ total and free testosterone levels
    - – Loss of diurnal variation
    - – Hypothalamic dysfunction
    - – Testicular atrophy

Adapted from: Fitz JG. *Sleisenger & Fordtran's Gastrointestinal and Liver Disease: Pathophysiology/Diagnosis/Management* 2006; pg. 1982.

➤ Preventive care

- Give factors to consider in the **preventive care** of the patient with cirrhosis.
  - o Esophageal varices
    - – Prevention of first variceal hemorrhage: EGD q3 years, with banding or beta blockers (primary prophylaxis)
    - – Prevention of recurrent variceal hemorrhage (secondary prophylaxis)
      - ▪ Beta-blockers, non-specific (NSBB)
      - ▪ Banding
      - ▪ Sclerotherapy
      - ▪ Shunts (TIPS)
  - o Spontaneous bacterial peritonitis
    - – Prevention of bacterial infections after GI bleeding (antibiotic prophylaxis
    - – Prevention of SBP (antibiotics for previous SBP)
  - o Hepatic encephalopathy
    - – Assess for minimal (subclinical) HE (grade 0), and treat appropriately; testing for driving competence

264

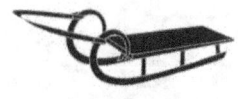

- o Diet
  - – Nutrition assessment and treatment
  - – Normal protein intake
  - – 2 g salt diet if indicated
- o Drugs
  - – Avoid
    - ▪ Alcohol
    - ▪ Viagra ®
    - ▪ Vasodilators
    - ▪ NSAIDs
    - ▪ Opioids
    - ▪ Hepatotoxic herbs
    - ▪ Benzodiazepines
    - ▪ ACE inhibitors
- o Vaccination
  - – Influenza, Pneumococcus, HAV, HBV
- o Screening
  - – CEA, DM, HBP, HCC, osteoporosis, diabetes, hypertension; usual screening for breast, prostate, cervix, colon
  - – Medialert bracelet
- o Regular follow up and evaluation for possible liver transplantation
- o Education, family counselling

➢ Treatment

- Give the mechanism(s) of action of drugs used to treat portal hypertension (PHT).

Drugs used for treatment of PHT generally are selected to act to
  - – ↓ portal blood flow, or
  - – ↓ intrahepatic resistance

- ↓ Portal Blood Flow → ↓ PP (Portal Pressure)
  - o Octreotide
    - – ↓ glucagon
      - ▪ ↑ splanchnic vasoconstriction
      - ▪ ↓ portal and azygous blood flow
      - ▪ ↓ postprandial splanchnic blood blow
    - – ↓ GT-1-dependent contraction of HSC (hepatic stellate cells)

265

- o β-adrenergic blocking agents (non-selective)
  - – ↓ cardiac output (CO)
  - – Vasodilation of mesenteric circulation
  - – ↑ "unopposed action of α1-adrenergic receptors →
    - ▪ ↓ portal flow
    - ▪ ↓ intrahepatic resistance
- o Vasopressin
  - – Splanchnic vasoconstriction
  - – ↓ PV (portal vein) inflow
  - – ↓ CO (inotropic)
  - – ↓ HR (chronotropic)
- ↓ Intrahepatic Resistance
  - o Nitrates
    - – Venodilation from ↓ $Ca_i^{2+}$ in smooth muscle in venous wall
  - o Under study
    - – α1-adrenergic antagonists
    - – ARBs (angiotensin II receptor type I blockers)

## Coagulopathy

- Give factors which contribute to the **coagulation disorders** in cirrhosis.
  - o ↓ synthesis of procoagulant factors
    - – Vitamin K-dependent factors II, VII, IX, X
    - – Factor V
    - – Factor XI
  - o Thrombocytopenia in cirrhosis
    - – Hypersplenism
    - – ↓ hepatic synthesis of thrombopoietin
    - – Bone marrow toxicity
      - ▪ HCV
      - ▪ Alcohol
    - – ↓ thrombin produced by platelets
  - o Dysfibrogenemia
    - – Altered production of activators/inhibitors of fibrolysis
    - – Endotoximemia-associated activation of coagulation cascade
    - – ↓ clearance of fibrinolytic proteins
    - – ↑ D-dimer
    - – ↑ fibrinogen degradation products
    - – ↑ clot lysis time

266

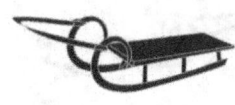

A Practice Curiosity

In cirrhosis, the increase in INR predicts a bad prognosis, but the risk of spontaneous bleeding is not increased by ↑ INR (of course ↑ INR is associated with serious bleeding, if and when bleeding occurs from a pathological cause, such as bleeding esophageal varices.

So what is the curiosity? The evidence is not strong that the severity of bleeding esophageal varices is reduced by giving

- o Vitamin K

- o FFP (fresh frozen plasma)

- o rVIIa (recombinant factor VIIa)

- o Platelets

- o Desmopressin

So, why do we sometimes do this in common everyday practice?

- – Well, because it "makes sense", or "it's the local standard of care", or "if I don't, the lawyers will eat me alive"!

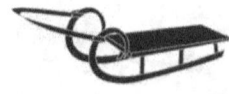

## Idiopathic Portal Hypertension (IPH) and Hepatoportal Sclerosis (HPS)

- o   IPH and HPS are associated with ↑PP (portal pressure) and no obstruction of the extrahepatic portion of the PV (portal vein).

- •   Give the distinctive hepatic histopathological feature of IPH versus HPS seen on liver biopsy.
  - o   IPH
    - –   Normal
  - o   HPS
    - –   Intrahepatic portal veins show
      - ▪   Subendothelial thickening
      - ▪   Thrombosis
      - ▪   Recanalization

## Hereditary Hemorrhagic Telangiectasia (HHT) / Osler-Weber-Rendu Disease (OWRD)

- o   HHT/OWRD may be associated with portal hypertension and bleeding esophageal varices.

- ➢   Clinical

- •   Give the diagnostic criteria for HHT/OWRD.

The diagnostic criteria for HHT/OWRD include

- o   Epistaxis
- o   Telangiectasias        ⎫
- o   AV fistulas (lung, liver)   ⎬   diagnostic criteria
- o   Positive family history   ⎭
- o   Intrahepatic shunts
  - –   In hereditary hemorrhagic telangiectasic (HHT) liver disease, clinical manifestations are the result of the development of shunts between the hepatic artery (HA), hepatic vein (HV), or portal vein (PV).

- Give the different clinical presentations arising from shunting between HA (hepatic artery), HV (hepatic vein) and PV (portal vein) in HHT (hereditary hemorrhagic telangiectasia).

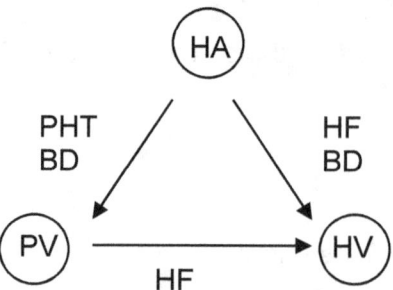

Abbreviations: BD, biliary disease; HF, heart failure; PHT, portal hypertension

- o High-output heart failure (HF) (hepatic artery [HA] and/or portal vein[PV] to hepatic vein [HV] shunt)
    - – Shortness of breath on exertion
    - – Orthopnea
    - – Ascites
    - – Edema
- o Portal hypertension (PHT) (hepatic artery [HA] to portal vein [PV] shunt)
    - – Esophageal varices
    - – Nodular regenerative hyperplasia (NRH)
- o Biliary disease [BD] (hepatic artery [HA] to hepatic vein [HV] and/or portal vein [PV] shunt)
    - – Severe cholestasis
    - – Recurrent cholangitis
- o Hepatic disintegration

Abbreviation: BD, biliary disease;  HA, hepatic artery; HV, hepatic vein; PHT, portal hypertension ; PV, portal vein.

Adapted from: Sabbà C, Pompili M. Review article: The hepatic manifestations of hereditary hemorrhagic telangiectasia. *Aliment Pharmacol Ther* 2008;28(5):523-33.

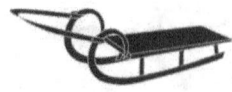

# ASCITES

➢ Clinical

Clinical Examination

- Give the volume of ascites fluid which must be present to detect flank dullness on percussion.

  o 500 – 100 mL
    - If there is no flank dullness, there is a 90% likelihood that there is no ascites.

- Give the options to increase the diagnostic yield.

  o Test for shifting dullness, or perform an abdominal ultrasound.

➢ Pathophysiology
   o The peritoneal surface absorbs up to 500 mL/day of ascitic fluid.
   o Excessive use of diuretics above this physiological level of mobilization of ascitic fluid of 500 mL/day causes depletion of fluid from intravascular spaces.
   o Contraction alkalosis develops, together with prerenal azotemia.
   o Prerenal azotemia is diagnosed from
     - $Na^+ < 10$ mmol/L

- Give the current theory of the pathogenesis of ascites.

  o PHT → ↑ NO → vasodilation → ↓ effective arterial BP

    → ↑ vasoconstrictors

    → ↑ vasopressin

    → ↑ renin-aldosterone

    → ↑ sympathetic nervous system (SNS) activity

    → ↑ Na+ -retaining hormones

→ ↑ renal vasoconstriction → ↓ renal function → ↑ retention of $Na^+$ / $H_2O$ → Ascites

270

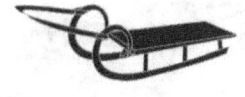

➢ Laboratory

Serum ascites albumin gradient (SAAG)

- o In NA (North America, Canada and USA), the usual cause of ascites is cirrhosis, but don't forget that "…approximately 5% of patients have two causes of ascites…." (Feldman M., et al. Sleisenger and Fordtran's Gastrointestinal and Liver Disease. 9th Edition. Saunders/Elsevier, Philadelphia, 2010, page 1527).

- • Give the use of the serum ascites albumin gradient (SAAG) and ascites protein to determine the cause of ascites.

| SAAG | Ascites Protein < 2.5 g/dL | Ascites Protein > 2.5 g/dL |
|---|---|---|
| >1.1 | o Portal hypertension due to cirrhosis<br>o "Cardiac cirrhosis" | – Portal hypertension due to hepatic venous outflow obstruction (including right heart failure) |
| <1.1 | o Nephrotic syndrome | – Malignancy, tuberculosis |

Abbreviation: SAAG, serum ascites albumin gradient

➢ "When the SAAG sags"

- o The SAAG (serum-ascites albumin gradient" is an index of portal pressure: if the SAAG is ≥ 1.1 g/dL, there is a 97% accuracy of the test for the patient having portal hypertension (↑ hydrostatic pressure gradient between portal blood and ascitic fluid).

- o A "falsely low" SAAG may be caused by

  - – Hyperglobulinemia ( > 5 g/dL)

  - – During diuretics for cardiac cirrhosis

- o The commonest cause of a ↓ SAAG is peritoneal carcinomatosis, but the low SAAG is not diagnostic for this condition.

Please see Sleisenger and Fordtran's Gastrointestinal and Liver Disease. 10th Edition. Saunders/Elsevier, Philadelphia, 2016, Box 91.3, Box 93.1, page 1559.

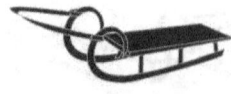

- In both cirrhotic and cardiac ascites, SAAG > 1.1. Give an approach to distinguish between hepatic and cardiac causes of ascites:

| Sample | Cirrhotic | Cardiac |
|---|---|---|
| ○ Ascitic fluid | | |
| – Protein | ↓ | ↑ |
| ○ Blood | | |
| – Hematocrit < 32 | Yes (in 32%) | No |
| – PbNP median concentration (pg/mL) | 166 | 6100 |

Abbreviation: pbNP, pro-brain-type naturetic peptide

- ○ Pointers on ascites
  - – ↑ ascitic fluid amylase (> 2000 U/L, or 5x > serum amylase) suggests
    - Acute pancreatitis
    - Intestinal perforation
  - – If ascitic fluid contains ↑ lymphocytes (not PMNs), suspect
    - Tuberculous peritonitis
    - HCC / hepatic metastases
    - Pancreatitis
  - – Chylous ascites
    - Ascitic fluid becomes creamy coloured (chylous) when the concentration of triglyceride in ascites > 200 mg/dL.
    - Chylous ascites occurs with cirrhosis, rupture of the intra-abdominal lymphatics (e.g., malignancy surgery – retroperitoneal, radical pelvic)
  - – Dark brown ascites
    - Dark brown (not pink or red) ascitic fluid (bilirubin concentration in ascitic fluid > 6 mg/dL) suggests perforation of
    - Biliary tree
    - Duodenum/jejunum
  - – Cloudy ascites
    - ↑ neutrophils, or fat (chylous ascites) makes ascetic fluid cloudy
    - In a patient with chronic renal failure on hemodialysis, look hard for causes of ascites before diagnosing idiopathic (nephrogenous) ascites.

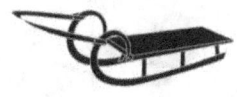

- In the context of the patient with ascites, give the meaning of "ovarian hyperstimulation syndrome" (OHS), "Poems syndrome", and "hemophagocytic syndrome".

    o OHS                        – ↑ stimulation of the ovaries with sexual activity may lead to ascites

    o Poems syndrome             – Polyneuropathy, organomegaly, endocrinopathy, M component, skin changes → may be associated with ascites

    o Hemophagocytic syndrome    – Leukemia or lymphoma associated with ascites

➤ Treatment

　o Salt restricton, 2 g/day

　o Diuretics

　　　– Furosimide blocks active $CL^-$ reabsorption from the loop of Henle, aldactone blocks active $Na^+$ reabsorption in the distal renal tubule

　　　– Too aggressive diuretic therapy may be complicated by renal failure, hepatic encephalopathy, and electrolyte disturbances (↑$Na^+$, ↑ or ↓ $K^+$)

　o LVP (large volume paracentesis)

　　　– Large volume paracentesis (> 5 L) is safe as long as 6-8 g albumin are given per liter fluid removed

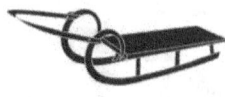

Clinical Pearls

- o The cirrhotic patient often will have a systolic blood pressure (SBP) of ~ 70 mmHg, and as long as there has been
  - – No recent further drop in SBP
  - – No Azotemia
  - – No confusion

  There is no need to stop the once daily dosage of furosemide and aldactone.

- o Remember, "….complete remission of ascites should not be a prerequition for discharge from the hospital" (Sleisenger and Fordtran's Gastrointestinal and Liver Disease. 10th Edition. Saunders/Elsevier, Philadelphia, 2016, page 1573).

274

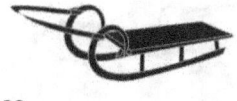

- Give which laboratory value predicts an ascitic patient's likely response to diuretics.

  - When a patient has ascites and the SAAG is > 1.1 g/dL, there is likely to be a response to diuretics.

  - TIPS
    - Decreases sinusoidal portal pressure, and decreases $Na^+$ reabsorption in the proximal renal tubules, producing a diureses
    - Will modulize ascites in 70% of persons with diuretic-resistant ascites, but there is a 50% risk of the TIPS precipitating hepatic encephalopathy, and the shunt may become stenotic, requiring angiography and dilation of the shunt
    - Should not be performed for ascites mobilization in the patient who already has hepatic encephalopathy, whose MELD score is greater than 20 points

- Give examples of non-diuretic treatments for ascites.

  - Peritoneal carcinomatous from ovarian cancer
    - Surgical debulking

  - Tuberculous ascites
    - Appropriate antituberculous therapy

  - Chlamydia ascites
    - Tetracycline

  - Lupus
    - Glucocorticosteroids

  - Nephrogenous ascites
    - Hemodialysis

  - Alcoholic cirrhosis
    - Stop drinking alcohol

  - NASH
    - Weight loss
    - Treatment of metabolic syndrome
    - Vitamin E (possibly)

  - AIH
    - Corticosteroids / immune suppression

  - Portal hypertension
    - Low salt/fluid restriction

  - HBV
    - Interferon, or oral nucleoside

  - HCV
    - Interferon plus ribavirin plus third agent

  - Pre-operative
    - Change IV from normal saline

  - Paracentesis
    - Continue regular paracentesis, including large volume paracentesis (LVP)

  - TIPS
    - Doppler ultrasound to exclude possible vascular obstruction (e.g., Budd-Chiari syndrome)
    - Consider inserting new stent

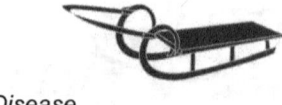

## Refractory Ascites

➢ Definition and diagnostic criteria

- o Diuretic-resistant ascites
  - Ascites that is difficult to mobilize, as defined by a failure to lose at least 1.5 kg/week of fluid weight, despite maximal diuretic therapy with spironolactone (400 mg/day) and furosemide (160 mg/day) or an equivalent dose of a distal-acting and loop-acting diuretic respectively.
  - ".....ascites unresponsive to a sodium-restricted diet [ 2 gm per day, 88 mEq per day ] and high-dose diuretic treatment [e.g., furosemide 160 mg/day and aldosterone 400 mg/day]) (Sleisenger and Fordtran's Gastrointestinal and Liver Disease. 9th Edition. Saunders/Elsevier, Philadelphia, 2010, page 1538).
  - Ascites that is not eliminated even with maximum and optimal diuretic therapy, or
  - Ascites that is not eliminated because maximum dosages of diuretics cannot be attained, given the development of diuretic induced complications (renal failure)
  - 1 year mortality rate for ascites refractory to medical care ~ 68%

- o Diuretic-intractable ascites
  - Ascites that is difficult to mobilize, as defined above, due to the inability to effectively dose diuretics because of diuretic-induced adverse effects e.g., azotemia, hyponatremia, etc.

- o Prerequisites
  - Treatment duration
    - Patients must be on intensive diuretic therapy (spironolactone 400 mg/day and furosemide 160 mg/day) for at least 1 week and on a salt-restricted diet of less than 90 mmol/day

  - Lack of response
    - Mean weight loss of <0.8 kg over 4 days and urinary sodium output less than the sodium intake

  - Early ascites recurrence
    - Reappearance of grade 2 or 3 ascites within 4 weeks of initial mobilization

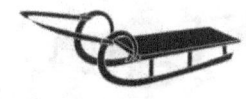

- Diuretic-induced complications
  - Diuretic-induced hepatic encephalopathy is the development of encephalopathy in the absence of any other precipitating factor
  - Diuretic-induced renal impairment is an increase of serum creatinine by >100% to a value >2 mg/dl (177 mol/L) in patients with ascites responding to treatment
  - Diuretic-induced hyponatremia is defined as a decrease of serum sodium by >10 mmol/L to a serum sodium of <125 mmol/L
  - Diuretic-induced hypo- or hyperkalemia is defined as a change in serum potassium to <3 mmol/L or >6 mmol/L despite appropriate measures

Printed with permission: European Association for the Study of the Liver. EASL clinical practice guidelines on the management of ascites, spontaneous bacterial peritonitis, and hepatorenal syndrome in cirrhosis. J Hepatol. 2010;53(3):397-417, Table 3.

➢ Treatment

• Give a management strategy for refractory ascites.

  o Recommended therapy
    - Total paracentesis plus IV albumin (6-8 g of albumin per liter of ascites removed)
    - Note recent recommendation:
      ▪ "Consider albumin infusion [10 g albumin per L ascitic fluid drained] optional after taps of a larger volume [> 5 L] in patients with diuretics-resistant ascites" (Feldman M., et al. Sleisenger and Fordtran's Gastrointestinal and Liver Disease. 9th Edition. Saunders/Elsevier, Philadelphia, 2010, page 1540)
      ▪ If < 5 L of ascites is removed, a synthetic plasma volume expander may be used instead of albumin
      ▪ Continue with salt restriction and diuretic therapy, as tolerated

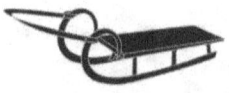

- Give the pros and cons of **albumin infusion** being given in conjunction with a therapeutic paracentesis.

  - Pros      – Prevents post-paracentesis ↑ renin concentration and development of paracentesis-induuced circulation dysfunction

  - Con      – No benefit on survival
    - ↓ opsonin in ascitic fluid
    - Considerable cost
    - Increasing serum albumin concecntration leads to
      - ↑ breakdown of albumin
      - ↓ synthesis of albumin

- Give an alternative therapy to therapeutic paracentesis plus albumin.

  - TIPS for patients who require frequent paracentesis (every 1-2 weeks) and whose MELD score is <11

  - Peritoneovenous shunt for patients who are not suitable for TIPS or liver transplantation

- When using a coated stent for the treatment of refractory ascites (in patients with low or high MELD, there is
  - No survival advantage
  - ↑ HE (hepatic encephalopathy)
  - Consistent superiority over TIPS

Abbreviations: TIPS, transjugular intrahepatic portosystemic shunt

Printed with permission: Garcia Tsao, et al. *The American Journal of Gastroenterology* 2009; 104:1816.

---

SO YOU WANT TO BE A HEPATOLOGIST!

- In the context of refractory ascites, give the meaning of "paracentesis-induced circulation dysfunction" (PICD).

  - Paracentesis-induced circulatory dysfunction is an ↑ renin concentration in the blood after a paracentesis.

  - Associated with ↓ life expectancy

---

278

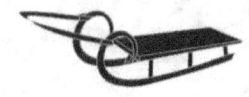

## Malignancy-Associated Ascites

- Give causes of malignancy-associated ascites.
    - Peritoneal carcinoma (1°, 2°)
    - Massive liver metastases
    - Peritoneal carcinomatosis with massive liver metastases
    - Hepatocellular carcinoma (HCC)
    - Malignant lymph node obstruction
    - Malignant Budd-Chiari syndrome (BCS, from tumour emboli in hepatic veins)

Please see: Sleisenger and Fordtran's Gastrointestinal and Liver Disease. 10th Edition. Saunders/Elsevier, Philadelphia, 2016, page 1563.

- Give tumours which commonly metastasize to the peritoneum.

    - Adenocarcinoma    -    GI
        - Stomach
        - Colon
        - Pancreas

    - Lymphoma    -    Non-GI
        - Ovary
        - Lung
    - Sarcoma

---

SO YOU WANT TO BE A GASTROENTEROLOGIST!

- Give mechanisms by which tumours may cause ascites.
    - Peritoneal carcinomatosis
    - Extraperitoneal carcinomatosis
        - Hepatic 1° (HCC)
        - Hepatic 2° (metastases)
    - Lymph node obstruction
    - Budd-Chiari syndrome ± IVC obstruction

    Abbreviation: HCC, hepatocellular cancer; IVC, inferior vena cava

---

279

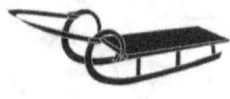

SO YOU WANT TO BE A GASTROENTEROLOGIST!

Tumours which commonly metastasize to the peritoneum include adenocarcinomas (stomach, colon, pancreas; ovary, lung) , lymphoma and sarcomas.

- In this context, give the meaning of "**pseudomyxoma peritonei**".

  o Pseudomyxoma peritonei is a metastatic mucinous cyst adenocarcinoma of the appendix or ovary which results in a jelly-like tumour implant on the peritoneum, and may cause malignant ascites.

- Give the features which help to distinguish between peritoneal carcinomatosis (CA) versus tuberculous peritonitis (TB) as causes of high-lymphocyte-count ascites.

|  | CA | TB |
| --- | --- | --- |
| o Prevalence | +++ | + |
| o Fever | + | - |
| o Ca125 (ovary) | + | + |
| o AD | - | + |

Abbreviation: AD, adenosine deaminase

---

Diagnostic Tip

  o Cytology of ascitic fluid is ~ 100% sensitive to detect peritoneal carcinomatosis, but the sensitivity to detect 1°/2° liver tumour is low.

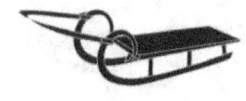

# SPONTANEOUS BACTERIAL PERITONITIS (SBP)

- ➤ Demography
  - ○ In the cirrhotic with ascites admitted to hospital
    - – About 1/3 have bacterial peritonitis
    - – 2/3 SBP, 1/3 MNB
    - – Commonest monomicrobial organisms: E. Coli, Streptococci (pneumococci), Klebsiella
  - ○ In the cirrhotic patient who is hospitalized for GI bleeding, 40% develop SBP (that's why treatment of all cirrhotics with GI bleeding and ascites are given prophylactic antibiotics).
  - ○ SBP is present in at least 20% of cirrhotics at the time they are admitted to the hospital
  - ○ SBP worsens vasodilation, and thereby contributes to early variceal rebleeding and to the development of renal failure (HRS, hepatorenal syndrome)
  - ○ Persons at risk of developing SBP include those with a previous episode of SBP, SBP occurring with variceal hemorrhage, or low protein ascites
  - ○ Once SBP has occurred, the one year mortality rate is 50-70%
  - ○ Early treatment of SBP is associated with a mortality rate (MR) of (only) 5%, with higher MR with creatinine > 350 µmol/L, or if shock has developed.
  - ○ Initiation of the beta-blocker nadolol in cirrhotic patients with high risk esophagealvarices delays or prevents the first occurrence of ascites seen in patients who had an improvement by 10% or more from baseline HVPG pressure.
  - ○ Consider SBP and perform diagnostic paracentesis if:
    - - Symptoms/signs (abdominal pain, fever, chills)
    - - Patient is in emergency room or admitted
    - - Worsening renal function or development of hepaticencephalopathy

- ➤ Clinical
  - ○ In the cirrhotic patient with ascites, suspect SBP when there is
    - – Abdominal pain
    - – Abdominal tenderness
    - – Rebound tenderness
    - – Unexplained fever
    - – Change in mental status
    - – Clinical deterioration
    - – On hospitalization (all ascitic admitted to hospital should have a peritoneal tap to exclude SBP)

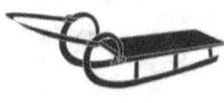

> Laboratory

  o The median colony count of bacteria in the ascitic fluid in SBP is only 1 organism per mL

  o When ascitic fluid contains $10^4$ organisms per mL, the gram stain becomes positive.

  o Ascitic fluid gram stain may be useful in 2° BP (bacterial peritonitis [2°] to intestinal perforation), but not in SBP.

  o In neutrocytic ascites, bed-side inoculation of ascitic fluid placed in blood culture bottles demonstrates bacterial growth in ~ 80%

  o Ascitic fluid concentration < 2.5 g/dL protein reflects a low opsonin concentration, and a low opsonin concentration increases the risk of SBP (the concentration of opsonin in ascitic fluid is directly related to its total protein concentration).

- Give the types of spontaneous bacterial peritonitis (SBP).

| | >250 neutrophils | Ascitic culture |
|---|:---:|:---:|
| o Classical SBP (culture-positive neutrocytic ascites) | + | + |
| o Culture-negative neutrocytic ascites (CNNA) | + | - |
| o Monomicrobial nonneutrocytic bacterial ascites (MNB; aka bacterascites) | - | + |
| o Polymicrobial non-neutrocytic* ascites (aka secondary bacterial peritonitis [2° BP]) | - | + |

*Usually from needle perforation of the gut, is associated with

  – Severe symptoms and signs
  – ↓ ascitic fluid glucose (< 50 mg/dl)
  – ↑ ascitic fluid LDH
  – Polymicrobial anaerobic infection
  – Strictly speaking, this is not included in the term "spontaneous" BP

Abbreviations: SBP, spontaneous bacterial peritonitis; TIPS, transjugular intrahepatic portosystemic shunt

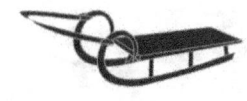

**False-positive** neutrocytes in ascitic fluid

- o An ascitic fluid neutrocyte count > 250 mm³ is diagnostic of neutrocytic ascites. Give the condition under which this count may be falsely elevated.

- o "during diuretics in patients with cirrhotic ascites, the WBC count can concentrate to more than 1000 cells/mm³ (Sleisenger and Fordtran's Gastrointestinal and Liver Disease. 9th Edition. Saunders/Elsevier, Philadelphia, 2010, page 1523).

- • Give how to diagnose neutrocytic ascitic fluid in the presence of blood.

  - o If there are RBC in the tap (pink colour, RBC > 10,000/mm3; red, RBC > 20,000 mm3), for each 250 RBCs, subtract 1 PMN in order to achieve a corrected count to diagnosis neutrolytic ascites.
    - – Caution: if a blood contaminated tap has sat for some time, or if the leakage of blood into the ascitic fluid occurred at a time in the distance, the PMNs will have disappeared (lysis), and when the correction formula is used, the count may be low or even negative.

- • Give how to diagnose secondary bacterial peritonitis (2° BP).

  - o Secondary bacterial peritonitis from bowel perforation is polymicrobial, but unless gene probes are used for rapid diagnosis, a serious time delay will ensure.

  - o Measure the ascitic fluid total protein, glucose and LDH; if 2 or 3 of these are abnormal, the patient likely has secondary rather than spontaneous BP excluded perforation rather than diagnosing neutrocytic spontaneous bacterial peritonitis (SBP).
    - – Total protein > 1 g/dL
    - – Glucose < 50 mg/dL
    - – LDH > ULN for serum

  - o PMNs contain LDH, so when PMNs increase in SBP, there is ↑ LDH; in secondary BP, there is ↑↑↑ PMNs, so ↑↑↑ LDH (LDH in ascites > serum LDH)

---

Clinical Pearls

- o If you think the patient might have ascites from secondary peritonitis, don't play around with measuring ascitic fluid concentrations of glucose or LDH (lactate dehydrogenase): do diagnostic imaging (such as CT scan) to find the source of the suspected perforation, or laparoscopy to find and biopsy metastatic deposits.

---

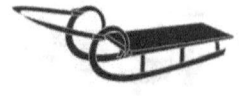

> Treatment

❖ SBP and CNNA

- Give the indications for treatment of spontaneous bacterial peritonitis(SBP), including recurrent SBP.

  - o Indications
    - – Prior history of SBP
    - – GI bleeding without ascites
    - – GI bleeding, with ascites (even without SBP [PMN > 250; WBC > 500]), acute treatment)
    - – Low ascitic fluid protein concentration
  - o Culture negative neutrocytic ascites (CNNA) Rx
    - – Treatment is the same as that for SBP

Please see: Swan MG. Chapter 58. In: Therapeutic Choices. Grey J, Ed. 6th Edition, Canadian Pharmacists Association: Ottawa, ON, 2011, Table 2: Spontaneous Bacterial Peritonitis, page 774.

  - o General management
    - – Avoid therapeutic paracentesis during active infection
    - – Intravenous albumin (1.5 g/kg of body weight for 3 days, then 1 g/kg) if BUN >30mg/dl, creatinine >1mg/dl, bilirubin >4 mg/dl, and repeat at day 3 if renal dysfunction persists
    - – Avoid aminoglycosides

  - o Emperical antibiotics
    - – Ceftriaxone (2g IV q 24 h) or
    - – Cefotaxime (2 g IV q 6-12 h) (98% of organisms are susceptible), or
    - – Ampicillin/clavulanate (2g/1g i.v q 6 h)
    - – Continue therapy for 7 days
    - – Repeat diagnostic paracentesis at day 2
    - – If ascites PMN count decreases by at least 25% at day 2, intravenous therapy can be switched to oral therapy (quinolone such as ciprofloxacin or levofloxacin 250 mg po bid) to complete 7 days of therapy
    - – Oral norfloxacin 400 mg p.o q.d (preferred) or
    - – Oral ciprofloxacin 250-500 mg q.d* or
    - – Oral levofloxacin 250 mg q.d*
    - – TMP-SMX 1 double strength tablet p.o q.d
    - – (Patients who develop quinolone resistant organisms may also have resistance to TMP-SMX)

284

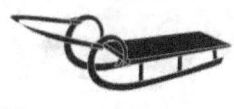

- o Duration     –    Prophylaxis should be continued until the disappearance of ascites or until liver transplantation

- o IV albumin

\* Empirical doses

Abbreviations: BUN, blood urea nitrogen; PMN, Polymorphonuclear (neutrophil) cell count; PO, orally; QD, once daily; RBC, Red blood cell count; SBP, spontaneous bacterial peritonitis; TMP-SMX, trimethoprim sulfamethoxazole

Printed with permission: Garcia-Tsao G, et al. Management and treatment of patients with cirrhosis and portal hypertension. *The American Journal of Gastroenterology:* page 1811.; and adapted from: Rimola A, et al. *J Hepatol* 2000;32(1):142-53.

- Give the rational for using IV albumin (1.5 g/kg BW at diagnosis, then 1 g/kg on day 3) together with an empirical antibiotic when treating SBP).

  - o SBP is associated with type I HRS in about 1/3 of patients, and this is associated with an ↑ risk of mortality

|  | Cefotaxime alone | Cefotaxime plus albumin |
|---|---|---|
| HRS type 1 | 30% | 10% |
| Mortality | 29% | 10% |

  - – This positive outcome was obtained in patients with jaundice (serum bilirubin ≥ 68 µmol/L) and renal failure (serum creatinine ≥ 88 µmol/L.
  - – Until more information is available, it is recommended that persons develop SBP should be treated with broad spectrum antibiotics and intravenous albumin (EASL Clinical Practice Guidelines, J. Hepatol 2010; 53: 399-417).

- MNB (monomicrobial non-neutrocytic bacterial ascites)

  - o Repeat diagnostic paracentesis, and if

    - – Neutrophils > 250/mm$^3$, treat as for classical SBP or CNNA

    - – Neutrophils < 250/mm$^3$, follow patient

  - o "Paracentesis should be repeated after 48 hours of treatment if the [clinical] course is atypical" (Feldman M., et al. Sleisenger and Fordtran's Gastrointestinal and Liver Disease. 9th Edition. Saunders/Elsevier, Philadelphia, 2010, page 1534).

285

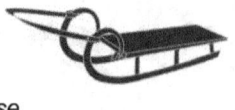

o "….spontaneous ascitic fluid infection is a good marker of end-stage liver disease" [ESLD] and has been proposed as an indication for liver transplantation in a patient who is otherwise a candidate" (Feldman M., et al. Sleisenger and Fordtran's Gastrointestinal and Liver Disease. 9th Edition. Saunders/Elsevier, Philadelphia, 2010, page 1534).

---

## SO YOU WANT TO BE A GASTROENTEROLOGIST!

The most common causative organisms of SBP are gram-negative aerobes such as E.Coli, and these should be sensitive to first line use of quinolones such as ciprofloxacin.

- Give circumstances when you would **avoid quinolones** for an empiric diagnosis of SBP, and instead start with
  - o Cephataxime, 4 g / day IV for 5 days, or
  - o Amoxicillin / clavulanic acid IV, then po
    - Previously taking quinolones for prophylaxis of SBP
    - High prevalence of quinolone-resistant bacterial in practice area
    - SBP developing in hospital (nosocomial SBP)

---

➤ Prophylaxis

  o Indications

    – Primary prevention of SBP with norfloxacin or ciprofloxacin has survival advantage and is recommended for
      ▪ Previous SBP
      ▪ Variceal bleeding
    – Ascitic fluid protein < 1g/dL

  o First line        – Oral ciprofloxacin 250-500 mg qd* or
                      – Oral levofloxacin 250 mg q.d*

  o Alternative       – TMP-SMX 1 double strength tablet po qd
    therapy           – Patients who develop quinolone resistant organisms may also have resistance to TMP-SMX

  o Duration          – Prophylaxis should be continued until the disappearance of ascites or until liver transplantation

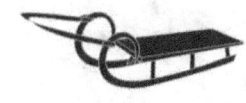

Abbreviations: po: Orally; SBP: Spontaneous bacterial peritonitis; TMP-SMX: Trimethoprim sulfamethoxazole, q.d: Once daily

*Empirical doses

Source: Garcia Tsao et al. *Am J Gastroenterol* 2009; 104:1806-1829.

SO YOU WANT TO BE A GASTROENTEROLOGIST!

The most common causative organisms of SBP are gram-negative aerobes (GNA) such as E.Coli, and these should be sensitive to first line use of quinolones such as ciprofloxacin.

- Give the reason why selective intestinal decontamination with norfloxacin (400 mg / 12 h po for 7 days) is no longer recommended for the prophylaxis of SBP in patients with cirrhosis who develop bleeding from the GI tract.
  - This is a kind of a trick question
    - Prophylaxis is needed of course, but there is
      - ↑ incidence of quinolone resistant gram-negative bacteria (GNB)
      - ↑ incidence of gram-positive bacteria in SBP (likely related to endoscopic procedures)
    - Ceftriaxone is more effective than norfloxacin in prevention of SBP in the cirrhotic with GI bleeding, especially if they have 2 or more of the following
      - Ascites
      - Severe malnutrition
      - Hepatic encephalopathy
      - Bilirubin > 3 mg / dL

Clinical Alert
  - Once SBP has developed, the patient's prognosis is poor, and they should be referred for consideration of liver transplantation
    - While awaiting LT, give prophylactic antibiotics to prevent recurrent SBP:
    - Cotrimazole (800 mg sulfamethoxazole and 160 mg trimethoprim po od.
    - If the total protein concentration of the ascitic fluid is < 15 g/L in the patient with severe liver disease, norfloxacin 400 mg/day po ↓ risk of SBP and death.

287

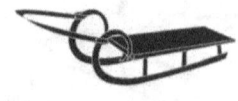

MASTERING THE BOARDS
Hepatology & Pancreaticobiliary Disease

A.B.R. Thomson

**Spontaneous Bacterial Hydrothorax** (SBH)

- o SBH may develop in cirrhotic pleural effusion (hydrothorax) with/without ascites.

- o Perform DP (diagnostic paracentesis) of hydrothorax

- o If hydrothorax fluid

  - \- > 250/mm$^3$ neutrophils, plus positive culture → treat> 500/mm$^3$ but negative culture (in the absence of pneumonia) →

- o Why ascites matters

  - \- Once ascites develops in the patient with cirrhosis, the 2 year mortality rate is 50%

  - \- Ascites may become complicated by SBP (spontaneous bacterial peritonitis), which may cause or worsen decompensation.

---

Clinical tips

- o Cirrhotic ascites plus pleural infusion(s)
  - \- L. – side
    - ▪ Suspect TB
  - \- R. – side
    - ▪ Likely "sympathetic" to ascites

- o Cirrhotic ascites plus hernia of abdominal wall
  - \- Elective surgical repair after drainage of ascites to ↓ complications of strangulation, or perforation.

- o Recurrence of abdominal hernia when preoperative drainage of ascites is
  - \- Performed, 14%
  - \- Not performed, 73%

---

"What is not started today is never finished tomorrow."

Johann Wolfgang von Goethe

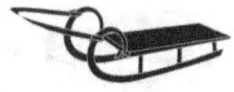

# HEPATORENAL SYNDROME (HRS)

➢ Definition

- A functional and potentially reversible form of prerenal azotemia with .....
  a cascade of events associated with intense dilation of the splanchnic
  arterial vasodilation in the setting of cirrhosis or acute liver injury and
  resulting in profound renal arterial vasoconstriction and progressive renal
  failure" (Sleisenger and Fordtran's Gastrointestinal and Liver Disease. 9th
  Edition. *Saunders/Elsevier* 2010, page 1546).

- Functional renal failure in the person with cirrhosis and ascites

- Practical definition
  - Consider HRS in a patient with cirrhosis and ascites and
  - Creatinine level of >1.5 mg/dl

➢ Other important definitions

- Most cirrhotics with renal dysfunction do not have HRS (only 15-20%
  have HRS)

- Hypnatremia may preceed the development of HRS

- Type I HRS is associated with intense vasoconstriction, which may cause
  the HRS to progress to ATN

- Parenchymal renal disease as defined by
  - Proteinuria < 0.5 g/day
  - No microhematuria (<50 red cells/high powered field), and
  - Normal renal ultrasonography

- Absence of hypovolemia as defined by no sustained improvement of
  renal function (creatinine decreasing to <133 mol/L) following at least 2
  days of diuretic withdrawal (if on diuretics), and

- If renal dysfunction persists despite stopping diuretics and correction of
  hypovolemia, diagnose HRS

- No or insufficient improvement in serum creatinine level (remains > 1.5
  mg/dL) 48 hr after diuretic withdrawal and adequate volume expansion
  with intravenous albumin

- Consider the possibility of HRS in any patient with cirrhosis and ascites,
  as well as a serum creatinine level of >1.5 mg/dl (133 mmol/L)

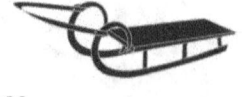

- ➢ Demography
  - ○ HRS occurs in cirrhotics with ascites, ~8% per year
    - – Admitted for SBP or other infections, 30%
    - – Needing large volume paracentesis, 10%
  - ○ Severe alcoholic hepatitis, HRS develops in ~25%
  - ○ Reduces 3 year survival from liver transplant to 60% versus ~75% when there is no HRS

Printed with permission: EASL clinical practice guidelines on the management of ascites, spontaneous bacterial peritonitis, and hepatorenal syndrome in cirrhosis. *J Hepatol*. 2010;53(3):397-417, Table 8.

- ➢ Types

- • Give features to distinguish between Type 1 and Type 2 HRS.

| Characteristics | Type 1 | Type 2 |
|---|---|---|
| ○ Progression | Fast (< 2 wks) | Slow |
| ○ Serum creatinine | > 2.5 mg/dL | < 2.5 mg/dL |
| ○ Triggers | Bacterial infection (SBP) GI bleeding Surgery | Diuretic resistant ascites |
| ○ ↓ Sys BP | ↓↓↓ ALF | ↓ |
| ○ Adrenal insufficiency with sepsis | Common (80%) | Uncommon |
| ○ Cross-over | No, but may progress to ATN | Yes (HRS 2 → HRS 1) |

Abbreviations: ALF, acute liver failure; ATN, acute tubular necrosis; MAP, mean arterial pressure; SBP, spontaneous bacterial peritonitis; SBP, systolic blood pressure

Please see: Swan MG. Chapter 58. In: Therapeutic Choices. Grey J, Ed. 6th Edition, Canadian Pharmacists Association: Ottawa, ON, 2011, Table 1: Ascites, pg 773.

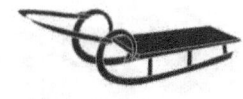

➢ Pathophysiology

• Give the pathophysiology of renal arterial vasoconstriction leading to HRS.

• When there is no

• When there is cirrhosis
- Infection
- Inflammation
- Vasoactive mediators

↓

o Fluid loss
 – Diarrhea
 – GI bleeding
 – Diuresis
 – Serial large volume paracentesis
 – SBP
 – Sepsis

Splanchnic and peripheral vasodilation ⟵ Vasodilates
 – NO
 – CO
 – Glucagon
 – Prostacyclin
 – Adenomedullin
 – Endogenous opiates

↓

EBCV ⟵ - - - -

↑ plasma ADH
 – ↓ clearance
 – ↑ activity
 – ↑ ADH regulated water channel

Ascites
SBP
↓ Na$^+$

o CBV - - - - - - - →

↑ production / action
 – Endothelins
 – Kalikreins
 – F2-isoprotanes

↑

o Renal
 – ↑ RAAS
 – ↑ plasma ADH
 – ↑ Na$^+$ / H$_2$O retention

 – Lower setpoint for renal response to ↓ SBP and cardiac output
 – ↑ blood norepinephrine and ↑ plasma renin activity

Renal

↑

o CVS
 – ↓ systemic BP
 – ↑ HR / ↑ cardiac output
 – ↑ SNS activity
 – Hyperdynamic circulation

o Cirrhotic cardiomyopathy
 – Hyperdynamic circulation → LV hypertrophy → diastolic dysfunction → ↓ B-adrenergic signaling
 – ↓ cardio-myocyte function
  ▪ ↑ QTC

o Drugs
 – NSAIDs
 – ARBs
 – ACEIs
 – Diuretics
 – Lactulose
 – Nephrotoxic antibiotics
 – Cyclosporine
 – Tacrolimus

⟶

o Renal arterial vasoconstriction

↓

↓ GFR
↓ renal perfusion
↓ HRS (inappropriate and intense vasoconstriction)

Abbreviations: ACEIs, angiotensin-converting enzyme inhibitors; ADH, antidiuretic hormone; ARBs, angiotensin receptor blockers; BP, blood pressure; CBV, circulating blood volume; CC, cirrhotic cardiomyopathy; CO, carbon monoxide; ECBV, effective circulating blood volume; GFR, glomerular filtration rate; NO, nitric oxide; RAAS, renin-antgiotensin-aldosterone system; SBP, systemic blood pressure

➢ Diagnosis

• Give the major and minor criteria for the diagnosis of the hepatorenal syndrome, and distinguish this from acute tubular necrosis (ATN).

• Major criteria

    o Presence of cirrhosis
        – Renal failure (creatinine >1.5mg/dl); if no previous renal impairment, or a serum a ↑ by 50% over baseline

    o Lack of improvement in serum creatinine after ≥48 hrs of diuretic withdrawal and volume expansion with 1.5 L of normal saline
        – Sepsis
        – Volume depletion
        – Use of vasodilators

    o Absence of:
        – Shock
        – Use of nephrotoxic drugs (eg: aminoglycosides)
        – Parenchymal renal disease (urine protein > 500 mg/day, granular or red cell casts, hematuria, urinary obstruction by sonography)

• Minor criteria (suggests HRS, or prerenal failure)

| Parameter | Osmolarity mOsm/Kg | Urine (Na) mmol/L | Sediment | Protein mg/day |
|---|---|---|---|---|
| o Prerenal | | | | |
| – Hypovolemia | >500 | <20 | Normal | <500 |
| – Hepatorenal | >500 | <10 | Normal | <500 |
| o Renal | | | | |
| – Acute tubular necrosis | <350 | >40 | Granular casts | 500-1500 |
| – Interstitial | <350 | >40 | WBC eosinophils | 500-1500 |

Adapted from: Sleisenger and Fordtran's Gastrointestinal and Liver Disease. 10th Edition. Saunders/Elsevier, Philadelphia, 2016, Box 94-2, page 1581

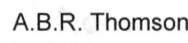

- Give the laboratory variables used differentiate between prerenal azotemia (PRA), hepatorenal syndrome (HRS) and acute renal failure (ARF) diagnosis for HRS.

| Variable | PRA | HRS | ARF |
|---|---|---|---|
| o Urinary sodium concentration, mEq/L | <10 | <10 | >30 |
| o Urine to plasma creatinine ratio | >30:1 | >30:1 | <20:1 |
| o Urine osmolality | At least 100m Osm >plasma osmolality | At least 100m Osm> plasma osmolality | Equal to plasma osmolality |
| o Urine sediment | Normal | Normal | Casts, debris |

Abbreviation: Osmp, osmolality of plasma; Osmu, osmolality of urine

➢ Treatment

- o NSAIDs, diuretics, other nephrotoxic drugs

- o Diuretics should be discontinued, and intravascular volume expanded with IV albumin, 1 g/kg per day, up to a maximum of 100 gm albumin per day

- o SBP may precipitate type I HRS, and this risk can be reduced by using albumin with the initial antibiotic therapy for SBP

- o Vasopressin vasoconstrictor therapy
  - – Terlipressin 1 mg / 4-6 hr intravenous bolus, plus IV albumin, to ↓ serum creatinine
    - ▪ < 133 µmol/L ( 1.5 mg /dL)
    - ▪ > 25% over 3 days (partial response)
    - ▪ Increase terlipressin to 2 mg / 4 hr if there is not a partial or complete response over 3 days treatment.
    - ▪ If serum creatinine does not fall or normalize within 14 days of terlipressin, stop therapy.
    - ▪ If HRS recurs after terlipressin is stopped, repeat course of Rx.
    - ▪ There is less date for the efficacy of norepinephrine or midodrine, plus octreotide plus albumin.

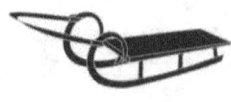

- o Vasoconstrictors plus albumin for ≥ 7 days (Alternative [bridging therapy])

  - Octreotide
  
    PLUS
  
  - Midodrine, or
  - Terlipressin[a]

  100-200 mcg SC t.i.d

  5-15 mg p.o t.i.d
  0.5 – 2.0 mg IV, q4-6 hr
  50-100 g IV q.d

  Goal : ↑ MAP by 15 mmHg

- o 35-50% of type I HRS responds to vasoconstrictors (midodrine, terlipressin, norepinephrine)
- o Renal dialysis ("support") for type I HRS may be a necessary bridge to liver transplantation
- o Liver transplant (priority dependent on MELD score)
  - Liver transplantation is the definitive treatment for type I HRS
  - If patient is not on transplant list, packet should be prepared urgently
  - If patient is on transplant list, MELD score should be updated daily and communicated to transplant center

- ➢ Prevention
  - o Severe alcoholic hepatitis – pentoxifylline
  - o Severe cirrhosis – Norfloxacin ↓ risk of HRS
  - o SBP
    - Antibiotics + albumin
  - o Drugs avoid
    - NSAIDs
    - ACEI
    - Antibiotics
  - o Combined kidney-liver transplantation
    - HRS, non-response to vasopressors, prolonged renal support > 12 weeks

Abbreviations: I.V., intravenous; HRS, hepatorenal syndrome; MAP,mean arterial pressure; MELD, model for end stage liver disease; t.i.d thrice a day; s.c subcutaneously

Adapted from: Garcia Tsao et al. *The American Journal of Gastroenterology* 2009; 104:1802-1829.

- o Transjugular intrahepatic portosystemic shunt (TIPS)
  - Role unproven: "TIPS may be considered in appropriately selected patients who meet criteria similar to those of published randomized trials" [for the prevention of HRS] (Runyon BA. Hepatology 2009; 49: 2087-2107, Table 4).

Printed with permission:  Garcia-Tsao, et al. *Am J Gastroenterol* 2009;104: 818.

294

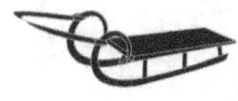

## HEPATIC ENCEPHALOPATHY (HE)

➤ Demography
- ○ HE occurs in ½ to ¾ of cirrhotics
- ○ Effects of HE non-transplanted mortality rate > 50% in 3 year

➤ Definition
- ○ A clinically diagnosed disorder of brain function due to impaired hepatic function resulting in "AtoD LMPS"
  **A**ffect behavious confusion
  **D**rowsiness/disorientation

  **L**earning
  **M**emory
  **P**ersonality
  **S**leep

➤ Pathophysiology

● Give the contribution of the small and large intestine, liver, skeletal muscle, kidney and brain in patients with HE.

- ○ Small bowel and large intestine
  - – Dietary amino acids and urease-positive bacteria → glutamine

  > glutaminase (deamination)
  > glutamine    →    glutamate + $NH_3$
  >           ←    glutamine synthetase (amination)

  - – Activity of gut glutaminase increased in liver disease
  - – Uptake of glutamine
- ○ Liver
  - – Portosystemic shunting, by-passing portovenous system with less hepatic detoxification of ammonia via the urea cycle
  - – $NH_3$ → urea, periportal hepatocytes → glutamine, perivenous hepatocytes
  - – In presence of hyponatremia, myoinositol falls, with less compensation for ↑ intracellular glutamine
- ○ Skeletal muscle
  - – Normally responsible for uptake of 50% of $NH_3$
  - – In cirrhosis, atrophy of skeletal muscles → ↓ muscle synthesis of glutamine
- ○ Kidney
  - – ↑ $NH_3$ production in presence of hypokalemia

295

- o Brain
  - – Edema
    - ▪ $NH_3$ and glutamate are normally converted and detoxified to glutamine by glutamine synthetase in astrocytes
    - ▪ In cirrhosis
      - –↑ brain blood flow
        - –↑ BBB permeability → ↑ brain $NH_3$ and glutamate → asteocyte swelling
        - → ↑ $NH_3$ taken uptake into
          - –Cerebellum
          - –Basal ganglia
          - –↑ brain edema
          - –↑ swelling of astrocytes - ↑ neurosteroids → ↑ activity of GABA-benzodiazepine system
          - –↑ benzodiazepine system
          - –↑ production of glutamine by astrocytes
    - ▪ In presence of hypokalemia and metabolic alkalosis, $NH_4 \rightarrow NH_3$, which crosses BBB
    - ▪ Plasma $NH_3$ > 150 μmol is associated with brain herniation
    - ▪ Abnormal form and function of astrocytes, with reduced glutamine synthetase and peripheral type benzodiazepine receptors (PTBR)
      - –↑ mitochondrial permeability → ↑ astrocyte swelling → ↑ brain edema
  - – Neurotransmitters signal transduction pathway
    - ▪ ↑ $NH_3$ activates N-methyl-D-aspartate-nitric oxide-C-guanylate cyclase (NMDA-NO-C6MP) signal transduction pathway → impairment of
      - –Memory
      - –Learning
      - –Sleep

| Neurotransmitter System | Findings in HE |
|---|---|
| o ↑ GABA, ↑ serotonin | – ↑ astrocyte sensitivity |
| | – ↑ endogenous BZs |
| o ↓ glutamine receptors | |
| o ↓ dopamine/noradrenaline | – ↓ false neurotransmitters |
| o Glutamate (neuro-excitation) | – ↓ receptors → ↓ uptake of glutamate |
| | – ↓ glutamatergic neurotransmitter function |
| o ↑ nitric oxide (NO) | |
| o ↑ serotonin (arousal) | – ↑ serotonin turnover, synaptic defect |

Abbreviations: BZ, benzodiazepine; GABA-γ-aminobutyric acid

296

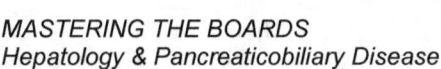

➢ Pathology

➢ Clinical

- Give a **grading stage** of the mental impairment of persons with HE.

Stage 0     – No clinical findings, but abnormal psychometric tests may progress to higher stages of HE (aka "minimal [preclinical] HE)

Stage 1     – Minor changes in
- Affect
- Sleep
- Concentration
– Trivial lack of awareness
– Euphoria or anxiety
– Shortened attention span
– Impaired performance of addition; sleep-wake disorder; tremor

Stage 2     – Drowsiness
– Disorientation
- Time or place
– Confusion
– Lethargy or apathy
– Subtle personality changes
– Inappropriate behavior
– Impaired performance of subtraction

297

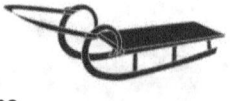

| Stage 3 | – Somnolence |
| | – Incoherence |
| | – Somnolence to semi-stupor, but responsive to verbal stimuli |
| | – Confusion |
| | – Gross disorientation |

Stage 4          – Coma (unresponsiveness to verbal or noxious stimuli), with
- Minimal response (4a)
- No response (4b)

Adapted from: Sleisenger and Fordtran's Gastrointestinal and Liver Disease. 10th Edition. Saunders/Elsevier, Philadelphia, 2016, Table 94.1, page 1579.

Patients with stage 0 to 2 HE and who can co-orperate with the physical examination will have tremor and asterixis. Patients with stage 3 or 4 may not be able to corporate for the clinical testing for these signs.

- Give the upper motor neuron (UMN) signs in stage 3 or 4 HE which can be demonstrated without the patient's co-orporation.

  o Hyperreflexia

  o Clonus

  o Hyperigidity

  o Positive Babinski sign

---

Clinical Tips when Assessing Risk of HE

"The absence of papilledema on fundoscopy and of typical features of cerebral edema on computer tomography (CT) of the head do not preclude the presence of cerebal edema complicating worsening encephalopathy" (Sleisenger and Fordtran's Gastrointestinal and Liver Disease. 9th Edition. Saunders/Elsevier 2010, page 1601).

---

➤ Laboratory
  o Blood concentrations of $NH_3$
    - Arterial or venous $NH_3$ concentrations are neither sensitive nor specific – please see Feldman M., et al. Sleisenger and Fordtran's Gastrointestinal and Liver Disease. 9th Edition. Saunders/Elsevier, Philadelphia, 2010, Table 92.1, for the Differential Diagnosis of Hyperammonemia.
    - Arterial hyperammonemia in 90% of HE
    - Arterial NH3 ≥ 200 mg/L predict brain edema and herniation of the brain stem
    - MRI based techniques

298

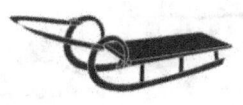

The finding of an elevated serum ammonia concentration is not specific for the diagnosis of hepatic encephalopathy.

- Give causes of hyperammonemia.
    - o Liver/GI tract
        - – Acute liver failure
        - – Cirrhosis
        - – Gastrointestinal bleeding
    - o Renal
        - – Chronic kidney disease
    - o Inborn errors of metabolism
        - – Proline metabolism disorders
        - – Urea cycle disorders (e.g carbamyl phosphate synthetase I deficiency, ornithine transcarbamylase deficiency, argininosuccinate lyase deficiency, *N*-acetyl glutamate synthetase deficiency)
    - o Medications
        - – Alcohol
        - – Diuretics (e.g., acetazolamide)
        - – Narcotics
        - – Valproic acid
    - o Muscle exertion and ischemia
    - o Blood sampling
        - – Tourniquet use
        - – High body temperature
        - – High protein diet
    - o Diet
    - o Cigarette smoking

Adapted from: *Sleisenger and Fordtran's Gastrointestinal and Liver Disease: Pathophysiology/ Diagnosis/ Management*. 10th edition, 2016, Box 94-1, page 1579.

- ➢ Diagnosis
    - o Exclude other causes of metabolic encephalopathy
    - o Exclude possible precipitating factors of HE
    - o Clinical examination

299

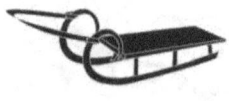

- o Altered neuropsychiatric testing
    - Number connection tests (Trail making)
    - Visuomotor skills
    - Mental tracking and concentration
    - Digit symbol test
    - Block design test
    - Standardized test battery, the psychometric HE score (PHES)
    - Digit span test (Weschler adult intelligence scale – passive auditory, working attention)
    - Critical flicker frequency (correlates with PHES [Psychometric hepatic encephalopathy score])
    - Quality of life measures: SE-36, chronic liver disease questionnaire (CLDQ)
- o Scoring systems
    - PSET (portosystemic encephalopathy syndrome test
    - Psychometric tests (Stage 0, minimal HE)
- o EEG abnormalities
    - Bilateral slow wave activity
    - Neither sensitive nor specific

---

Clinical caution:

- o Vitamin E deficiency is common in patients with cirrhosis (cholestasis → ↓ absorption of fat soluble vitamins → vitamin E deficiency

- o The neurological signs of vitamin E deficiency are similar to those of HE (hepatic encephalopathy).

- o Don't confuse the two; when in doubt, give vitamin E (tocopherol 1000 IU per day) to the patient with HE.

---

"We make a living by what we get, we make a life by what we give."

Winston Churchill

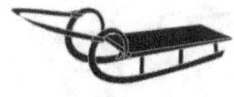

> Treatment

Diagnosis of hepatic encephalopathy

**Rule out other causes of encephalopathy**

- ❖ Drugs
  - ○ Sensitivity to CNS drugs
  - ○ Drug intoxication

- ❖ CNS
  - ○ Prior seizure or stroke (postictal confusion)
  - ○ Delirium tremens
  - ○ Wernicke-Korsakoff syndrome
  - ○ Intracerebral hemorrhage
  - ○ CNS sepsis
  - ○ Cerebral edema and/or intracranial hypertension*

- ❖ Lung
  - ○ Hypoxia
  - ○ Hypercapnia
  - ○ Acidosis

- ❖ Kidney
  - ○ Gross electrolyte changes
  - ○ Uremia

- ❖ Endocrine
  - ○ Hypoglycemia*
  - ○ Pancreatic encephalopathy

**Identify precipitating cause of hepatic encephalopathy**

- ○ Gastrointestinal hemorrhage
- ○ Constipation / dietary protein overload
- ○ Poor compliance with lactulose therapy
- ○ Recent anesthesia

- ○ Bowel obstruction or ileus

- ❖ Liver
  - ○ Prior portal decompression procedure (e.g., TIPS)*
  - ○ Superimposed hepatic injury*
  - ○ Development of hepatocellular carcinoma

- ○ Dehydration
- ○ Hypokalemia/alkalosis
- ○ Uremia

- ❖ CNS
  - ○ CNS active drugs
  - ○ Sepsis

**Initiate empiric treatment for hepatic encephalopathy**

- ○ Lactulose, oral dose of 1-30 ml twice daily
- ○ Rifaximin, oral dose of 550 mg twice daily
- ○ Neomycin, oral dose of 500 mg four times daily (use high doses with caution)
- ○ Metronidazole, oral dose of 250 mg four times daily
- ○ Vancomycin, oral dose of 250 mg four times daily
- ○ Sodium benzoate, oral dose 5 g twice daily (not approved for use in the USA)

- ○ Flumazenil, intravenous injection of 1-3 mg (potentially effective, but very short duration of action)

Abbreviation: AB, acid base

*Predominantly observed in patients with acute liver failure

301

- o Treat precipitants
  - Infections e.g., SBP, aspiration RTI
  - ↑ ammonia production
  - Excessive protein intake
  - Constipation
  - GI bleed (20%)
  - Azotemia (30%)
  - Hypokalemia
  - ↑ protein catabolism - surgery, diuretics, arterial hypotension/hypovolemia
  - Malnutrition
    - Skeletal muscle wasting (less muscle metabolism of $NH_3$ through muscle urea cycle)
    - Treat zinc deficiency
- Increased diffusion across BBB (alkalosis)
- Synergistic effects of cytokines – infection (SBP) (10%)
- Altered brain function – sedative drugs, psychotropics, analgesics, benzodiazepines; hyponatremia; astrocyte swelling
- Dehydration – fluid restriction, diuretics, excessive paracentesis, vomiting, diarrhea (mechanism unknown)
- Hypoxia, anemia, fever, sepsis
- Metabolic-:K+↓ (50%), hyperglycemia, alkalosis; ↓hypoxemia, thyroid, dehydration
- Drugs (30%) - benzodiazapines, analgesics, interferon, alcohol, NSAIDs, acetaminophen
- Surgery
- Shunting, anesthetic, TIPS
- Liver decompensation
  - HCC
  - PVT
  - BCS

Abbreviations: BBB, blood brain barrier; BCS, Budd-Chiari syndrome; HCC, hepatocellular cancer; PVT, portal vein thrombosis; RTI, respiratory tract infection; SBP, spontaneous bacterial peritonitis; TIPS, transjugular intrahepatic portosystemic shunt

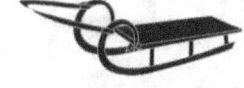

- Lactulose (beta-galactosidofructose), lacitol beta-galactosidosorbitol (traps NH₃)
  - Enters colon, broken down by colonic bacteria to lactic acid and acetic acid, with acidification of stool pH < 5

$$NH_3 \xrightarrow{pH < 5} NH_4^+ \text{ (non-absorbable)}$$

  - Lactulose enemas (300 mL in 1L of water) in patients who are unable to take lactulose po
  - Lactulose 30 mL p.o every 1-2 h until bowel evacuation, then adjust to a dosage that will result in 2-3 formed bowel movements per day (usually 15-30 mL po bid)
  - Lactulose can be discontinued once the precipitating factor has resolved
- Hyperosmolar purgation (including lactulose)
- ↑ stool volume
- ↑ loss of nitrogen compounds
- Acarbose
  - α-glucosidic inhibitor → ↓ glucose absorption → ↓ proteolytic urea producing luminal microbiotica → ↓ NH₃
- Antibiotics (pre-, pro- and synbiotics)
  - ↑ lactobacillus spp., ↓ urease-containing bacteria → ↓ NH₃ production
  - ↑ bacterial NH₃ utilization
  - ↓ pro-inflammatory response
  - ↓ gut permeability
  - ↓ bacterial translocation

---

SO YOU WANT TO BE A HEPATOLOGIST!

A patient with cirrhosis develops HE (hepatic encephalopathy) is treated with antibiotics, and their MELD score rises.

- Give the explanation for this deterioration in HE with antibiotics.
  - Antibiotic for HE reduce the intestinal microbiotica
  - This ↓ microbiotica → ↓ bacterial synthesis of vitamin K
  - With ↓ bacterial vitamin K available for absorption and production of coagulation factors (II, VII, IX, X, protein C), the INR rises
  - ↑ INR contributes points to ↑ MELD score

303

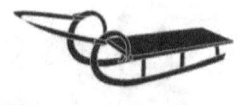

- L-ornithine-L-aspartate (LOLA)
  - Activate the urea cycle → ↑ $NH_3$ clearance
  - Improves grade 3 or 4 HE in ~ 25% of patients
- Neurotransmitters: flumazenil (a competitive GABA-benzodiazepine receptor antagonist) or bromocriptine
- Nutrition
  - Treat malnutrition, including EN (enteral nutrition), and TPN (total parental nutrition)
  - Treat associated zinc deficiency
  - Branched chain amino acids
  - Short term (< 72 hr) protein restriction may be considered in severe HE, but is not used for mild to moderate HE
  - No longterm protein restriction
- Intracranial pressure (ICP) monitoring
  - Transcranial Doppler
  - Jugular venous oximetry
  - 45° elevation of head of bed
  - Moderate hypothermia to
    - ↓ ICP and cerebral blood flow (CBF)
  - ↓ arterial $NH_3$
  - ↓ cerebral $NH_3$ uptake
  - IV mannitol
    - ↓ ICP
  - Hyperventilation
    - Vasoconstriction → ↓ CBF
  - Manage circulatory effects
  - Fluid management, consider central venous pressure (CVP) monitoring
  - Manage lactic acidosis and sepsis
  - Perform short synacthen test, and give glucocorticosteroids if adrenal insufficiency is present
  - Inotropes: terlipressin (a vasopressin analog) or norepinephrine
  - Albumin infusion
- Extracorporeal liver assist devices (ELADs)
  - MARS (molecular absorbent recirculating system): providing counter-current hemodialysis against albumin and bicarbonate circuits
  - SPAD (single-pass albumin dialysis): counter-current albumin dialysis against high blood flow in a fibre hemodin filter, and continuous veno-venous hemofiltration
  - Prometheus R system, direct albumin adsorption through a specific polysulfur filter
  - Enteral feeding/TPN

304

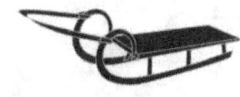

- o Orthoptic liver transplantation
  - – Removes shunted (non-detoxified blood)
  - – ↓ production of potentially toxic SCFA (proprionate, butyrate, violerate)

Adapted from: Sleisenger and Fordtran's Gastrointestinal and Liver Disease. 10<sup>th</sup> Edition. Saunders/Elsevier, Philadelphia, 2016, page 1579-1580.

- o Sedation (e.g., for EGD and EVL)
  - – Propofol safe in cirrhosis with no Δ cognition
  - – Midazolam or fentanyl worsens HE
    - ▪ NCT (number connecting time), i.e., ↑ severity of HE score
    - ▪ ↑ agitation
  - – Titrate sedation to point where patient's speech is slurred.
- o Note: osmotic agents (e.g., lactulose) and antibiotics (metronidazole, neomycin, rifaximin) helps symptoms, but do not change in mortality rate

**Minimal Hepatic Encephalopathy** (MHE; aka stage 0 HE, or preclinical HE))

- • Give reasons to treat MHE.
  - o ↑ cognitive function
  - o ↑ driving performance
  - o ↑ performance in workplace
  - o ↑ quality of life
  - o ↑ sleep
  - o ↑ survival
  - o ↓ development of overt clinically evident HE

Adapted from: Ortiz M, et al. *J Hepatol* 2005;42 Suppl(1):S45-53.

- • Give management options for MHE.
  - o Give same treatment as for stages 1 – 4 HE, e.g.,
    - – Reverse any precipitants (e.g., drugs)
    - – Cathartics: Lactulose
    - – Antibiotics: Flagyl, vancomycin, ampicillin, rifamycin
    - – Probiotics
    - – High calorie, high protein diet

Adapted from: Holstege A, et al. *Best Practice & Research Clinical Gastroenterology* 2007; 21(3): pg. 541.

305

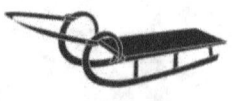

➤ Prognosis

• Give the survival rate and etiological factors for the 3 types of hepatic encephalopathy (acute liver failure, cirrhosis with precipitant, and chronic HE).

| Type of HE | Approximate Survival | Etiological Factors |
|---|---|---|
| o Acute liver failure | ~ 20% | – Viral hepatitis<br>– Alcoholic hepatitis<br>– Drug reactions and overdose |
| o Cirrhosis w/precipitant | ~ 80% | – Drugs/toxins<br>  ▪ Diuretics<br>  ▪ Alcoholic excess<br>  ▪ Sedatives<br>– Infection<br>  ▪ Any type, including SBP<br>– Volume loss<br>  ▪ Hemorrhage<br>  ▪ Paracentesis<br>  ▪ Diarrhea/vomiting<br>– Surgery<br>– Constipation |
| o Chronic HE | ~100% | – Portal-systemic shunting<br>– ↑ Dietary protein intake<br>– Intestinal bacteria |

"Success is liking yourself, liking what you do, and liking how you do it."
Maya Angelou

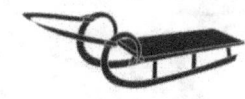

# PULMONARY COMPLICATIONS OF CHRONIC LIVER DISEASE

## Dyspnea

- Give potential causes of **increasing dyspnea** in a patient with chronic liver disease.
  - Cardiac failure (including cirrhotic cardiomyotomy, and tricuspid valve incompetence)
  - Pulmonary hypertension (portopulmonary hypertension syndrome, PPH)
  - Pleural/pericardial effusions
  - Atelectasis secondary to ascites
  - Pulmonary embolus
  - Pulmonary infection
  - Pulmonary fibrosis (methotrexate)
  - Interstitial lung disease
  - Acidosis
  - Severe anemia
  - Hepatopulmonary syndrome (HPS)
  - Liver disease caused by
    - Cystic fibrosis
    - $\alpha_1$ – antitrypin deficiency
    - Pulmonary fibrosis from use of methotrexate

Adapted from: Kim YK, et al. *Radiographics* 2009;29(3):825-37.

- Give the laboratory/radiological tests for the investigation of the pulmonary complications of cirrhosis.
  - CVS
    - ECG
    - Echocardiogram with Doppler
    - Right heart angiogram
  - Lung
    - CXR (chest x-ray; normal)
    - CT chest
    - ABG in erect and supine positions, for A-a O2 gradient
    - Hemoglobin concentration, electrolytes
    - PFTs (pulmonary function tests)
    - Echo bubble (shunting)
    - Pleural tap
  - Ascites
    - Radiolabeled ascites scan (technetium – labeled scan)
    - Methylene blue injection followed by tap of pulmonary fluid

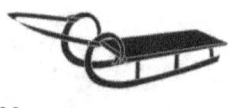

Adapted from: Sleisenger and Fordtran's Gastrointestinal and Liver Disease. 10th Edition. Saunders/Elsevier, Philadelphia, 2016, page 1584 – 1587.

**Hepatic Hydrothorax**

- Give characteristics of pleural fluid in hepatic hydrothorax.

  - Cell count < 250 polymorphonuclear cells mm$^3$ (uncomplicated)

  - Protein < 2.5 g/dL

  - Pleural fluid/serum total protein ratio <0.5

  - Pleural fluid/serum lactate dehydrogenase ratio >0.6

  - Pleural fluid/serum albumin gradient >1.1

  - Pleural fluid/serum bilirubin ration <0.6

  - pH >7.4

  - Glucose level similar to that of serum

  - Note: The pressure of hepatic hydrothorax indicates a bad prognosis

Printed with permission: Cárdenas A, and Arroyo V. *Best Practice & Research Clinical Gastroenterology* 2007; 21(1): pg. 69.


**Hepatopulmonary syndrome** (HPS)

➢ Definition

  - ↑ Aa PO$_2$ (age-corrected alveolar-arterial oxygen) gradient (< 64 years, 15 mmHg; > 64 years, 20 mmHg) arising from intrapulmonary vasodilation

  - Diagnostic approach if PO$_2$ from pulse oximeter is < 96, then there is likely moderate severe HRS (Pa O$_2$ < 70 mmHg; sensitivity 100%, specificity 88%)

  - Diagnosis made by transthoracic echocardiography with contrast (technetium-labeled macroaggregated albumin) to detect > 6% shunt fraction

  - Delay of microbubbles reaching the left ventricle on V echo bubble study

Abbreviations: AaPO$_2$, alveolar-arterial O$_2$ pressure gradient for oxygen; PaO$_2$, partial pressure gradient for oxygen; $^{99m}$Tc-MAA, perfusion body scan with $^{99m}$ Technetium-labeled macroaggregated albumin

Printed with permission: Pastor CM, and Schiffer E. Nature *Clinical Practice Gastroenterology & Hepatology* November 2007;4(11): pg 615.

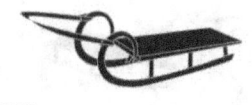

➢ Pathophysiology

    o Intra-pulmonary vasodilation and shunting occurring in the presence of chronic liver disease or pulmonary hypertension, resulting in acute or alveolar-arterial $O_2$ gradient > 15 mmHg (> 20 mmHg for persons > 64 yrs)

---

## SO YOU WANT TO BE A HEPATOLOGIST!

About half of patients with cirrhosis have intrapulmonary vasodilation, but only when this is severe does HPS occur. The increased production of nitric oxide (NO) and carbon monoxide are important in the pathophysiology of HPS.

- Give the mechanisms responsible for the increase in NO (nitric oxide) and CO (carbon monoxide) in cirrhosis complicated by hepatorenal syndrome.

    o NO   –  ↑ production / release of endothelin – 1 → ↑ endothelin – B receptors in pulmonary microvasculature → ↑ eNos (endothelin-1-mediated endothelial NO synthase → ↑ NO

        – ↑ bacterial translocation in gut → ↑ TNF-α → ↑ macrophages adhering to pulmonary vessels → ↑ iNos (inducible NO synthase) → ↑ NO

    o CO   –  The ↑ adherence of macrophages to pulmoandy vessels ↑ the production of CO through heme oxygenase-1

---

➢ Clinical

- Give the clinical changes which suggest that the patient with cirrhosis has developed HPS (hepatopulmonary syndrome).

    o Presence of cirrhosis plus
        – Platypnea (↑ SOB [shortness of breath] on sitting up)
        – Cyanosis (especially distal)
        – Clubbing
        – Permanent telangiectasias of the face (angiomas)

    o Hypoxemia (PaO2 < 70 mmHg) is usually present, together with cyanosis and clubbing

    o SOBOE
        – Mechanism of platynea (dyspnea worse when sitting up and better when lying down
        – The result of reduction of intra-pulmonary shunting when lying down, with improved oxygenation due to blood going to both lower and upper parts of the lungs.

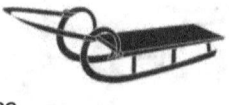

309

- Orthodeoxia (worsening of hypoxemia when person sits up or stands) is due to more blood going to the lower lungs when standing, more intra-pulmonary shunting, and a drop in blood gas arteria $PaO_2$ decreasing by more than 4 mmHg
- Orthodeoxia occurs in HPS, ASD (atrial septal defect) and recurrent pulmonary emboli; oxygen desaturation during sleep may occur with orthodeoxia
- Chronic liver disease patients with numerous spider angiomas are more likely to have HPS
- Suspect HPS if alveolar-arterial $PaO_2$ gradient on room air is > 15 mmHg, and if $PaO_2$ is < 70 mmHg, or if arterial blood gas $PaO_2$ falls by more than 4 mmHg on standing
- Seen in 4-24% of persons being evaluated for liver transplantation

---

### SO YOU WANT TO BE A HEPATOLOGIST!

Clubbing is common in persons with liver disease, but when it is associated with distal cyanosis, HPS is suspected. Neither the presence nor the severity of HPS reflect the severity of the associated liver disease and its dysfunction.

- In this setting, give the difference between platypnea and orthodeoxia.
  - Platypnia      – Dyspnea, which is
    - ↑ when upright
    - ↓ when supine
  - Orthodeoxia      – Hypoxia/hypoxemia, which is
    - ↑ when upright

---

➤ Laboratory
  - ↑ $AaPO_2$ and ↓ $PaO_2$
  - Orthodeoxia (↑ hypoxemia on sitting up)
  - Lung perfusion showing brain uptake > 40% (↑ intrapulmonary shunting)

➤ Diagnostic imaging
  - Pulmonary vascular dilation at contrast-enhanced echocardiography or $^{99m}$Tc-MAA
  - Pulmonary vasodilation on chest CT
  - Tests of pulmonary shunting
    - Using technetium macro-aggregated albumin

➤ Pulmonary function testing (PFT)
  - ↓ diffusion capacity on pulmonary function testing (PFT)

310

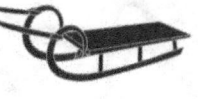

➢ Treatment

Therapies for hepatopulmonary syndrome have only been tested in small and uncontrolled trials.

- o Oxygen therapy
  - Oxygen therapy (0.5 l/min at rest and 2 l/min during exercise) prevents the deleterious consequences of hypoxemia
  - Treatment for 1 year had a beneficial effect on liver function in two patients (their Child-Pugh score markedly improved (Fukushima et al).

- o Transjugular intrahepatic portosystemic shunt
  - The placement of a transjugular intrahepatic portosystemic shunt (TIPS) to relieve portal hypertension that might participate in the pathophysiology of HPS has failed to improve patient outcome.

- o Cavoplasty and coil emboli
  - In some patients with Budd-Chiari syndrome (BCS), cavoplasty reversed HPS.
  - The injection of coil emboli that preferentially distribute to dilated vessels might also decrease hypoxemia by obstructing flow to these areas.

- o Pentoxifylline
  - Pentoxifylline inhibits tumour necrosis factor-α overproduction and is effective in attenuating HPS in rats with ligated common bile ducts. The drug has not been tested in patients with HPS.

- o Nitric oxide inhibition
  - ↑ production of nitric oxide (NO) causes pulmonary vascular dilatation
  - Therapies that reduce pulmonary NO levels or control its effects have been tested.
  - By blocking the NO-induced activation of guanylate cyclase in smooth muscle cells, methylene blue has been shown to improve pulmonary vascular dilatation and hypoxemia.
  - Inhalation of the NO synthase inhibitor $N^G$-nitro-arginine methyl ester, reduces intrapulmonary vascular dilatation, also improved by the $PaO_2$ and decreases the associated dyspnea in some patients
  - It is disputed whether there is any benefit from inhibiting the NO-cyclic guanosine monophosphate pathway (Almeida *et al).*

- o Liver transplantation
  - $O_2$, TIPS, liver transplantation
  - Prolonged post-operative mechanical ventilation may be needed
  - Mortality rate after liver transplantation is high

Printed with permission: Pastor CM, and Schiffer E. *Nature Clinical Practice Gastroenterology & Hepatology* 2007; 4(11): pg. 615.

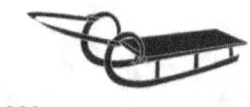

**Portopulmonary Hypertension** (PPH)

➤ Definition
- o Portal hypertension associated with hepatic cirrhosis

➤ Demography
- o Occurs in 0.25-4.0% of persons with end-stage liver disease, and usually within 4-7 years of the diagnosis of portal hypertension (PHT) (even though there is not a direct correlation between the development of PPH and PHT

➤ Pathogenesis
- o Cirrhosis causes ↑ PA (pulmonary artery) pressure due to
  - − Volume overload and ↑ cardiac output (from ↓ systemic vascular resistance and hyperdynamic circulation)
- o ↑ pulmonary vascular resistance in PPH →
  - − ↓ NO plus ↑ endothelin-1 → PA vasoconstriction
  - − Obliteration of pulmonary arterioles may occur from intimal proliferation, adventitial fibrosis, and thrombosis of pulmonary vasculature
  - − ↑ MPAP > 25 mmHg
  - − ↑ PVR > 240 dynes /s / cm$^{-5}$
  - − ↓ PCWP < 15 mmHg
- o ↑ mPAP (mean pulmonary arterial pressure)
  - − > 25 mmHg, at rest
  - − > 30 mmHg, with exercise
- o ↑ PVR (pulmonary vascular resistance) > 240 dynes / sec / cm$^{-5}$
- o The presence of
  - − PHT (pulmonary hypertension)
  - − Portosystemic shunts
  - − Hemodynamic abnormalities in portal vein
- o Severity
  - − Mild, mPAP of 25 to 35 mmHg
  - − Moderate, mPAP of 35 to 50 mmHg
  - − Severe, mPAP of > 50 mmHg (prohibitive operative mortality from liver transplantation

Abbreviations: MPAP, mean pulmonary artery pressure; AVR, pulmonary vascular resistance; PCWP, pulmonary capillary wedge pressure

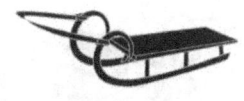

- Clinical
  - Fatigue, SOBOE, orthopnea, hemoptysis, palpitations
  - Hypoxemia and cyanosis are absent
  - PPH is more common in persons with cirrhosis and refractory ascites, and in 12% of persons evaluated for liver transplantation

- Differential

- Give how to distinguish between hepatopulmonary syndrome (HPS) and portopulmonary hypertension (PPH).

| Clinical | Hepatopulmonary syndrome (HRS: AV shunts) | Portopulmonary hypertension (PPH: constriction of pulmonary vessels) |
|---|---|---|
| Prevalence in cirrhotics evaluated for LT | - ~ 25% | ▪ 5% |
| Symptomatology | – Progressive dyspnea SOB on sitting up | ▪ Chest pain<br>▪ SOB on lying down |
| Pathophysiology | - ↑ VEGF → ↑ angiogenesis<br>- ↓ gas exchange – hypoxemia<br>- Intrapulmonary vasodilation in precapillary and capillary PA circulation due to vasoactive mediators | ▪ Vasoconstriction<br>▪ Remodeling of resistance vessels<br>▪ ↑ PAP<br>- Medial proliferation and hypertrophy<br>- Arteriopathy<br>- Thrombosis<br>- ↑ endothelin – 1 |
| Production of NO and CO | - ↑ (↑ iNos, ↑ HO-1) | ▪ Normal |
| Clinical examination | - Platypnea<br>- Cyanosis<br>- Finger clubbing<br>- Spider angiomas | ▪ No cyanosis<br>▪ RV heave<br>▪ Pronounced P2 component |
| ECG findings | - None | ▪ RBBB, rightward axis<br>▪ RV hypertrophy<br>▪ No/mild hypoxemia |
| Arterial blood gas levels | - Moderate-to-severe hypoxemia | |

313

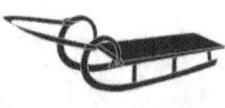

| Clinical | Hepatopulmonary syndrome (HRS: AV shunts) | Portopulmonary hypertension (PPH: constriction of pulmonary vessels) |
|---|---|---|
| ○ Chest radiograph | - Normal | ▪ Cardiomegaly<br>▪ Hilar enlargement |
| ○ CEE | - Tri-regurg; Always positive; left atria opacification for >3-6 cardiac cycles after right atrial opacification > 6% | |
| ○ 99mTcMAA shunting index ("bubble study") | - Normal/low PVR | ▪ Usually negative. Positive for <3 cardiac cycles; if arterial septal defect or patent foramen ovale<br>▪ < 6% roatrial opacification<br>▪ Elevated PVR<br>▪ Normal mPAOP<br>▪ Large pulmonary arteries |
| ○ Pulmonary hemodynamics | - Normal/spongy appearance (type I) | ▪ Distal arterial pruning |
| ○ Pulmonary angiography | - Discrete arteriovenous communications (type II) (usually lower lobe) | ▪ Only indicated in mild-to-moderate stages |
| ○ OLT | - Always indicated in severe stages | ▪ Late contraindication |
| ○ MELD exception points | - Yes | ▪ No |
| ○ Role of LT | - Reverses HPS in 80% | ▪ Nuclear |

Abbreviations: 99mTcMAA, technetium-99 m-labelled macroaggregated albumin; CEE, contrast enhanced echocardiography; ECG, electrocardiogram; HPS, hepatopulmponary syndrome; OLT, orthotopic liver transplantation; PAOP, mean pulmonary artery occlusion pressure; PAP, pulmonary arterial pressure; PVR, pulmonary vascular resistance; RBBB, right bundle branch block; SOB, shortness of breath (aka dyspnea)

Printed with permission: Herve P, et al. *Best Practice & Research Clinical Gastroenterology* 2007; 21(1): pg. 142.

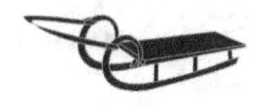

- ➢ Treatment
  - ○ Bosentan (anti-endothelin activity) plus sildenafil (a phosphodiesterase – inhibitor) and prostacyclin reduce PA pressure
  - ○ Anticoagulation plus long-term $O_2$ therapy
  - ○ Liver transplantation
  - ○ Liver transplantation only offered when MPAP > 25 but < 35 mmHg

Abbreviations: PA, pulmonary artery; PHT, portal hypertension; PPH, portopulmonary hypertension; SOBOE, shortness of breath on exertion

- ➢ Prognosis
  - ○ Median survival for persons with PPH is only 2 years without liver transplantation, but 91% 1 year survival from liver transplantation

---

MCQ TIPS: "Buzz Word" Associations

| | | |
|---|---|---|
| ○ | NASH | – Ballooning hepatocytes |
| | | – Mallory bodies |
| | | – Portal and lobular inflammation |
| | | – Chicken-wire fibrosis |
| ○ | PBC | – Florid duct lesion |
| | | – Ductopenia |
| | | – Granulomas |
| ○ | PSC | – "onion-skinning" obliterative fibrosis |
| | | – Infiltration of limiting plate |
| | | – Interface hepatitis |
| ○ | Congestive hepatopathy aka "nutmeg liver" | – Speckled appearance |
| | | • Dark areas (Dilated blood-filled hepatic venules) |
| | | • Light areas (Normal hepatic parenchyma) |
| ○ | α-1 AT | – PAS-positive, diastase resistant globules in the ER (endoplastic reticulum) of hepatocytes |
| ○ | HBV "ground glass" hepatocytes | – HBsAg in ER of hepatocytes giving dull appearance of hepatocytes in chronic HAV. |

  - ○ The laparoscopic appearance suggestive of peritoneal TB
    - – "millet-seed"
    - – "violin-string"

Abbreviations: α-1 AT, alpha-1 antitrypsin deficiency; HBV, hepatitis B virus; MCQ, multiple choice questions; NASH, non-alcoholic steatohepatitis; PBC, primary biliary cholangitis; PSC, primary sclerosing cholangitis

---

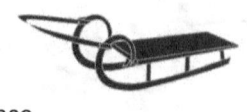

# PREGNANCY AND THE LIVER

- ➤ Incidence
    - ○ 1/200
        - – Hyperemesis gravidarium
        - – HELLP (hemolysis, elevated LFTs, low platelets)
    - ○ 1/1000 ICP (intrahepatic cholestasis of pregnancy)
    - ○ 1/10,000 AFLD (acute fatty liver of pregnancy)

- ➤ Clinical
    - ○ Palmar erythema and spider angiomas occur in two thirds of women with normal pregnancies

- ➤ Laboratory
- • Give which liver enzymes/tests of liver function increase, decrease, or remain unchanged in normal pregnancy.
    - ○ Unchanged
        - – AST, ALT
        - – INR
        - – Bilirubin
        - – GGT
    - ○ Increased
        - – Alkaline phosphatase (↑ 2-400%)
        - – Fibrinogen (↑ 50%)
        - – α- and ß- globulins
        - – Alpha-fetoprotein*
        - – Leukocytes
        - – Ceruloplasmin
        - – Cholesterol
        - – Triglycerides
    - ○ Decreased
        - – γ- globulin
        - – Platelets (>50,000)
        - – Hemoglobin
        - – Albumin

* Moderate increase, especially with twins

Abbreviations: ALT, alanine aminotransferase; AST, aspartate aminotransferase

Adapted from Hay E. *Mayo Clinic Board Review* 2008: pg. 419.

316

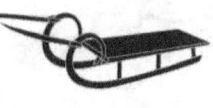

## Drugs in Pregnancy

- Give physiological mechanisms which contribute to the altered metabolism of some drugs during pregnancy.

    - ↑ maternal blood volume (50%)

    - ↓ maternal serum albumin concentration (20%)

    - Progesterone → proliferation of SER

    - Estrogen → proliferation of RER

    - ↑ cytochrome P-450 gene products

    - Increased maternal nitric oxide (NO) release during pregnancy causes maternal vasodilation, ↓ systemic vascular resistance, mean arterial blood pressure, reduced responsiveness to vasoconstrictors, resulting in maternal cardiac output rising 30-50%, sixth activation of the rennin-angiotensin system, and increased GFR as well as renal blood flow.

- Give the FDA category and risk of liver disease-treating drugs during pregnancy and lactation.

| Drug | FDA Class | Risk in Pregnancy | Risk with Nursing |
|---|---|---|---|
| Adefovir | C | Low risk | + |
| **Anti-rejection drugs** | C | **Not recommended** | |
| B blockers | C 1st trimester | IUGR, fetal brachycardia, hypoglycemia | - |
| **Cyclosporine** | **D** | | + |
| **D-penicillamine** | **X** | **Teratogenic** | |
| **Interferon** | C | **Not recommended** | + |
| Lamuvidine | C | Low risk | - |
| **Methotrexate** | **X** | **Contraindicated** | |
| Metronidazole | B | | |
| **Octreotide*** | **B** | Uterine ischemia | + |
| **Penicillamine** | **D** | **Significant embryopathy** | - |
| **Ribavirin** | **X** | **Contraindicated** | + |
| **Thalidomide** (IBD) | **X** | **Contraindicated** | |
| Trientine | C | Alternative to penicillamine | - |
| Ursodiol (UDCA) | B | Low risk | + |

- Octreotide is useful to stop the bleeding from esophageal varices (EV) in males and in non-pregnant females
- In the setting of a pregnant woman with
  - Bleeding EV, infusion of octreotide may result in ischemia of the uterus, and the induction of premature labor, so do **not** use.

Note: Avoid the "X" medications for 6 months before conception.

Printed with permission: Katz PO. *2008 ACG What's New in Pharmacology Course:* pg. 50.

- Give medications used in gastroenterology and hepatology which have an FDA (food and drug administration, USA) "X" category of fetal risk.
  - Ribavirin (HCV)
  - Thalidomide
  - D-penicillamine
  - Methotrexate (IBD)
  - Cyclosporine

- Give the FDA class and risk of liver transplantation-treating drugs during pregnancy and lactation.

| | Drug | FDA Class | Risk in Pregnancy | Risk with Nursing |
|---|---|---|---|---|
| o | Antithymocyte globulin | C | Low risk | UN |
| o | Mycophenolate | C | Do not use | + |
| o | OKT3 | C | Probably low risk | - |
| o | Sirolimus | C | Do not use | - |
| o | Tacrolimus | C | Use if necessary | - |

Abbreviation: UN, unknown

Printed with permission: Katz PO. *2008 ACG What's New in Pharmacology Course:* pg. 50; and Mahadevan U. *Best Practice & Research Clinical Gastroenterology* 2007; 21(5): pg. 867.

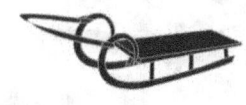

## Cholelithiasis in Pregnancy

- Give changes in bile acid metabolism which occur during pregnancy, and which increase the risk of **choletithiasis** (but not acute cholecystitis).

  o ↑ cholesterol

  o ↑ supersaturation of bile with cholesterol

  o ↑ bile acid pool size

  o ↑ cholic acid

  o ↓ chenic acid (chenodeoxycholic acid)

  o ↑ volume of gallbladder (fasting/fed states)

  o ↓ gallbladder contraction

A trick question

- Give the effect of pregnancy on the prevalence of cholelithiasis, and the incidence of acute cholecystitis.

  o Cholelithiasis ↑

  o Acute cholecystitis – no change from non-pregnant state

- Give factors associated with ↑ risk of recurrent cholestasis of pregnancy.

  o Further pregnancies

  o Use of oral contraceptive agents (OCAs)

  o Cholecystectomy for ↑ risk of cholelithiasis, cholecystitis, pancreatitis

  o Use of progesterone during subsequent pregnancy

319

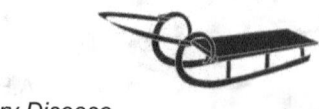

- o Use of estrogen
  - – The increased risk of biliary sludge (10-30%) and cholelithiasis (2-3% of all pregnant women) during pregnancy is due to
    - Estrogen-associated with increased transport of cholesterol into bile from the liver
    - solubilization of this cholesterol as the result of reduced hepatobiliary transport of bile acids and phosphoplipids
    - Slowing of gallbladder emptying contributes to the formation of stones
    - Pregnancy-associated increase in estrogens increases the risk of biliary pain in 28% of pregnant women who had pre-existing gallstones

**Viral hepatitis** may flare in pregnancy, and gallstones form in pregnancy, and both these as well as pre-existing gallstones may become symptomatic.

- Give how to differentiate between viral hepatitis versus symptomatic gallstones in pregnancy.

| Findings | Viral Hepatitis (flaring in pregnancy) | Gallstones |
|---|---|---|
| o Nausea/vomiting | Yes | Variable |
| o Abdominal pain | Variable | Variable |
| o Pre-eclampsia | No | No |
| o Cholestasis | Mild to marked | Marked |
| o AST/ALT elevation | High | Low |
| o Coagulopathy | Rare and late (acute fulminant) | No |
| o Hepatic failure | Rare | No |
| o U/S | Nonspecific | Dilated bile ducts, stones |
| o Management of mother and child | Support<br><br>HBV – Lamivudine for mother, $mT_3$ HBIG at birth for child; immunize child<br><br>HCV – none; check child at 18 weeks | Support, avoid cholecystectomy if possible |

Please see: Swan MG. Chapter 58. In: Therapeutic Choices. Grey J, Ed. 6th Edition, Canadian Pharmacists Association: Ottawa, ON, 2011, Table 4: Cholestatic Liver Disease, page 776-777.

320

## Cirrhosis in Pregnancy

- Give the complications of cirrhosis in the pregnant patient.

  - In the pregnant woman with cirrhosis, the maternal mortality rate is 10%, and there is a 3-25% risk of abortion, premature birth and perinatal death.

  - In the pregnant woman with portal hypertension, 18-50% will bleed during pregnancy from esophageal varices

## Liver Disorders seen only in Pregnancy

- Give the trimester (T) in pregnancy of the onset and treatment of liver diseases unique to pregnancy.

| Liver Disease | Onset | Treatment |
|---|---|---|
| o Hyperemesis gravidarum | T1 | – Supportive care, rehydration |
| o Intrahepatic cholestasis of pregnancy (ICP) | T2-3 | – Ursodeoxycholic acid (UDCA) or cholestyramine |
| | | – Preterm delivery if fetal compromised |
| o Pre-eclampsia and eclampsia | T2-3 | – Antihypertensive drugs, magnesium sulfate |
| o HELLP syndrome | T3 | – Induction of delivery |
| o Acute fatty liver of pregnancy | T3 | – Consider early induction of delivery |

HELLP, a syndrome characterized by hemolysis, elevated liver enzymes and a low platelet count; T, trimester

Printed with permission: Keller Jutta, et al. *Nature Clinical Practice Gastroenterology & Hepatology* 2008: 5(8): pg. 437.

- **T1-first trimester**

❖ Nausea and vomiting in pregnancy

  - Nausea and vomiting are common in pregnancy, usually beginning by week 4 to 6, and settling by week 20.

  - Hyperemesis gravidarum (HG) is severe, persistent vomiting which requires medical therapy

  - The PUQE score (pregnancy-unique quantification of nausea and emesis) may be used to assist in directing therapy for HG

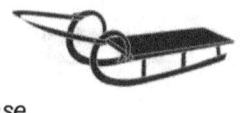

**Hyperemesis Gravidarium** (HG)

- Give mechanisms for the development of hyperemesis gravidarium (HG), and its associated conditions.

❖ Mechanisms
- o Gastroparesis – estrogen, progesterone
- o Obesity ($\uparrow$ estrogen)
- o Gastric infection –H. pylori
- o Hormone changes
  - HCG
  - Estrogen
  - Progesterone
  - Thyroid hormones
  - Leptin

❖ Associations
- o Female fetus
- o Multiple gestation
- o Trophoblastic disease
- o Trisomy 21 (Down syndrome)
- o Hydrops fetalis
- o Personal/family history

Abbreviation: HCG, human chorionic gonadotropin

- **T2 – Second Trimester**

❖ Intrahepatic cholestasis of pregnancy (ICP)

➤ Demography
- o Present in 2% of pregnancies in America, 6% in Chile and Scandinavia
- o 10-15% of first degree relatives of women with ICP also develop ICP
- o 3rd trimester

➤ Pathophysiology
- o Usual cholestatic effects of estrogen in pregnancy, plus
- o Genetic predisposition (imitations in canalicular transporters for bile acids, phospholipids and cholesterol [amino phospholipid flippase], as well as FXR, the nuclear regulator of bile acid synthesis)

322

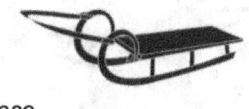

- ➢ Risk factors
  - o Previous ICP (50% recurrence)
  - o Multiple pregnancies
  - o Multiple gestations
  - o Descent
    - Chilean
    - Scandinavian

- ➢ Clinical
  - o Usual presentation is painless jaundice and pruritus, possibly due to elevated serum bile acid concentrations
  - o Generalized pruritus of skin especially on palms & soles but no rash
  - o Second or third trimester ($T_2$, $T_3$)
  - o Fetal complications
    - Usually occur after 32 weeks and include
      - Intrauterine growth retardation
      - Fetal distress
      - Premature labour
      - Stillbirth (fetal death rates in ICP are two-fold increased, usually occur between 37-40 weeks, are associated with much higher concentrations of serum bile acids, and may be sudden and intrauterine
    - For this reason the fetus should be delivered early [36-37 weeks of pregnancy]
    - The newborn may have meconium ileus
    - When serum bile acids > 40 µmol/L, ↑ risk of complications
    - Increase risk for
      - Prematurity
      - still birth
      - spontaneous preterm labour and delivery,
      - fetal compromise,
      - fetal cardiac dysrhythmias
      - meconium stained amniotic fluid, and intrauterine fetal death
  - o Maternal complications
    - Vitamin K deficiency
    - Coagulopathy postpartum hemorrhage
    - Pruritus and abnormal laboratory tests resolve with delivery
    - Recurs 40-60%)with subsequent gestations

323

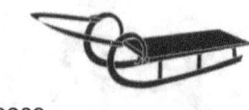

- Increased risk for cesarean delivery due to fetal compromise
- Can recur with subsequent use of oral contraceptives (OCAs) and hormonal fluctuations
- Recurrence of ICP (~50%)
- ↑ risk of need for Cesarean section delivery
- ↑ risk of
  - Cholelithiasis
  - Cholestasis with use of OCAs
  - Cholecystitis
  - Pancreatitis

Schutt VA, and Minuk GY. *Best Practice & Research Clinical Gastroenterology* 2007; 21(5): pg. 778.

➢ Laboratory

  ○ ↑↑↑ serum alkaline phosphatase, bilirubin, and serum bile acids > 10 µmol/L

  ○ ALT/AST may be ↑ 20x

  ○ LEs/LFTs fluctuate

Abbreviations: Les, liver enzymes; LFTs, liver function tests

➢ Histopathology

  ○ Liver biopsy is not necessary to make the diagnosis, but would show intrahepatic centralobular cholestasis, with bile plugs in cannaliculi and hepatocytes

➢ Prognosis

• Give the fetal and maternal outcomes of intrahepatic cholestasis of pregnancy.

| Maternal Outcome | Fetal Outcome |
| --- | --- |
| ○ Pruritus and abnormal laboratory tests resolve with delivery | - Increase risk for<br>  ▪ Prematurity |
| ○ Recurs 40-60%) with subsequent gestations | ▪ Still birth |
| | ▪ Spontaneous preterm labour and delivery, |
| ○ Increased risk for cesarean delivery due to fetal compromise | ▪ Fetal compromise, |
| ○ Can recur with subsequent use of oral contraceptives (OCAs) and hormonal fluctuations | ▪ Fetal cardiac dysrhythmias, |
| | ▪ Meconium stained amniotic fluid, and intrauterine fetal death |

324

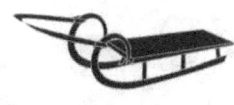

> Treatment

- Give the **medical treatment** of cholestatic disorders during pregnancy.

| Indication/Drug | Fetal Risk (FDA Category) | Use and Safety |
|---|---|---|
| o Immune-mediated disorders | | |
| - UDCA | B | Low risk after T1 |
| - Prednisolone | C | Low risk: increased risk of cleft palate, adrenal insufficiency |
| - Azathioprine | **D** | Low risk |
| o Bacterial cholangitis | | |
| - Ampicillin | B | Low risk |
| o Sedation and analgesia | | |
| - Fentanyl | C | Use in low doses |
| - Meperidine | B | Use in low doses |
| - Midazolam | **D** | Use in low doses |
| - Propofol | B | Avoid in first (and second) trimester |
| o Replacement of any deficiency, e.g., fat soluble vitamins | | |

> Fetal risk categories (FDA): A – no risk; B – risk in animal studies, but not in humans; C – human risk cannot be excluded; D – risk; X – absolute contraindication.

Abbreviation: UDCA, ursodeoxycholic acid

Printed with permission: European Association for the Study of the Liver. EASL Clinical Practice Guidelines: Management of cholestatic liver diseases. J Hepatol 2009; 51(2), Table 7: 237–267.

- Give benefits of UDCA in the management of cholestasis of pregnancy.

  o ↓ concentration of bile acids in maternal serum and amniotic fluid

  o ↑ transport of bile acids in placenta

  o ↓ cholestatic potential of progesterone during pregnancy

  o ↓ pruritus

  o ↓ fetal distress, premature delivery, stillbirth

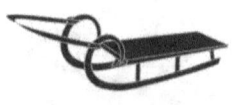

- Give the role of SAM (S-adenosyl – L- methoionine) in the treatment of cholestasis of pregnancy.
  - SAM may enhance the benefit of UDCA (ursodeoxycholic acid) in cholestasis of pregnancy.

- Give the different types of drugs used for the treatment of pruritus in patients with cholestatic liver disease.
  - Decrease degree of cholestasis: UDCA
  - Non-absorbable anion exchange resins: cholestyramine
  - Changes in opioidergic neurotransmission : naloxone, natrexone
  - Hepatic enzyme (cP452) inducers: rifampicin, metronidazole, phenobarbital
  - Cannabinoid agonist
  - Serotonin antagonists: ondansetron
  - Changes in threshold to experience nociception: dronabinol
  - Antidepressants (SSRIs)
  - Sedation (antihistamines)
  - Invasive procedures: plasmapheresis, MARS (extracorporeal albumin dialysis), biliary drainage
  - IV propofol
  - Gabaergic changes: gabapentin
  - UV light
  - Liver transplantation – removes cause of cholestasis

Adapted from: Kremer AE, et al. *Drugs* 2008;68(15):2163-82.

"The only thing that stands between you and your dream is the will to try and the belief that it is actually possible."

Joel Brown Denis Waitley

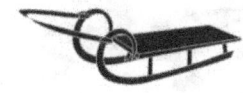

- **T3 – Third Trimester**

❖ ICP, ALF and HELLP

Acute fatty liver of pregnancy (AFLP), the HELLP syndrome* and intrahepatic cholestasis of pregnancy (ICP) occur only in pregnant women.

- Give the distinguishing characteristics between ICP, HELLP and AFLD.

| | ICP | AFLP | HELLP |
|---|---|---|---|
| • Mother | | | |
| ○ % Pregnancies | 0.1–1.0 | 0.005–0.01 | 0.2–0.6 |
| ○ Time of onset in pregnancy | T3 | Second half of pregnancy, or postpartum | Second half of pregnancy, or postpartum |
| ○ Trimester | (2 or) 3 | 3 or postpartum | 3 or postpartum |
| ○ Maternal mortality (%) | 0 | 7–18 | 1–25 |
| ○ Presence of preeclampsia | No | 50% | Yes |
| ○ Typical clinical features | Pruritus Elevated serum ALT/AST fasting bile acids | Liver failure with mild jaundice, coagulopathy, encephalopathy, hypoglycemia, DIC | Hemolysis Elevated serum liver tests Thrombocytopenia (often <50,000/µL) |
| ○ Nausea/ vomiting | Rare | Yes (80%) | Yes |
| ○ Abdominal pain | Rare | Yes (60%) | Yes (100%) |
| • Laboratory | | | |
| ○ Cholestasis | Marked | Modest and late | Mild or absent |
| ○ ALT | Mild to 10–20-fold ↑ | 5–15-fold, ↑ variable | Mild to 10–20-fold ↑ |
| ○ Bilirubin | <5 mg/dL (<85 µmol/l) | Often <5 mg/dL (<85 µmol/l) | Mostly <5 mg/dL (<85 µmol/l) |
| ○ Fetal/perinatal mortality (%) | 0.4–1.4 | 9–23 | 11 |
| ○ Recurrence in subsequent pregnancies (%) | 45–70 | 20–70 (carriers of LCHAD mutations) Rare (others) | - 4–19 |

327

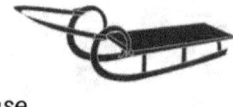

|  |  | ICP | AFLP | HELLP |
|---|---|---|---|---|
| o | Coagulopathy | No | In severe cases, late | Early: thrombocytopenia<br><br>Late: DIC |
| o | Hepatic failure | No | Yes (70% when severe) | Rare |
| • Imaging |  |  |  |  |
| o | U/S | Normal | No change or fatty liver | Areas of necrosis, infarction , or hematoma |
| • Liver biopsy |  | Cholestasis | Microvesicular fatty infiltration | Periportal patchy, hemorrhagic necrosis,<br><br>Fibrin deposition<br><br>Perisinusoidal mild microvesicular fat |
| • Treatment |  |  |  |  |
| o | Management of mother and child | UDCA, vitamin K | Early delivery (cesarian section) increased risk of AFLP in next pregnancy, check LCHAD in fetus(unknown risk of recurrence of AFLD) | Early delivery (cesarian section) for severe uncontrolled pre-eclampsia (hemolysis, seizures) |

UDCA is low risk after first trimester and is effective for cholestasis of pregnancy.

Abbreviation: LCHAD: α-subunit, long-chain 3-hydroxyacyl-CoA dehydrogenase; HELLP, hemolysis, elevated serum liver enzymes, low platelets

Adapted from: EASL Clinical Practice Guidelines: Management of cholestatic liver diseases. J Hepatol 2009; 51(2), 237–267 and Myers RP,et al. *First Principles of Gastroenterology* 2005. pg. 652.

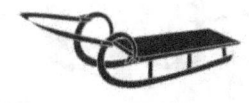

328

**HELLP** (Hemolysis, Elevated LFTs, Low Platelets) **Syndrome**

➤ Definition

- o The HELLP (<u>h</u>emolysis, <u>e</u>levated <u>l</u>iver enzymes, <u>l</u>ow <u>p</u>latelet) syndrome is a form of pre-eclampsia liver disease.

---

Danger sign!

A woman in the second trimester of pregnancy with RUQ (right upper quadrant) pain, nausea and vomiting, should be suspected of having HELLP always consider this possibility, rather than focusing just on gallbladder disease.

---

➤ Demography

- o Pre-eclampsia occurs in 5-10% of pregnancies, and accounts for 20% of maternal deaths (Van Dyke 09)
- o Preeclampsia occurs in about 4% of pregnancies, and HELLP occurs with about 12% of women with severe eclampsia
- o Pre-eclampsia and the HELLP syndrome usually occur in the 3rd trimester, but in 28% HELLP occurs in the early postpartum period.

➤ Pathophysiology

- o Both HELLP and AFLP may be associated with maternal defects in the mitrochondrial oxidation of fatty acids arising from deficiency of **LCHAD** (long-chain 3- hydroxyacyl- CoA dehydrogenase).
- o ↓ LCHAD in fetus: "AFLP may develop regardless of maternal genotype if the fetus is deficient in LCHAD and carries at least one allele for the G 1528C LCHAD mutation" (*Sleisenger & Fordtran's gastrointestinal and liver disease* 2010, page 635)..." In cases of AFLP the mother, father and child should be tested for the G1528C LCHAD mutation" (*Sleisenger & Fordtran's gastrointestinal and liver disease* 2010, page 636)
- o ↓ carnitine palmitoyltransferase
  - Both HELLP and AFLD are associated with defects in fatty acid oxidation and prenatal genetic diagnosi may be performed in pregnant women in affected families

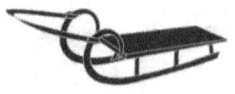

- Give the role of deficiency of the mitochondrial fatty acid oxidation enzyme LCHAD (long-chain 3-hydroxyacyl-coenzyme A dehydrogenase) in AFLD.

  - ↓ ability of fetus to oxidize long-chain fatty acids (LCFA), sometimes from a mutation causing ↓ LCHAD activity.

  - LCFA from fetus are transferred from fetus to placenta to mother.

  - If the mother is heterogeneous for LCHAD, she will accumulate LCFA as microvesicular fat, and will develop
    - Hepatic steatosis
    - HE (hepatic encephalopathy)
    - ALF (acute liver failure)

  - If the newborn child has LCHAD deficiency, she/he has ↑ risk of fatal, fasting non-ketotic hypoglycemia over next several months – <u>must check</u> the newborn for their LCHAD levels.


- Give the maternal and fetal factors implicated in the pathogenesis of HELLP.

  - Mother
    - ↑ sFlt1 (soluble form-like tyrosine kinase 1 (an antagonist of VEGF [vascular endothelial growth factor] and an antagonist of PIGF [placental growth factor])
    - ↑ sEng (soluble endoglin, which reduces the formation of capillaries)
    - ↑ procoagulant (eg, factor V Leiden, anticardiolipin antibody)
    - ↑ systemic vascular resistance
    - ↓ plasma volume
    - ↓ LCHAD (long-chain 3-hydroxyacyl – CoA dehydrogenase), which when reduced leads to ↓ mitochondrial oxidation of fatty acids)

  - Fetus
    - On the fetal side, the high capacity low resistance placental vessels do not develop, which leads to ↓ blood flow to the fetus from the placenta, fetal ischemia and intrauterine growth retardation
      - ↓ trophoblast invasion of wall of uterus
      - Dilation of spiral arteries
      - ↓ uteroplacental perfusion

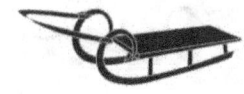

- Pathophysiology relates to the fetal and maternal sides of the placenta
- Even if there are no signs of preeclampsia at the time of delivery, about 30% of cases of HELLP will develop eclampsia after delivery
- On the maternal side,
  - ↑ release of anti-angiogenic and ↓ release of pro-angiogenic factors → maternal vessel vasoconstriction
  - ↑ sensitivity to vasoconstrictors and vasoconstriction → damage to the endothelium of the maternal blood vessels and deposition of fibrin.
  - Deposition of fibrin → ischemic infarcts, including acute hepatic necrosis in 10-20% of pre-eclamptic women.

- Clinical
  - Associations
    - Hyperreflexia
    - Peripheral edema
    - DIC (disseminated intravascular coagulation)
    - Abruption placentae
    - Budd-Chiari syndrome (hepatic vein thrombosis)
  - Often associated with preeclampsia
    - ↑ SBP (systolic blood pressure)
    - Proteinuria
    - Peripheral edema
  - Mortality rate
    - Mother 20%
    - Fetus 20%
  - Recurs
    - 1/3 of future pregnancies
  - There is an increased risk of **recurrence** of HELLP in women with severe
    - Hypertension
    - Chronic renal disease
    - Lupus anticoagulant, or
    - Women with a liver transplantation (or other organ transplantation)

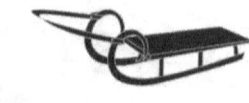

➢ Diagnosis

o Required for diagnosis
  – Hypertension (sustained systolic blood pressure of ≥ 140/90 after week 20 of pregnancy, in a women whose blood pressure was previously normal)
  – Hypertension-associated end organ damage (eg, liver damage in HELLP syndrome)

o Proteinuria (≥ 300 mg urinary protein per 24 hr, or 30 mg/dL urine [dipstick #1])

o While abdominal ultrasound may be reliable to detect intrahepatic complications of HELLP, imaging is not reliable to prove the absence of AFLP (the liver must contain > 30% before the abdominal ultrasound becomes reliably positive for steatosis).

---

SO YOU WANT TO BE A GASTROENTEROLOGIST!

Using the presence of elevated serum values of AFP (alpha-fetoprotein) is **not** widely recommended as a screening test for hepatocellular cancer (HCC).
o In the setting of a pregnant woman with cirrhosis or chronic HBV infection who has been found to have an increased serum AFP, what are the differential possibilities besides HCC?

    o Mother     – Physiological (↑ AFP in normal pregnancies)
                          – Hydatidiform mole

    o Fetus      – Down syndrome
                          – Neural tube defects

---

➢ Laboratory

o The extent of laboratory abnormalities does not reflect the severity of HELLP

o Lab' abnormalities
  – Hemolysis (from microangiopathic hemolytic anemia) unconjugated hyperbilirubinemia
    ▪ ↑ LDH
    ▪ ↓ haptoglobulin
  – ↑ ALT, AST
  – ↓ platelets

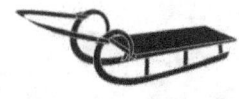

- In keeping with the hemolysis ("H") in HELLP
  - The peripheral blood smear may show schistocytes
  - There may be increased serum LDH (lactate dehydrogenase)
  - Although transaminases are often increased 6x (median, 249 U/L for serum aspartate aminotransferase), values > 1000 may occur.
- In HELLP, there are:
  - The usual laboratory findings of hemolysis (H).
  - The elevated liver tests (EL) include a wide range of changes in ALT/AST, further increased in alkaline phosphatase, and jaundice in 5-40% depending on the extent of patchy ischemic necrosis and fibrin deposition, and hemolysis.
  - The thrombocytopenia (LP) may be associated with low fibrinogen, increased fibrin degradation products and renal dysfunction.
- Fetal hypoxia may develop quickly, with sudden intrauterine death, so early delivery of the fetus is recommended. Fetal mortality is 3-23%, and maternal mortality is up to 3.5%.

---

Clinical Alert

In the pregnant woman with Wilson disease who develops hemolysis and acute liver disease at the time of delivery, in addition to suspecting the HELLP syndrome, consider and exclude acute Wilson disease.

---

➢ Histopathology
- The usual patchy hepatic necrosis may lead to confluent necrosis, hepatic hematoma, and even hepatic rupture requiring surgical intervention or hepatic artery embolization.
- Fibrin deposit in sinusoids → focal ischemic necrosis → periportal hemorrhage subcapsular hematoma hepatic rupture.
- Maternal and fetal mortality from a free rupture is 50-100%.

➢ Treatment
- Urgent delivery of the fetus

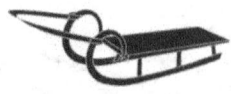

**Acute Fatty Liver in Pregnancy** (AFLP)

- ➤ Demography
  - ○ Seen in 1/1000 pregnancies
  - ○ AFLP accounts for 16-70% of severe liver disease as well as maternal and fetal deaths during pregnancy

- ➤ Pathophysiology
  - ○ Impaired mitochondrial beta-oxidation or oxidative phosphorylation of fatty acids, resulting in mitochondrial damage, ↓ ATP production, and destruction of hepatocytes
  - ○ Associated with pre-eclampsia in 30%, genetic abnormality in LCHAD (long chain 3-hydroxyacyl-CoA-dehydrogenase) in 20%, possibly other as yet unknown genetic mutations, and the use of drugs such as ASA/NSAIDs
  - ○ When mother is LCHAD heterozygote but fetus is homozygote, the risk of AFLP is 43%; when the fetus is a heterozygote or normal, the risk of AFLP is 2.7%

- ➤ Pathophysiology
  - ○ Both HELLP and AFLP may be associated with maternal defects in the mitrochondrial oxidation of fatty acids arising from deficiency of **LCHAD** (long-chain 3- hydroxyacyl- CoA dehydrogenase).
  - ○ ↓ LCHAD in fetus: "AFLP may develop regardless of maternal genotype if the fetus is deficient in LCHAD and carries at least one allele for the G 1528C LCHAD mutation" (*Sleisenger & Fordtran's gastrointestinal and liver disease* 2010, page 635)..." In cases of AFLP the mother, father and child should be tested for the G1528C LCHAD mutation" (*Sleisenger & Fordtran's gastrointestinal and liver disease* 2010, page 636)
  - ○ ↓ carnitine palmitoyltransferase
    - Both HELLP and AFLD are associated with defects in fatty acid oxidation and prenatal genetic diagnosi may be performed in pregnant women in affected families

- • Give the role of deficiency of the mitochondrial fatty acid oxidation enzyme LCHAD (long-chain 3-hydroxyacyl-coenzyme A dehydrogenase) in AFLD.
  - ○ ↓ ability of fetus to oxidize long-chain fatty acids (LCFA), sometimes from a mutation causing ↓ LCHAD activity.
  - ○ LCFA from fetus are transferred from fetus to placenta to mother.
  - ○ If the mother is heterogeneous for LCHAD, she will accumulate LCFA as microvesicular fat, and will develop
    - – Hepatic steatosis
    - – HE (hepatic encephalopathy)
    - – ALF (acute liver failure)

334

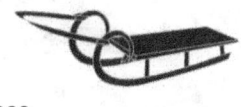

- o If the newborn child has LCHAD deficiency, she/he has ↑ risk of fatal, fasting non-ketotic hypoglycemia over next several months – <u>must check</u> the newborn for their LCHAD levels.

---

Clinical Gem
- o After an episode of AFLP, the microvesicular steatosis may progress!

---

➤ Clinical
- o The presentation is that of acute liver failure, including hepatic encephalopathy, coagulopathy, jaundice, ascites, hypoglycemia, renal impairment and pancreatitis
- o Intrauterine fetal mortality may be as high as 32%, and maternal mortality rates of 5-26%.

➤ Laboratory
- o The level of the altered serum transaminases do not reflect the severity of the liver damage and failure. In addition to an elevated INR, anti-thrombin III levels are often increased as well

➤ Differential

---

Ticks and Treats
- o Overlap - questions are often asked of candidates to distinguish between AFLP (acute fatty liver of pregnancy) and HELLP.
- o It is helpful that AFLP does not usually have thrombocytopenia.
- o In groups of patients, ALT/AST may be increased in AFLP; although this increase may not be as high as in HELLP, and in the individual patient this relative elevation of differences in ALT/ AST is not useful.
- o Beware, AFLP is not considered to be a preclamptic liver disease, but about 50% of AFLP may actively have associated pre-eclampsia.
- o Both HELLP and AFLP may be associated with inherited defects in the beta oxidation of fatty acids.
- o And don't forget: AFLP is associated with severe pericentral (zone 3) microvesicular fat, and HELLP may be associated with fatty liver, albeit not as severe as the pericentral microvesicular fat of AFLP.

---

335

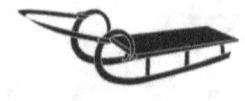

> Treatment

  o Urgent delivery of the fetus is required; test the mother and infant for LCHAD mutations

Abbreviations: AFLP, acute fatty liver of pregnancy; LCHAD, long chain 3-hydroxyacyl-CoA-dehydrogenase

- **Liver Diseases occurring in Pregnancy which are not unique to pregnancy**

- Give the cautions to be considered when treating the following liver conditions during pregnancy.

  o **HAV**
    – Hepatitis A has low risk in pregnancy, and only requires supportive care for the mother

  o **HBV**
    – Hepatitis A has low risk in pregnancy
    – Lamivudine is low risk treatment for HBV infection in pregnancy
    – **Interferon** and **ribavirin** are <u>contraindicated</u> in pregnancy (use lamivudine, tenofovir if necessary)
    – Adefovir and entecavir have no data in human pregnancy
    – Hepatitis B vaccine has low risk in pregnancy
    – Vertical transmission from mother to child is the commonest route for HBV infection, and depending upon the viral load, may be 80-90%.
    – Babies born to HBV positive mothers should receive HBIG and HB vaccine at birth, and further vaccine at one and six months of age. at 18 months of age, the child born to the HCV positive mother should have HCV RNA testing.

  o **HCV**
    – HCV infections are the result of vertical transmission rarely transmitted to fetus
    – Risk of 30% if the mother is both HCV and HIV positive.
    – HCV – do not treat in pregnancy

  o **HDV**
    – HDV may be transmitted at the same time as HBV.

  o **HEV**
    – HEV hepatitis in pregnant women is associated with a high rate of fulminant hepatic failure, and maternal as well as fetal death. Transmission of HEV is vertical, and the HEV vaccine will soon be available.

336

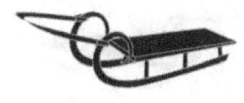

- HEV – often fatal in Africa and Asia
  - Underlying chronic liver disease
    - Rare to become pregnant
    - Prognosis variable
    - Stillbirths increased
    - High bilirubin → kernicterus
- **HSV**
  - The risk of herpes simplex hepatitis is increased during pregnancy, and may present with markedly elevated transaminases or with fulminant hepatic failure.
- **Autoimmune hepatitis** (AIH)
  - Maintenance medications for autoimmune hepatitis (AIH) should not be stopped during pregnancy, and even with these being continued, there is an increased risk of spontaneous abortion (12%) and perinatal deaths (7%)
- **Wilson disease** (WD)
  - Penicillamine should be avoided, or dose reduced durung pregnancy
  - If necessary, switch to oral zinc, or trientine
  - The woman of child bearing potential who has WD is usually not able to conceive because of associated amenorrhea and infertility.
  - If the couple wishes to become pregnant, the planned mother should be switched from a chelator to oral zinc before the planned pregnancy.
  - If conception occurs without prior stoppage of the chelation therapy and switching to zinc, then reduce the dose of the chelator currently being used.

- Give the reason why some form of copper-lowering therapy should be continued when D-penicillamine is teratogenetic in humans.
  - When therapy for Wilson disease is stopped during pregnancy, the sudden release of copper causes RBC hemolysis, with possible acute liver failure and death.
  - If a woman with Wilson disease is planning/hoping to become pregnant, switch her from D-penicillamine to trientine (not teratogenic in humans).
- **PBC/PSC/ICP**
  - UDCA has low risk after first trimester and is effective for intrahepatic cholestasis of pregnancy and for primary biliary cholangitis (PBC)
    - UDCA us not of benefit in primary sclerosing cholangitis (PSC), and is not indicated anytime.
- **Portal hypertension**
  - Propranolol -avoid after first trimester (fetal cardiotoxicity)
  - Nadolol has a long half-life- should be avoided

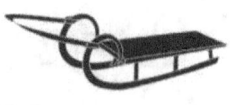

# JAUNDICE/HYPERBILIRUBINEMIA

➢ Pathophysiology

• Give the pathophysiology of the development of hyperbilirubinemia and jaundice.
  o RBC heme is broken down by RE (reticuloendothelial system), largely in the spleen.
  o Heme oxygenase converts heme to biliverdin.
  o Biliverdin reductase converts biliverdin to bilirubin.
  o Lipid soluble unconjugated bilirubin (UB) is made water soluble by the binding of UB to albumin (albumin – UB complex).
  o The albumin-UB complex passes through the fenestrations in the endothelium of the hepatic sinusoids and into the space of Disse.
  o In the space of Disse the UB dissociates from the albumin.
  o UB is transported by OATP (organic anion transport protein) across the SM (sinusoidal membrane) of the hepatocyte.
  o In the cytosol of the hepatocytes, UB binds to glutathione S- transferase.
  o UDP – GT (uridine – 5' – diphosphate glucuronyl transferase) in the ER.
    – Binds to UB to prevent its back flux across the SM and into portal blood
    – Conjugates UB to glucuronic acid
  o The CB (conjugated bilirubin) is a mono- and diglucuronic
  o The CB is transported across the CM of the hepatocyte by ATP-dependent MRP2 (multiple rug resistance-associated protein 2)
  o CB enters the bile, and passes along the length of the small intestine and into the colon.
  o The bacteria in the liver of the distal ileum and colon contain B-glucuronidases bacterial B-glucuronidases hydrolyze CB to UB.
  o UB is reduced further by intestinal bacteria to urobilinogen.
  o The fate of urobilinogen includes
    – Passed in stool
    – Oxidized to urobilin and passed in urine
    – Absorbed in the distal, ileum and colon, to be re-secreted
      ▪ By liver into bile
      ▪ By renal glomerulus into urine
    – CB is water soluble, and when the bilirubin level is high in serum and bile, not all CB is hydrolyzed to UB.
    – CB tea-coloured urine occurs only in conjugated hyperbilirubinemia urine. Urine turns to colour of tea.
    – In unconjugated hyperbilirubinemia, all UB is bound to albumin and does not enter the urine so the urine is not tea-coloured.

338

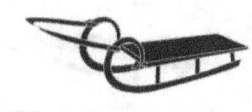

➢ Causes/associations

• Give the clinical processes which contribute to the development of hyperbilirubinemia.

  o Increased bilirubin production (indirect hyperbilirubinemia; AP/ALT often normal)
    – Destruction of transfused erythrocytes
    – Hemolysis secondary to pre-existing hemolytic conditions (eg: G6PD deficiency, hemoglobinopathies)
    – Hemolysis secondary to mechanical heart valve prostheses
    – Reabsorption of hematomas
    – Multiple blood transfusions

  o Hepatocellular Injury (predominant serum ALT elevation with or without hyperbilirubinemia)
    – Inhalational anesthetics-halothane, others
    – Ischemic hepatitis (shock liver)
    – Hepatic artery thrombosis
    – Other drugs-antihypertensives (eg: labetalol), heparin
    – Acute post-transfusion hepatitis
    – Unrecognized previous chronic liver disease-NASH, HCV etc.
    – Hepatic allograft rejection

  o Cholestastic Jaundice (elevated serum alkaline phophatase, GGT, direct hyperbilirubinemia)
    – Benign postoperative cholestasis
    – Cardiac bypass of prolonged duration
    – Sepsis
    – Acalculous cholecystitis
    – Common bile duct obstruction-gallstones, pancreatitis
    – Cholangitis
    – Bile duct injury-post-cholecystectomy, post-liver transplantation
    – Microlithiasis (biliary sludge)
    – Prolonged total parenteral nutrition
    – Hemobilia
    – Drugs-amoxicillin-clavulanate. chlorpromazine, erythromycin, telethromycin, trimethoprim-sulfamethoxazole, warfarin, others

Adapted from: Sleisenger and Fordtran's Gastrointestinal and Liver Disease. 10th Edition. Saunders/Elsevier, Philadelphia, 2016, Table 21-1, page 338; and Faust TW, et al. *Clin Liver Dis* 2004;8(1):151-66.

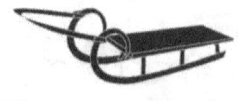

➢ Differential diagnosis

• Give major intrahepatic and extrahepatic causes of cholestasis leading to jaundice.
  ○ Intrahepatic
    – Liver
      ▪ Drugs (DILI)
      ▪ Alcoholic hepatitis ± cirrhosis
      ▪ PBC
      ▪ Viral hepatitis
      ▪ Chronic hepatitis ± cirrhosis
      ▪ Cholestasis of pregnancy

    – Non-liver
      ▪ Sepsis
      ▪ TPN
  ○ Extrahepatic
    – Biliary tree
      ▪ Common bile duct stone(s)
      ▪ Benign biliary stricture
      ▪ PSC, SSC (secondary sclerosing cholangitis)
      ▪ Bile duct carcinoma Pancreatic/periampullary cancer

    – Pancreas
      ▪ Pancreatic/periampullary cancer
      ▪ Benign pancreatic disease
      ▪ Extrinsic duct compression

Adapted from: Heathcote J. *First Principles of Gastroenterology* 2005: pg. 590.

• Give factors contributing to **physiological jaundice** in the neonate.
  ○ Absence of placental bilirubin metabolism
  ○ Reduced hepatic blood flow via ductus venosus shunting
  ○ Decreased red blood cell survival
  ○ Proportionally increased red blood cell mass
  ○ Reduced enteric bacterial flora
  ○ Presence of intestinal β-glucoronidase
  ○ Immature liver function
  ○ Delayed oral feeding

Printed with permission: Machida H. *First Principles of Gastroenterology* 2005: pg. 725.

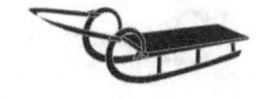

- Give causes of unconjugated hyperbilirubinemia in the neonate.
  - Increased bilirubin production (hemolytic disease)
    - Blood group incompatibility (Rh, ABO, minor groups)
    - Membrane defects (spherocytosis, elliptocytosis, infantile pyknocytosis)
    - Enzyme deficits (G6-PD, hexokinase, pyruvate kinase)
    - Drugs (oxytocin, vitamin K)
  - Increased RBC breakdown
    - Infection
  - Hematoma, Extrahepatic biliary obstruction
    - Bile duct ligation/injury
    - Choledocholithiasis
    - Acalculous cholecystitis
    - Post cholecystectomy, post liver transplantation
    - Microlithias (biliary sludge)
    - Postoperative pancreatitis
    - Extrinsic compression of common bile duct or common hepatic duct
    - Hemobilia
  - Pre-existing Abnormalities in Bilirubin Metabolism/Excretion
    - Chronic liver disease
    - Gilbert's syndrome
    - Swallowed maternal blood
  - Increased RBC mass
    - Polycythemia (maternal diabetes, delayed cord clamping, small for gestational age, high altitude)
  - Decreased bilirubin metabolism
    - Reduced uptake
      - Portacaval shunt, hypoxia, sepsis, acidosis, congenital heart disease
    - Decreased conjugation (unconjugated)
      - Crigler-Najjar type I, II
      - Gilbert syndrome
      - Lucey-Driscoll syndrome
      - Hypothyroidism
      - Panhypopituitarism
  - Altered enterohepatic circulation
    - Breastfeeding
      - Free fatty acids, steroids, breast milk β-glucuronidase
    - Intestinal hypomotility
      - Retained meconium
    - Reduced intestinal flora
      - Newborn antibiotic use

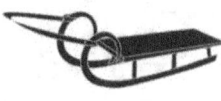

## Congenital Syndromes of Hyperbilirubinemia

- Give the defect causing congenital syndromes of conjugated hyperbilirubinemia (Crigler-Najjar types 1 & 2 [CN-T$_1$, CN-T$_2$], Dubin-Johnson (DJ), and Rotor syndrome).

| Name | Defects |
|---|---|
| ○ Unconjugated | |
|    – Gilbert syndrome | ▪ "a mutation in the TATAA element in the 5' promoter region of the UDP glucuronyl transferase gene" |
| | ▪ ↓ UDP-GT activity ~ 30% of normal. |
|    – Crigler-Najjar – type II | ▪ ↓ UDP-GT activity < 10% of normal |
|          – type I | ▪ UDP-GT is zero (risk of kernicterus) |
| ○ Conjugated hyperbilirubinemias ( > 15% of total bilirubin is conjugated) | |
|    – Dubin | ▪ Johnson syndrome |
| | ▪ Defect in MRP$_2$ gene |
|    – Rotor syndrome | ▪ Defect unknown |

Adapted from: Sleisenger and Fordtran's Gastrointestinal and Liver Disease. 9th Edition. Saunders/Elsevier, Philadelphia, 2010, page 1228; and 10th edition, 2016, Table 21.2, page 339

- Give the variables to differentiate between Gilbert syndrome, Crigler-Najjar type-1 and -2, Dubin Johnson (DJ) syndrome, and Rotor syndrome.

| Variables | Gilbert | CN-T1 | CN-T2 |
|---|---|---|---|
| ○ Prevalence | 7% of population | Very rare | Uncommon |
| ○ Inheritance (all autosomal) | Dominant | Recessive | Dominant |
| ○ Serum bilirubin concentration | <100 µmol/L (conjugated) | >400 µmol/L (conjugated) | <100 µmol/L (~ ½ conjugated) |
| ○ Diagnostic features | Bilirubin ↑ with fasting ↓ with phenobarbital | Bilirubin No response to phenobarbital | Bilirubin conc' ↓ with phenobarbital |
| ○ Treatment | None needed | Liver graft | Phenobarbital |

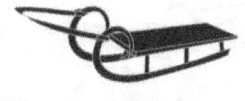

| | | |
|---|---|---|
| o Prognosis | Normal | Early death from kernicterus | Usually normal |

| Variables | Dubin Johnson (DJ) | Rotor Syndrome |
|---|---|---|
| o Prevalence | Uncommon | Rare |
| o Inheritance (all autosomal) | Recessive | Recessive |
| o Serum bilirubin concentration (µmol/L) | <100 (~ 1/2 conjugated) | <100 (~ 1/2 conjugated) |
| o Diagnostic features | Coproporphyrin excretion (>80% isomer !)<br><br>Pigment in centrolubular hepatocytes | Normal gallbladder visualization on oral cholecystography |
| o Prognosis | Normal | Normal |
| o Treatment | Avoid estrogen | None available |

- Give categories of causes of conjugated hyperbilirubinemia in the neonate, and for each give examples.

  - o Infection
    - Bacterial urinary tract infection/sepsis
    - Cytomegalovirus
    - HSV, type 6
    - Rubella
    - Syphilis
    - Toxoplasmosis
    - Other viruses: adenovirus, Coxsackie virus, echovirus, parvovirus B19

  - o Metabolic
    - Bile acid synthesis disorders
    - Cystic fibrosis
    - Endocrine disorders: hypopituitarism, hypothyroidism
    - Fructosemia
    - Galactosemia
    - Neonatal hemochromatosis
    - Niemann-Pick disease
    - Peroxisomal disorders
    - Progressive familial intrahepatic cholestasis
    - Tyrosemia
    - $\alpha_1$-antitrypsin deficiency

  - o Bile duct disorders

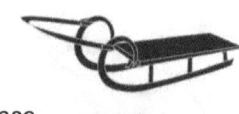

343

- Extrahepatic
  - Bile duct perforation, stenosis
  - Biliary atresia
  - Choledochal cyst
  - Cholelithiasis
  - Inspissated bile/bile plug
  - Intra/extrahepatic masses
  - Neonatal sclerosing cholangitis
- Intrahepatic
- Alagille syndrome
  - Byler disease (familial progressive disorder)
  - Nonsyndromic bile duct paucity

o Miscellaneous
  - Parenteral nutrition
  - Intestinal obstruction
  - Shock
  - Trisomy 21

Printed with permission: Robertson M, and Martin SR. *Principles of Gastroenterology* 2005: pg. 728.


- Give causes of jaundice in patients with lymphoma.

  o Related to lymphoma
    - Hepatic infiltration
    - Jaundice without infiltration
    - Intrahepatic cholestasis
      - Rare
      - Hodgkin's disease
      - Stauffer's syndrome-like [renal cell Ca]
    - Extrahepatic obstruction
      - Usually hilar
      - Usually non-Hodgkin's lymphoma
    - Autoimmune hemolytic anemia, DIC
    - Hepatic artery clots

  o Related to therapy
    - Chemotherapy (can cause acute liver failure)
    - Hepatic irradiation
    - Infection
      - Post-transfusion HCV
      - HBV reactivation
      - Opportunistic infections

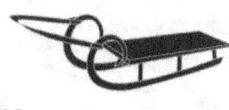

Adapted from: Sherlock S, and Dolley J. *Diseases of the Liver and Biliary System* (Eleventh Edition) 2002: pg. 60.

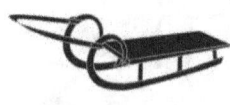

# CIRRHOTIC CARDIOMYOPATHY

➤ Definition

 o A cardiac dysfunction in patients with cirrhosis characterized by impaired contractile responsiveness to stress and/or altered diastolic relaxation with electrophysiological abnormalities in the absence of other know cardiac disease.

➤ Demography

 o Seen in 60% of persons with cirrhosis correlates with the severity of the liver disease

 o Predisposes the person to ventricular arrhythmias

➤ Pathophysiology

 o ↑ arterial vasodilation → hyperdynamic incubation → ↑ HR/ ↑ CO → ↓ SVR / ↓ BP → ↑ $IVV_p$

 o Note: While there is ↑ $IVV_p$, there is no ↑ central intravascular volume

Abbreviations: BP, arterial blood pressure; CO, cardiac output; HR, heart rate; $IVV_p$, intravascular volume (peripheral); SVR, systemic vascular resistance

• Give hepatic conditions associated with cardiac abnormalities, such as arrhythmias and heart failure (HF).

 o HH (hereditary hemochromatosis)

 o Alcoholic cardiomyopathy

 o Cardiac cirrhosis from right-sided HF

 o Drugs, e.g., amiodarone toxicity

➤ Diagnosis

❖ Diagnostic criteria

 o Systolic dysfunction

  – Blunted ↑ cardiac output on exercise, volume challenge or pharmacological stimuli

  – Resting ejection fraction <55%

 o Diastolic dysfunction

  – E/A ratio <1.0 (age-corrected)

  – ↑ deceleration time (>200 ms)

  – ↑ isovolumetric relaxation time (>80 ms)

346

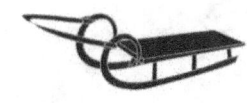

❖ Supportive criteria
  o Electrophysiological abnormalities
    – Abnormal chronotropic response
    – Electromechanical uncoupling/dys-synchrony
    – Prolonged Q-T$_c$ interval
  o Diagnostic imaging
    – Enlarged left atrium
  o Laboratory
    – ↑ myocardial mass
    – ↑ BNP and pro-BNP
    – ↑ troponin I

Abbreviations: BNP, brain natriuretic peptide; E/A ratio, ratio of early to late (arterial) phases of ventricular filling

Printed with permission: Møller S, and Henriksen JH. *Gut* 2008; 58: 274.

- Give the diagnostic tools in the assessment of systolic and diastolic dysfunction in persons suspected of having cirrhotic cardiomyopathy.

❖ Systolic function
  o Echocardiography/MRI:
    – Volumes
    – Fractional shortening
    – Velocity of fractional shortening
    – Ejection fraction (planimetry)
    – Response to stress (dobutamine)
    – Wall motion
  o Exercise ECG
    – Exercise capacity
    – Oxygen consumption*
    – Pressure x heart rate product
  o Radionuclide angiography (MUGA)
    – Ejection fraction
    – Cardiac volumes
    – Pattern of contractibility

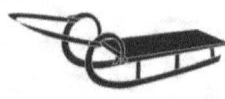

- o Myocardial perfusion imaging with gating
  - Regional myocardial perfusion
  - Cardiac volumes
  - Ejection fraction
  - Wall motion and wall thickening

- ❖ Diastolic function
  - o Echocardiography/MRI/MUGA (radionucleotide angiography)
    - E/A ratio
    - Deceleration time
    - A and E waves
    - Relaxation times

Printed with permission:  Møller S, and Henriksen JH. *GUT* 2008; 58: pg. 276. *training program in gastroenterology.*

- ➤ Treatment
  - o Left heart failure is rare because of the ↓ systemic vascular resistance, and no afterload reduction
  - o Preload reduction
    - $O_2$
    - Diuretics
    - Sodium restriction)

"Knowledge speaks, but wisdom listens."

Jimi Hendrix

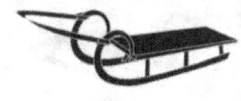

## HEPATIC MASSES

➤ Classification

- Give a classification of hepatic masses seen on abdominal ultrasound.
    - Primary and secondary (metastases)
    - Benign (usually require no further treatment)
        - Cavernous hemangioma
        - Focal fatty liver areas
        - Focal nodular hyperplasia (reaction to an arterial malformation; the telangiectatic subtype of FNH is associated with estrogen use; 10% multiple, 20% associated with cavernous hemangioma)
        - Hepatic adenoma (associated with the use of OCA; require further follow-up)
    - Malignant
        - Cholangiocarcinoma (↑ CA 19-9)
        - Cystadenocarcinoma
        - Epithelioid angiomyolipoma
        - Hemangioendotheliomatosis
        - Liver metastases
        - Lymphomas
        - Mixed epithelial and stromal tumours
        - Mixed hepatocellular-cholangiocarcinoma
        - Primary hepatocellular carcinoma
        - Sarcomas
    - Abscesses
        - Amebic liver abscess
        - Biliary cystadenoma
        - Echinococcal cysts
        - Granulomatous abscesses
        - Inflammatory pseudotumour
        - Nodular regenerative hyperplasia
        - Pyogenic liver abscess

Abbreviation: OCA, oral contraceptive agent

Adapted from: Roberts LR. *2008 AGA Annual Postgraduate Course Syllabus*: pg 245.

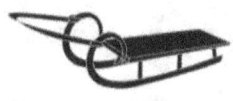

- ➢ Diagnostic imaging
  - o When a mass is identified in the liver of a person with or without chronic liver disease, a triple phase CT or MRI with gadolinium is performed

  - o Nuclear scintigraphy with sulphur colloid is
    - - ↑ uptaken up by Kupffer cells
      - ▪ Metastatic lesions (thyroid, breast, lung, pancreas, colon)
      - ▪ Hemangioma
      - ▪ Cysts
    - - ↓ uptake
      - ▪ Hepatic adenomas
      - ▪ HCC
    - - RBC
      - ▪ Identifies an hepatic mass, such as an hemangioma

- • Give the diagnostic workup of a liver mass in a patient with chronic liver disease.
  - o The sequence of events needed to make the radiological diagnosis depends on the size of the lesion.

| o Mass <1 cm | - Diagnosis | ▪ Low likelihood of being HCC, therefore no specific diagnostic tests | | |
|---|---|---|---|---|
| | - Follow up | ▪ Repeat imaging study every 3 months | | |
| | | ▪ If no growth in 1-2 years, no HCC; continue screening every 6 months | | |
| | | ▪ If growth, treat as HCC | | |
| o Mass 1-2 cm | - Diagnosis | ▪ Two dynamic imaging studies (US, CT scan, or MRI) | - Both with typical vascular pattern<br>- One typical and the other atypical | - Treat as HCC |
| | - Follow up after biopsy | ▪ Biopsy confirms HCC | - Both atypical<br>- Treat as HCC | - Consider biopsy of mass |
| | | ▪ Non diagnostic biopsy | - Repeat imaging study every 3 months:<br>- If no growth in 1-2 years- no HCC<br>- If growth, treat as HCC | o Consider biopsy of mass vs close follow up |

350

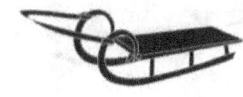

| Mass >2 cm | – Diagnosis | • One dynamic imaging study (US, CT scan, or MRI) | - Typical vascular pattern | - Treat as HCC |
|---|---|---|---|---|
| | | | - Atypical vascular pattern | |
| | – Follow up after biopsy | • Biopsy confirms HCC | - Treat as HCC | - Biopsy of mass |
| | | • Non diagnostic biopsy | - Repeat imaging study every 3 months: | |
| | | | - If no growth in 1-2 years- no HCC | |
| | | | - If growth, treat as HCC | |

- Note
  - The contrast enhanced imaging studies of computed tomography (CT) and magnetic resonance imaging (MRI) use the unique dynamic radiological behaviour of hepatocellular carcinoma (hypervascular on the arterial phase and washout on the delayed venous phase).

Abbreviations: CT, computerized tomography; HCC, hepatocellular carcinoma; MRI, magnetic resonance imaging; US, ultrasound

Printed with permission: Garcia Tsao, et al. The *American Journal of Gastroenterology* 2009; 104:1822.

- Give the diagnostic imaging characteristics on CT/MRI/PET scan/nuclear medicine of hemangioma, focal nodular hyperplasia (FNH), adenoma, HCC, and metastases.

  - Hemangioma – nodular, no washout at periphery; RBC scan, triphasic CT scan (arterial phase); MRI

  - Focular nodular hyperplasia
    - Central vessel
    - Stellate central scar
    - Homogenous

  - Adenoma
    - Heterogeneous
    - Hemorrhage
    - Fat
    - Necrosis
    - Impaired arteriole (no bile duct) "feeding" lesion

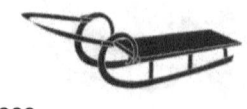

o HCC
  - Tumour thrombus in vessel
  - Fat
  - Cirrhosis
  - Capsule heterogeneous
  - Bile production
  - Extrahepatic involvement

o Metastases
  - Washout at periphery
  - Ring enhancing
  - Fat
  - Blood
  - Calcification
  - New or increasing size – may be hyper/hypo-vascular

Adapted from: Hussain SM, and Semelka RC. *Magn Reson Imaging Clin N Am* 2005;13(2):255-75.


➢ Diagnostic approach

• Give an algorithm for evaluation of hepatic mass in a patient without chronic liver disease (low pretest probability of hepatocellular cancer [HCC]).

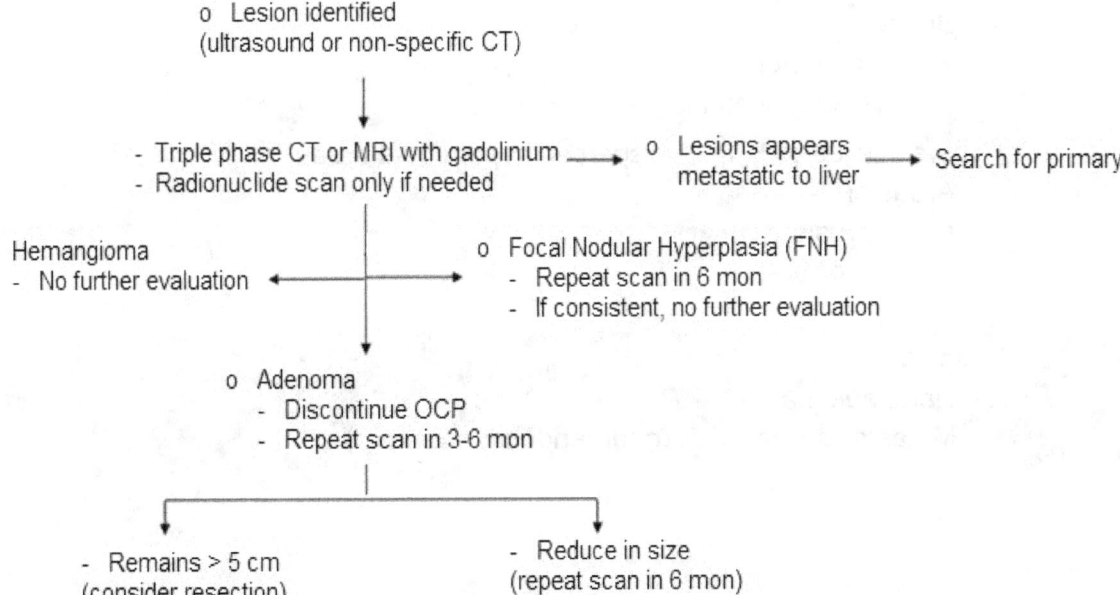

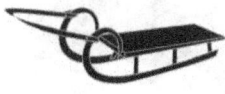

**Hepatic Cysts**

➤ Classification

- Give a classification of hepatic cysts.
  - Simple hepatic cysts
  - < 5 cm, and up to 3 cysts before PCLD (polycystic liver disease) needs to be considered
  - Polycystic liver disease
  - ADPKD (autosomal dominant polycystic kidney disease)
  - Biliary microhamartomas
  - Caroli disease (type V choledochal cyst)
  - Congenital hepatic fibrosis
  - Type IV choledochal cysts

➤ Diagnostic imaging

- Give features on diagnostic imaging which may help to differentiate the nature of the hepatic tumour/cyst.
  - Cysts containing daughter cysts (hydatid)
  - Partly cystic and partly solid
    - Biliary
      - Cystadenoma
      - Cystadenocarcinoma
  - Hyperechic lesion with interspersed hypoechoia areas
    - Areas of
      - Necrosis
      - Hemorrhage
      - Fat
  - Vascular
    - Hemangiomas
    - Metastasis from NET (neuroendocrine tumour)

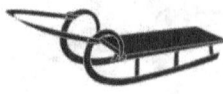

**Peliosis Hepatis** (PH)

- ➢ Definition
  - o Multiple blood-filled cavities distributed randomly throughout the parenchyma of the liver

- ➢ Types
  - o Parenchymal
    - – Cavities lined by hepatocytes
  - o Phlebectatica
    - – Cavities lined by hepatocytes
  - o May progress to
    - – Fibrosis
    - – Regenerative nodules
    - – Cirrhosis
    - – Tumours

- ➢ Causes/associations
  - o Anabolic steroids
  - o Asymptomatic
    - – About 1/3 of PH patients with severe disease will have asymptomatic, harmless ↑ ALT.
  - o Infection
    - – Bartonella infection in HIV-immunosuppressed patients
  - o Drugs/toxins
    - – Azathioprine
    - – OCA (oral contraceptive agent)
    - – Vitamin A
    - – Hydroxyurea

**Cavernous Hemangioma**

- ➢ Definition
  - o Common congenital malformation with ↑ hepatic capillaries of the liver vasculature
    - – Leads to tortous, ectactic blood vessels and statis
    - – No malignant potential
    - – Not affected by oral contraceptive hormones
    - – Thrombosis and pain

354

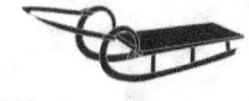

➢ Causes/associations

   o Congenital malformation

   o Hamartomatous change

   o Enlarges under influence of estrogens/pregnancy

➢ Diagnostic imaging

   o Abdominal ultrasound
     – Echogenic

   o Bolus-enhanced CT with sequential scans
     – Periphery – enhanced
     – Margin – corrugated
     – Centre – hypodense

   o SPECT (single photon emission computed tomography) with colloid $^{99M}$Tc –labelled red blood cells

   o MRI
     – Enhance slowly with dynamic studies because the ↑ vascularity is from capillaries
       ▪ Ring – or C-shaped configuration
       ▪ Centre – fibrous, with no uptake (avascular) and pathognomic changes

• Give the findings of diagnostic imaging tests which suggest that a hepatic mass is a cavernous hemangioma.

   o CT or MRI contrast enhanced   – Centipedal filling of contrast (from the periphery to the centre)
                   – well circumscribes

   o RBC nuclear scan with technetium   – ↑ Uptake of labelled RBC on the venous phage
                   – ↑ retention on delayed films

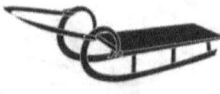

- Give the diagnostic features of hepatic hemangioma.

| | |
|---|---|
| o Ultrasound | – Hyperechoic<br>– Well defined borders |
| o Triple phase CT | – Pre contrast: hypodense<br>– Centripital globular enhancement<br>– Retained contrast in delayed images |
| o MRI | – T1: well circumscribed low signal<br>– T2: Hyperintense signal |
| o Gadolinium enhanced MRI | – Irregular enhancement with delayed washout |
| o Radionuclide scan (tagged RBC) | – ↓ uptake compared to surrounding liver |

Source: Shiffman ML. *2009 ACG Annual Postgraduate Course*:167-171.


## Adenoma

➢ Demography

- o Usually seen in $1/10^6$ women in their childbearing years, and especially if they are on OCA (3 x increased risk)
- o Premalignant, with risk of malignancy increasing with size of adenoma

➢ Pathology

- o 90% single, 10% multiple
- o Circumscribed, but not encapsulated
- o Vascular channels of various sizes

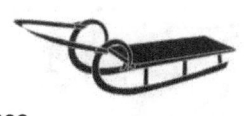

356

- ○ Thrombi in vascular channels
- ○ Mast cells within hemangiomas
- ○ Sclerosis
- ○ Sheets of normal or near normal looking hepatocytes
- ○ No triads, central vein or bile ducts
- ○ Adenomatosis may occur
- ○ May undergo malignant transformation

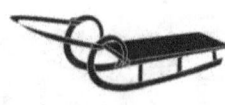

*MASTERING THE BOARDS*
*Hepatology & Pancreaticobiliary Disease*

A.B.R. Thomson

- ➢ Clinical
  - ○ Estrogen and/or progesterone oral contraceptive drugs
  - ○ Anabolic steroids
  - ○ Type I glucagon storage disease
  - ○ Clinical course
    - – May enlarge
    - – When ≥ 5 cm may
      - ▪ Bleed
      - ▪ Undergo malignant degeneration
  - ○ Associated with use of OCA (oral contraceptive agent)
    - – Large, subcapsular lesions may rupture and bleed
    - – Resect if > 5 cm
    - – No malignant potential

- ➢ Genetic alterations
  - ○ HNF 1α inactivation ,through biallelic mutations of the TCF1 gene
  - ○ B-catenin activation
  - ○ Acute inflammation

- ➢ Diagnostic imaging
  - ○ Multiphase, helical CT or MRI
    - – Definite margin (pseudocapsule)
    - – Vessels enter adenoma at the periphery and pass in a spoke-wheel manner to the centre
    - – Focal avascular areas
  - ○ Technitium sulfur colloid scan
    - – Features on triphasic CT or gadolinium enhanced MRI may be difficult to distinguish from HCC
    - – A technitium sulfur colloid scan may be needed to show the typical cold lesions (no sulfur colloid uptake)
    - – Serum AFP may become positive when hepatic adenomas becomes malignant

358

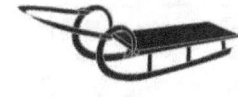

- Give the diagnostic imaging features of adenoma.
  - Ultrasound     -   Non diagnostic

  - Triple phase CT    -   Pre contrast: Hypo or isodense
    - Irregular enhancement
    - Delayed peripheral arterial enhancement during venous phase

  - MRI       -   T1: Low signal intensity with well defined capsule
    - T2: Heterogenous enhancement

  - Gadolinium enhanced MRI   -   Irregular enhancement with delayed washout

  - Radionuclide scan (tagged RBC)   -   ↓ uptake compared to surrounding liver

Source: Shiffman ML. *2009 ACG Annual Postgraduate Course*:167-171.


**Focal Nodular Hyperplasia** (FNH)

➢ Definition
  - "Focal nodular hyperplasia is a circumscribed, usually solitary lesion [of the liver] composed of nodules of benign hyperplastic hepatocytes surrounding a central stellate scar" (Sleisenger and Fordtran's Gastrointestinal and Liver Disease. 10th Edition. *Saunders/Elsevier* 2016, page 1622).

➢ Demography
  - 2nd only to hemangiomas as a cause of a benign tumour of the liver
  - Common congenital malformation of the liver vasculature

➢ Histopathology
  - With hyperplasia of hepatocytes around the vascular abnormality, leading to a central scan
  - Hyperplastic regenerative nodules separated by fibrosis septae.

359

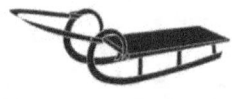

> Causes/associations

  o Adenomas

  o Cavernous hemangiomas (20%)

  o HHT (hereditary hemorrhagic telangiectasia)

  o Epithelial hemangioendothelioma

---

MCQ Trick

• Give whether FNH is caused by or affected by OCAs (oral contraceptive agents).

  o Caused by OCA     No

  o Affected by OCA     Yes

  o Not caused by OCA (oral contraceptive agents), but may enlarge under the influence of OCA

---

> Diagnostic imaging

  o Contract-enhanced CT (triphasic)

    – Hypodense

    – Arterial phase

      ▪ Enhanced

    – Single lesion

    – Subcapsular

    – Enhancement of mass during arterial phase

    – Fibrous septa

    – Centre

      ▪ No enhancement

      ▪ Central stellate scar

      ▪ Hemorrhage/necrosis

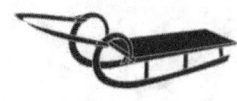

- Give the diagnostic imaging features of focal nodular hyperplasia.

    - Ultrasound  -  Variable appearance well defined borders

    - Triple phase CT  -  Pre contrast: Hypo or isodense
        - Homogenous arterial enhancement
        - Hypodense central scar
        - Isodense in delayed imaging
    - MRI
        - T1: low signal
        - T2: Hyperintense signal with central scar

    - Gadolinium
      enhanced MRI
        - Homogenous arterial enhancement
        - Hypodense central scar
        - Contrast accumulates in scar on delayed T1

    - Radionuclide scan  -  Equal or ↑ uptake compared to surrounding liver
      (tagged RBC)

Source: Shiffman ML. *2009 ACG Annual Postgraduate Course*:167-171.

> Differential

- Give an approach to distinguish between focal nodular hyperplasia (FNH) and hepatic adenoma (HA).

| | Characteristic | FNH | Adenoma |
|---|---|---|---|
| o | Gender | Female | Female |
| o | Hormone therapy | -* | +++ |
| o | Symptoms | Rare | Occasional |
| o | Multiple | About 30% | 12-30% |
| o | Pathological associations | Hemangiomas | Glycogenoses androgens, peliosis |
| o | Central arterial scar | Yes Static | No; If stimulated (estrogens, OCA) |
| o | Treatment | Conservative | Resection if symptomatic |
| o | Malignant potential | - | + |

*the telangiectatic subtype of FNA is associated with estrogen use

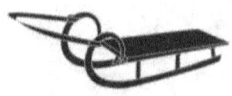

- Give clinical, laboratory and diagnostic imaging differences between FNH and FLHCC (fibrolamellar hepatocellular cancer).

| Feature | FLHCC | FNH |
|---|---|---|
| o Associated with cirrhosis | - | - |
| o Normal hepatic synthetic function | + | - |
| o Treated by surgical resection | + | Depends |
| o Diagnostic imaging | | |
|   - Central scar | + | + |
|   - Calcification | + | - |
|   - ↓ Intensity (dark, hypointense) on T2-images of MRI | + | - |
|   - Progressive enlargement | + | - |
| o Histology | | |
|   - Large, granular cells | + | - |
|   - Pale bodies | + | - |
|   - Bands of fibrosis | + | - |
| o Bile duct proliferation | - | + |
| o Malformed blood vessels in central scan | - | + |

➤ Treatment

- o No malignant potential

- o No treatment needed

## Nodular Regenerative Hyperplasia (NRH)

➤ Definition

- o Regenerative nodules without fibrosis

➤ Pathology

- o Injury to the hepatic vasculature from
  - Autoimmune disorders
  - Myeloproliferative syndromes
  - Antineoplastic medications → remodeling of surrounding liver tissue into a nodule around portal triads, which contains liver tissue and no fibrosis

362

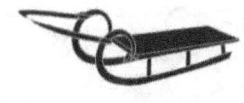

➢ Clinical
  o The nodules of regenerative liver tissue may
    - Compress adjacent hepatic vasculature, leading to non-cirrhotic portal hypertension
    - Compress bile ducts, leading to jaundice
  o Associated conditions
    – Hematological
      ▪ Hypercoagulable states
      ▪ Myelopreliferative disorders
      ▪ Lymphoproliferative disorders
    – Drugs
      ▪ Azathioprine
      ▪ Chemotherapeutic agents

➢ Diagnosis
  o MRI is the best diagnostic imaging test to distinguish HCC from a large cirrhotic nodule

➢ Treatment
  o Stop offending drug
  o Treat associated hematological disorders

## Focal Fatty Liver

  o Patchy process of fat accumulation which may look like a hepatic mass on diagnostic imaging

  o Typical appearance on CT scan which helps to distinguish FFL from metastatic lesion:
    – Density close to water
    – Not spherical in shape
    – No mass effect

  o The FFL may regress without treatment

➢ Diagnostic imaging
  o Abdominal ultrasound
    – Hyperechoic lesion       ▪ CT
    – Hypodense lesion          ▪ MRI
    – T1-weighted images positive
Note: No distortion of surrounding architecture

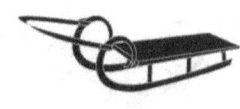

**Polycystic Liver Disease**

➤ Definition

o PCLD alone, or PCLD plus ADPKD (autosomal dominant polycystic kidney disease), or PCLD plus cysts in pancreas or spleen, arise from ductal plate malformation

➤ Histopathology

o May transform to squamous cell carcinoma

➤ Clinical associations

o CNS
   – Berry aneurysms

o CVS
   – Mitral valve prolapse

o Biliary tree
   – Biliary microhamartomous

o Liver
   – Congenital hepatic fibrous

o Colon
   – Colonic diverticulosis

o Inguinal hernias

➤ Clinical

o Associations
   – Congenital hepatic fibrosis
   – Caroli disease
   – Autosomal dominant polycystic kidney disease (ADPKD); aka PCLD, polycystic liver disease

o May undergo malignant degeneration to cholangiocarcinoma

➤ Diagnostic Imaging

o MRI
   – T2 – weighted image – bright fluid-filled cysts

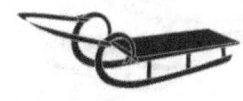

**Biliary Microhamartomas** (aka Von Meyenburg Complexes)

➤ Definition

   o Malformation of ductal plate leading to "cystically dilated intra- and interlobular bile ducts embedded in a fibrous stroma" in or near portal tracts

(Sleisenger and Fordtran's Gastrointestinal and Liver Disease. 10th Edition. *Saunders/Elsevier* 2016, page 1625)

**Hepatocellular Cancer** (HCC)

Clinical Pearls

   o Any mass in the liver of a patient with cirrhosis is considered to be malignant until proven otherwise.

➤ Demography

   o Hepatocellular carcinoma (HCC) is one of the most common malignant tumours worldwide and its incidence is increased in industrialized countries

   o M:F 2:1-4:1; increased BMI, androgenic hormones

   o 70-90% of HCC occur against the background of hepatic fibrosis grades 3 to 4, or cirrhosis, 1-4% per year (El-Serag HB, Rudolph KL. *Gastroenterology* 2007:2557-2576); the remainder are associated with HBV and hemochromatosis (HCV in Japan)

   o Risk of developing HCC in person with HBV infection
   
   – ~ 4/100 patient years

➤ Causes/associations

   o 70-90% of HCC occur against the background of hepatic fibrosis grades 3 to 4, or cirrhosis, 1-4% per year (El-Serag HB, Rudolph KL. *Gastroenterology* 2007:2557-2576); the remainder are associated with HBV and hemochromatosis (HCV in Japan)

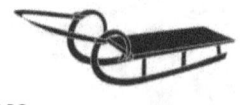

- Give risk factors for developing hepatocellular cancer ( HCC).
    - Patient
        - M:F 2:1 – 4.1
        - Africans > 20 years (HBV⁺)
        - Asian males> 40 years (HBV⁺)
        - Asian females >50 years (HBV⁺)
        - Family history of HCC
        - Dietary aflatoxin exposure
        - Obesity
        - Alcohol > 50 g/d
        - Tobacco
        - Marijuana
        - Oral contraceptive pill
        - Androgenic hormones
    - Inherited
        - Congenital/familial
    - Infection
        - HBV, HCV, HDV
    - Inflammation
        - AIH
    - Infiltration
        - HH
        - Adenoma
        - NASH
        - Previous HCC
    - Toxins
        - Alcohol
        - Tobacco
        - Alfatoxins
    - Metabolic
        - Diabetes mellitus
    - HBV + HIV coinfection
        - Older age of inset/diagnosis of HCC
        - Long duration of HCV > 25 yr
        - Failure to respond to treatment
            - Coinfection HCV + HDV and possibly HIV
            - Active

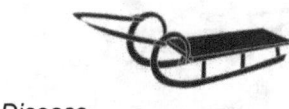

- o With cirrhosis
  - – HCV
  - – HCV +ALD + obesity (accelerated)
  - – EtOH
  - – Hemochromatosis- dietary Fe overload in persons of African ancestry; hereditary hemochromatosis
  - – PBC
  - – Alpha-1-antitrypsin deficiency
  - – NASH
  - – Autoimmune hepatitis
  - – Wilson disease
  - – Type 1 hereditary tyrosinemia
  - – Type 1 and type 2 glycogen storage disease
  - – Hypercitrulinemia
  - – Ataxia-telangiectasia
- o Medications
  - – Exposure to OCAs (oral contraceptives)

Abbreviations: ALD, alcoholic liver disease; FH, family history; NASH, non-alcoholic steatohepatitis; PBC, primary biliary cholangitis

Adapted from: Gores GJ. *AGA Institute Postgraduate Course Book* 2006: pg. 257.; Lai S-W, et al. Am J Gastroenterol 2012; 107: 46-52; and Sleisenger and Fordtran's Gastrointestinal and Liver Disease. 10th Edition. Saunders/Elsevier, Philadelphia, 2016, page Box 96.1, page 1604.

- • Give the mechanism for the ↑ risk of **HCC** in **HBV**, with or without the presence of cirrhosis.
  - o HBV is incorporated into cellular DNA (in 90% of HCC patients)
  - o Chromosomal insertion is random
  - o HBV is indirectly and directly carcinogenic
    - – Cis-activation of cellular genes
    - – Transcriptional activation of HBV x protein
    - – Viral mutations
    - – Activation of
      - ▪ MAP (mitogen-activated protein kinase)
      - ▪ JAK/STAT pathways (Janus kinase-signal transducer and activator of transcription)

367

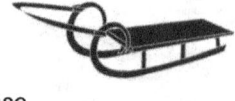

- Give the risk factors for HCC in HBV.
  - o Liver
    - – Degree of hepatic fibrosis
    - – Associated iron overload (hereditary hemochromatosis)
  - o Infection
    - – Failure of HCV to respond to IFN (interferon)
    - – Absence of previous HCV treatment
    - – Co-infection with HCV, HDV, and possibly HIV
    - – Active replication of HBV
    - – Genotype C
    - – Long duration of active disease

Adapted from: Gores GJ. *AGA Institute Post Graduate course book* 2006: pg. 251-2.

➢ Clinical
  - o Usually seen in the patient with cirrhosis
  - o Also occurs in non-cirrhotic
    - – HBV
    - – HCV (in Japan)
    - – Hereditary hemochromatosis
    - – α-AT deficiency
    - – NAFLD/NASH
    - – Hemochromatosis

---

SO YOU WANT TO BE A HEPATOLOGIST!

Auscultating an arterial bruit in the RUQ of a patient with cirrhosis suggests HCC.

- Give the significance of auscultating a friction rub.
  - o A friction rub auscultated in the RUQ of the abdomen suggests
    - – HCC (hepatocellular cancer)
    - – Liver metastasis
    - – Liver abscess

---

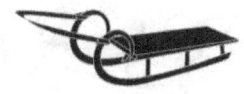

- Give paraneoplastic syndromes associated with hepatocellular carcinoma (HCC).

  - CNS          – Neuropathy

  - Endocrine    – Sexual changes- isosexual precocity, gynecomastia, feminization
    - Hypoglycemia
    - Hypercalcemia
    - Thyrotoxicosis

  - MSK         – Carcinoid syndrome
    - Hypertrophic osteoarthropathy
    - Osteoporosis
    - Polymyositis
    - Thrombophlebitis migrans

  - CVS         – Systemic arterial hypertension
  - Skin          – Porphyria
  - GI            – Watery diarrhea syndrome

  - Hematology  – Polycythemia (erythrocytosis)

Adapted from: *Sleisenger and Fordtran's Gastrointestinal and Liver Disease: Pathophysiology/ Diagnosis/ Management.* 10th edition, 2016, Box 96.3, page 1606.

---

**SO YOU WANT TO BE A GASTROENTEROLOGIST!**

Paraneoplastic syndromes are common in HCC.

- Give the name of the **substances secreted** by the HCC tumour, which result in paraneoplastic syndromes.

  | Syndrome | HCC-secreted substance |
  | --- | --- |
  | o Hypoglycemia | – Pre-IGF II (insulin-like growth factor) |
  | o Polycythemia | – Erythropoietin (or erythropoietin-like substance) |
  | o Hypercalcemia | – PTHrP (parathyroid hormone related peptide) |

369

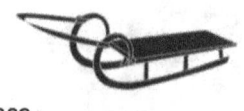

➤ Please also see

    o Sleisenger and Fordtran's Gastrointestinal and Liver Disease. 10th Edition. *Saunders/Elsevier* 2016, Box 96-1, page 1604; Table 92.2, page 1612; Table 96-3, page 1613

➤ Screening

- Give recommendations for **screening for HCC.**

    o Hepatitis B carriers
        – African >20 years
        – Asian males >40
        – Asian females >50
        – Family history of HCC
        – All patients with cirrhosis

    o Non HBV non-cirrhosis
        – Hepatitis C (in Japan)
        – Hereditary hemochromatosis
        – Alpha 1 antitrypsin deficiency
        – NASH
        – Autoimmune hepatitis

Adapted from: El-serag H.B. *2009 ACG Annual Postgraduate Course*: 39-43.

➤ Laboratory

---

**SO YOU WANT TO BE A GASTROENTEROLOGIST!**

- Give the circumstances when an elevated AFP (alfa fetoprotein) > 200 mg/mL is considered by AASLD guidelines to be diagnostic of HCC.

    o In the presence of cirrhosis or a mass in the liver (especially when > 2 cm)

---

    o In the presence of a liver mass in a person with cirrhosis and an AFP > 500 mg/mL, HCC is likely

        – Hepatic regenerative activity ↑AFP

    o Only 1/3 of HCC patients have AFP > 100 mg/ml, but values > 200 mg/ml are highly specific for HCC, 10.9 mg/ml, sensitivity 66% (Marrero JA, et al. *Gastroenterology* 2009.)

    o Diagnosis in a cirrhotic is usually made by diagnosticimaging, without liver biopsy (risk of seeding of tumour)

370

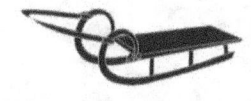

- A non-invasive diagnosis of HCC in a cirrhotic is suggested by
    - Nodule > 2 cm
    - AFP > 400 ng/mL
    - Diagnostic imaging
        - 1 of 2 tests, if AFP > 400 ng/mL
        - 2 of 2 tests, regardless of AFP

➢ Pathology

- Risk of seeding from tumour biopsy ~ 3%

\* Note: Not necessary to biopsy liver to diagnose HCC

- Give the pathology of hepatocellular (HCC).

    - Gross                – Nodules
        - Large circumscribed mass
        - Diffuse infiltration

    - Microscopic      – Well-differentiated
        - Trabecular form (thick trabeculae)
            - Hepatocytes – polygonal
            - Cytoplasm - ↓ eosinophilia
            - Nuclei
                - Large
                - Hyperdramatic
            - Nucleoli – prominent
            - Bile production
        - Acinar (pseudoglandular) form
            - Gland-lie structures arund a bile canaliculus
            - Bile canaliculus contains bile
        – Moderately differentiated
        - Pleomorphic, multinucleated giant cells
        - Cell nests
        - Central ischemic necrosis
        - Little bile connective tissue
        – Differentiated
        - Pleomorphic cells and nuclei
        - Bizz are giant cells
        - Globular hyaline

371

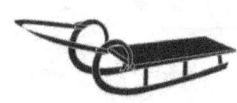

- Mallory hyaline

➢ Diagnostic imaging

- Give the **imaging criteria** applied for confirming HCC in patients with cirrhosis and a nodule detected by ultrasound.
  - o Ultrasound
    - Lesion has nodular configuration
    - Lesion is at least 1 cm in longest diameter*
    - Lesion shows arterial hypervascularization:
    - Hyper enhanced nodule in the arterial phase by two imaging techniques**
    - Hyper enhanced nodule in the arterial phase and as hypo enhanced nodule in the portal venous or delayed phase by one imaging technique**
    - In general terms, abdominal ultrasound has a sensitivity of 48% and a specificity of 97% for detection of HCC.

Algorithm for mass/nodule in cirrhotic liver on abdominal ultrasound (US) in persons at risk for HCC

| Diameter | Follow-up |
|----------|-----------|
| < 1 cm | US every 4 months for 1 year, then every 6 months longterm |
| > 1 cm | 4-phase CT / dynamic contrast enhanced MRI |

  - o Non-invasive criteria have been established by American and European groups (AASLD and EASL), and provide a similar sensitivity of about 80% in making a diagnosis of what turns out to be HCC.
  - o Hypervascularization in the arterial phase, followed by washout in the venous phase, suggestive of malignancy.
  - o CT scan
    - Arterial enhancement (hypervascular, supplied by hepatic artery) and washout, for HCC, sensitivity is 90% and specificityis 95%
    - ↓ HA, PV supply
    - Arterial neovascularization
    - Venous washout
  - o MRI
    - Similar performance characteristics as CT, but size of HCC is a factor, with accuracy of > 90% for > 20 mm lesion seen on MRI, but 30% for lesion < 20 mm
    - Biopsy under radiological guidance

| Test | Sensitivity | Specificity |
|------|-------------|-------------|
| • US | 90% | 91% |
| • CT | 92% | 98% |

- For hyper-enhanced nodule > 1 cm, suspect HCC
- Dynamic MRI using gadolinium contrast agents may be used in association with dynamic CT if the hepatic mass is 1 to 2 cm in size. The findings on the arterial phase of high signal intensity on T2-weighted images, on the venous and delayed phases finding central washout if contrast and capsular enhancement, have a sensitivity and specificity for HCC of 81% and 85%.
- MRI super-paramagnetic MRI
  - Iron oxide taken up by Kupffer cells, which are missing in HCC
  - Slows up as dark HCC on this test
  - Art phase gives sensitivity
  - Venous phase gives specificity

*apply to lesions emerged during Us surveillance. For lesions detected at first imaging examination, lesion diameter should be at least 2 cm to allow non-invasive diagnosis of HCC.

**imaging techniques include: contrast-enhanced US, contrast-enhanced spiral CT, and gadolinium enhanced MRI.

Source: El-serag H.B. *2009 ACG Annual Postgraduate Course*: 39-43.

➢ Staging

• Give the Okuda staging system of HCC.

| Criterion | Cut-off |
|---|---|
| o Tumour size | >50% (largest cross-sectional area of tumour to largest cross-sectional area of liver) = positive <br> <50% = negative |
| o Ascites | Clinically detectable = positive <br> Undetectable = negative |
| o Serum albumin | <3g/dL = positive <br> >3g/dL = negative |
| o Serum bilirubin | <3g/dL = positive <br> >3g/dL = negative |
| o Stage | |
| – I | No positive criterion |
| – II | positive criteria |
| – III | Three positive criteria |

Printed with permission: Nguyen MH, and Keeffe EB. *Best Practice & Research Clinical Gastroenterology* 2005;19(1):164.

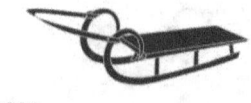

Accurate staging at the time of diagnosis, based on the Barcelona Clinic Liver Cancer classification (BCLC), is central to the choice of the appropriate therapeutic strategy

- Give the components of **BCLC** staging classification for HCC.
  - o Tumour size and spread
  - o Patient performance status
  - o Child-Pugh class

See Feldman M., et al. Sleisenger and Fordtran's Gastrointestinal and Liver Disease. 9th Edition. *Saunders/Elsevier* 2010, Figure 94.4, page 1576.

- Give the algorithm for staging and treating patients diagnosed as having hepatocellular carcinoma. This algorithm is based on the BCLC guidelines.

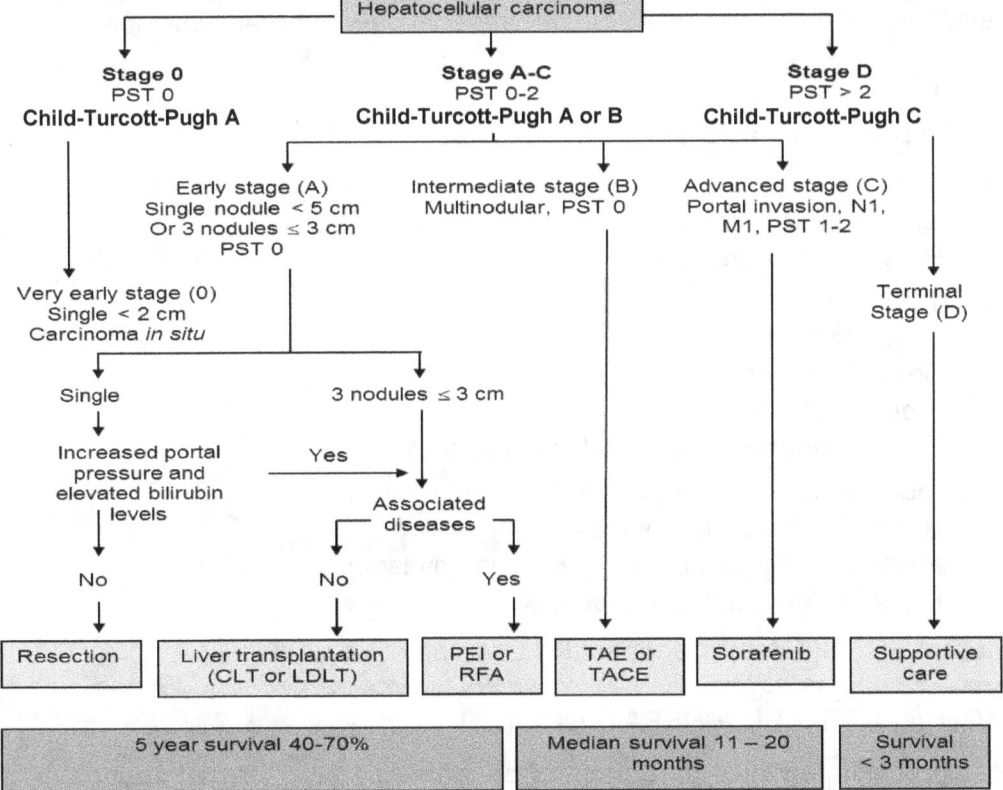

Abbreviations: CLT, cadaveric liver transplantation; LDLT, live donor liver transplantation; PEI, percutaneous ethanol injection; PST, performance status test; RFA, radiofrequency ablation; TACE; transarterial chemoembolization; TAE, transarterial embolization

Printed by permission: Cabibbo et al. *Nature Clinical Practice Gastroenterology and Hepatology* 2009;6(3): 159-169. and Bruix J, Sherman M. Hepatology. 2011; 53(3): 1020–1022.

374

- Give the differential of **hypervascularity** on ultrasound, in addition to HCC.
    - Arterial portal shunts
    - Atypical hemangiomas
    - Aberrant venous drainage
    - Dysplastic nodules
    - Confluent fibrosis
    - The most sensitive and specific imaging technique for the diagnosis of HCC is Gad-MR (gadolinium magnetic resonance). Other methods include contrast-enhanced ultrasonography, helical-computed tomography, and superparamagnetic iron oxide magnetic resonance.
    - Hepatic nodules < 2 cm in diameter may still contain a focus of HCC.

Abbreviation: LT, liver transplantation; RFA, radiofrequency ablation; TACE, transarterial chemoembolization; TACI, transarterial chemotherapy infusion

- ➢ Prognosis
- Give the prognostic factors in HCC.
    - Patient
        - ECOG classification
        - Presence of symptoms
    - Liver function
        - Child-Pugh class
        - Serum bilirubin
        - Albumin levels
        - Presence/absence of portal hypertension
    - Tumour status
        - Number and size of nodules
        - Presence/absence of macrovascular invasion
        - Presence/absence of extrahepatic spread

Abbreviation: ECOG, Eastern Cooperative Oncology Group

SO YOU WANT TO BE A HEPATOLOGIST!

- In approximately give proportion of patients with HCC or pancreatic cancer in whom investigations suggest that the primary lesion is resectable will the tumour turn out to be non-resectable as defined by diagnostic laparoscopy and laparoscopic ultrasound.

    - About one third of patient's with HCC or pancreatic cancer will have their respectability status down-graded to non-resectable by diagnostic laparoscopy and laparoscopic ultrasonography.

375

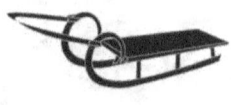

- ➤ Screening/surveillance
  - o Every 6 months AFP (alpha-fetoprotein) and abdominal ultrasound over 5 years improves survival from HCC in HBV-positive patients in China (42-5). Most of the detected HCC in the screened group were detected at an early stage; with 3 year survival rates after HCC resection of 53% in the screened group versus none in the non-screened group
  - o Improved survival from HCC screening depends of course on the availability of effective therapy for the early detected lesions
  - o HCC screening in persons awaiting liver transplantation is cost-effective

Abbreviation: AFP, alpha-fetoprotein; HCC, hepatocellular cancer

- • Give the category of patients with chronic liver disease who are recommended for surveillance for HCC.
  - o Non-cirrhotic
    - – HBV carriers with
      - ▪ Active hepatitis
      - ▪ Family history of HCC
    - – HCV chronic hepatitis plus fibrosis
  - o Cirrhotic
    - – C-P A and B
    - – C-P C awaiting liver transplantation

Abbreviation: C-P, Child-Pugh

- • Give the risk of cirrhosis, hepatocellular carcinoma (HCC) and mortality in hepatitis B and hepatitis C virus (HBV/HCV) monoinfected and coinfected patients.

|  | Cirrhosis[1] | HCC (OR)[2] | Mortality (SMR)[3] |
|---|---|---|---|
| HBV monoinfection | ~ 22% | 16-23 | 1.4-5.3 |
| HCV monoinfection | ~ 30% | 8-17 | 2.4-3.1 |
| HBV/HCV coinfection | ~ 50% | 36-165 | 5.6-49 |

Abbreviations: HBV, hepatitis B; HCC, hepatocellular carcinoma; HCV, hepatitis C; OR, odds ratio; SMR, standard mortality ratio

[1]Zarski et al, 1998
[2]Shi et al, 2005 Donato et al, 1998
[3]Amin et al, 2006 Di Marco et al, 1999

Printed with permission: Wursthorn, et al. *Best Practice Res Clin Gastroenterol* 2008;22:1063-1079.

376

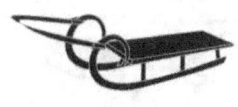

- Give precursor lesions of HCC (hepatocellular cancer) in the patient with hereditary hemochromatosis.
  - Males with iron overload and advanced fibrosis
  - Dysplastic lesions
  - Proliferative lesions
  - Increased number of iron free foci (IFF, >50% at risk to develop HCC)

Adapted from: Hytiroglou P, et al. *Gastroenterol Clin North Am* 2007;36(4):867-87.

---

**SO YOU WANT TO BE A HEPATOLOGIST!**

Multiphase, dynamic, helical CT is the imaging technique of choice for the diagnosis of HCC. The most helpful features are enhanced arterial phase in the involved area, washout (loss of central nodule enhancement composed with uninvolved liver), and enhancement of the capsule in the porto-venous and delayed phase. When the lesion is > 2 cm these diagnostic imaging changes.

- Give the reasons why the classical CT changes of HCC may disappear as the HCC enlarges
  - Arterial enhancement (neoangiogenesis causing hypervascularity)
  - Shift of blood from primarily portal artery

---

- Give non-histological diagnostic criteria for HCC (hepatocellular cancer).
  - Hepatic mass on ultrasound in cirrhotic
  - Focal lesion > 2 cm with evidence of cirrhosis (if <2 cm, on 2 imaging modalities – CT angiogram Arterial hypervascularization and venous washout MRI (contrast enhanced ultrasound; MRI – triphasic (hyper $T_2$, 150-$T_1$)
  - AFP > 200 ng/ml (normal AFP does not R/o HCC)
  - Sulphur colloid scan – old (Kupffer cells positive in FNH)
  - Non-cirrhotic HBV, HCV (Japan), hemochromatosis, αAT deficiency

Adapted from: Talwalkar JA, and Gores GJ. *Gastroenterology* 2004;127(5 Suppl 1):S126-32.

377

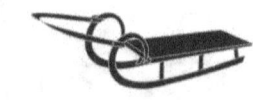

- Treatment
  - Accurate staging at the time of diagnosis, based on the Barcelona Clinic Liver Cancer classification, is central to the choice of the appropriate therapeutic strategy
  - Accurate staging at the time of diagnosis, based on the Barcelona Clinic Liver Cancer classification, is central to the choice of the appropriate therapeutic strategy
  - Therapeutic options for advanced HCC have improved considerably during the past few years and now include targeted therapy with sorafenib, an inhibitor of multiple tyrosine kinases
  - Novel therapeutic strategies are needed that will further improve survival of patients with HCC, especially for those who present with advanced disease at the time of diagnosis
  - Clinical trials should follow guidelines that define meaningful primary and secondary end points and should be coordinated by centres with expertise in the care of patients with HCC
  - Sorafanib, a mixed kinase inhibitor, prolongs survival in persons with metastatic HCC

---

SO YOU WANT TO BE A GASTROENTEROLOGIST!

- Give the management of the "**post-embolization syndrome**" (abdominal pain, nausea / vomiting, fever) associated with hepatic arterial embolization and chemoembolization for hepatic tumour (e.g., HCC, metastatic GIST).
  - Just provide supportive care.

---

- Give treatment options for the patient with HCC.
  - Staging, MRI – Barcellona criteria, Child's stage
  - Surgical resection
  - Partial hepatectomy (HBV) satisfying Milan criteria:
    - 1 tumour, < 5 cm
    - 3 tumours, each < 3 cm
    - Edmonton volume criteria <115 mm$^3$
    - No distant metastasis
    - No portal vein distension
    - Liver transplantation (LT)

378

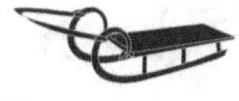

- Chemotherapy: po, iv, transarterial (TA) chemoembolization (TACE), TA chemotherapy infusion (TACI); drug eluting beads
- Percutaneous hepatic injection: ethanol or acetic acid injection
- Energy-mediated ablation: cryoablation, microwave or radiofrequency ablation (RFA), for < 2 cms potentially curative
- Radiotherapy: internal, external
- Palliative care
- Investigational: somastostatin, immune modulation, gene therapy, PDT
- Mixed tyrosine kinase inhibitors (sorafanib)

Adapted from: Nguyen MH,et al. *Best Pract Res Clin Gastroenterol* 2005;19(1): pg 164.; and Tranberg KG. *Best Pract Res Clin Gastroenterol* 2004;18(1): 127.

- Give the management strategy of HCC based on CTP class, size and performance status (PS).

| | | | |
|---|---|---|---|
| CTP A, PS-O | Single HCC <2cm | HVPG <10mmHg and bilirubin < 1.5 mg/dL | Surgical resection |
| | | Varices/collaterals or HVPG >10 mmHg or bilirubin >1.5mg/dL | Live transplant evaluation RFA/PEI |
| CTP A-B, PS, 0-2 | Single HCC 2-5 cm | HVPG <10mmHg and bilirubin <1.5 mg/dL | Surgical resection |
| | | Varices/collaterals or HVPG >10 mmHg or bilirubin >1.5mg/dL | Liver transplant evaluation RFA/PEI |
| | 2 or 3 HCC masses <3 cm (the largest) Intermediate stage (multinodular, PS,O) Advanced stage (portal invasion, metastases) | | Liver transplant evaluation Radiofrequency ablation Transarterial chemoembolization Sorafenib |
| CTP C, PS>2 | Terminal stage | | Symptomatic treatment |

Abbreviations: CTP, Child-Turcotte- Pugh; HCC,hepatocellular carcinoma; HVPG, hepatic venous pressure gradient; PEI,percutaneous ethanol injection; PS, performance status; RFA, radiofrequency ablation

Printed with permission: Garcia Tsao et al. *Am J Gastroenterol* 2009; 104:1802-1829.

379

- The BCLC staging system for HCC. M, metastasis classification; N, node classification; PS, performance status; RFA, radiofrequency ablation; TACE, transarterial chemoembolization.

- A cirrhotic patient with HCC has good hepatic reserve, and TACE (transarterial chemoembolization) is undertaken for downstaging of the tumour prior to liver transplantation (LT), as well as a bridge to LT. Unfortunately, hepatic decompensation may occur rapidly after TACE.

Compare and contrast the prevention and treatment of HCC in persons with HBV and HCV infection.

| | HBV | HCV |
|---|---|---|
| o New infection | – Neonatal vaccination | ▪ General infection control |
| o Existing infection | – Antiviral therapy (suppression) | ▪ Antiviral therapy (eradication) |
| | – Nucleos (t) ide analogues | ▪ Interferon plus ribavirin; role of proteinase inhibitors under study |
| o Treatment | – Early diagnosis and curative treatment | |
| o Prevent recurrence | – Transplantation | |
| | – Antiviral therapy (?) | |
| | – Molecular targeting drug | |

Abbreviations: HBV, hepatitis B virus; HCC, hepatocellular carcinoma; HCV, hepatitis C virus

Printed with permission: Masuzaki, et al. *Best Prac Res Clin Gastroenterol* 2008:1137-1151.

- Give the likely explanation for the severe and unfortunate adverse effect of TACE in a person with a portal vein (PV) thrombosis.

  - The TACE catheter is inserted into the HA (hepatic artery) which is the main source of blood supply to the liver, along with the PV (portal vein).

  - If the patient had a PV thrombosis associated with the HCC, the only residual blood supply to the liver is the HA, in which flow may have been partially compromised by TACE.

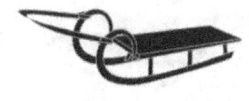

**Fibrolamellar HCC**

➤ Pathology

- Hepatocytes      – Large
  -                            – Eosinophilic

- Cytoplasm      – Large mitochondria
  -                            – Hyaline bodies

- Fibrous stroma      – Forming trabeculae or nodules

- Stain for cytokerain 19 to determine if the HCC is the even more aggressive progenitor cell variety arising from stems cells near the canals of Hering

➤ Differential

- Give the non-pathological characteristics with differentiate FLM (fibrolamellae HCC) from HCC.

  - Younger persons
  - Not associated with
    - Cirrhosis
    - HBV, HCV
  - No AFP secreted
  - Better prognosis

**Cholangiocarcinoma**

➤ Demography
  - Prevalence in North America, $1/10^5$
  - Cholangiocarcinoma is the second most common hepatic malignant tumour.

➤ Subtypes
  - Intrahepatic
  - Extrahepatic
  - Hilar (Klatskin tumour)
  - Distal bile duct
  - Bismuth - Corlette Classification (Sleisenger and Fordtran's Gastrointestinal and Liver Disease, 9th Edition. Sauders/Elsevier, Philadelphia, 2010, Table 69.3, page 1173 for details of Diagnostic Criteria for Cholangiocarcinoma.
  - Perihilar cholangiocarcinoma is extrahepatic in location, but the ICD classification considers that this an intrahepatic tumour

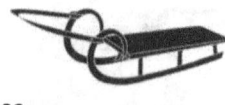

➤ Causes/associations

• Give factors/associations which increase the risk of cholangiocarcinoma.

| | | | |
|---|---|---|---|
| ○ | Infection | – | HCV-associated cirrhosis |
| | | – | Clonorchis viverrini and sinensis |
| ○ | Developmental | – | Caroli disease |
| | | – | Choledochal cyst |
| ○ | Cholelithiasis, intrahepatic | – | PSC (primary sclrosing cholangitis) |
| | | – | Caroli disease |
| | | – | Choledochal cyst |
| | | – | Thorotrast contract dye |

➤ Laboratory tests

• Give tests used to diagnose cholangiocarcinoma.

  ○ Diagnosis        – CA 19-9, CEA, CA 19-9 + CEA, CA-125

  ○ Tumour marker CA 19-9

    – False positives   ▪ Cancer   – Stomach
                                   – Pancreas
                                   – Colon
                                   – Gynecologic

                      ▪ Acute bacterial cholangitis

    – False negative   ▪ Lewis blood group-negative
                         – With PSC – CA 19-9 > 129 U/ml; sensitivity 79%; specificity 98%
                         – Without PSCs > 100 U/ml; sensitivity, 53%; specificity 89%

| CA 19-19 | Sensitivity | NPV | Specificity |
|---|---|---|---|
| ○ CA 19-9, biliary obstruction | | | |
| – Without PSC | 53% | 72 to 92% | |
| – With PSC | 38% to 89% | | 50% to 98% |

| ○ Cytology | Sensitivity |
|---|---|
| – Cytology | 30% |
| – Cytology, brushings and biopsies | 40% to 70% |

382

- ➢ Diagnostic Imaging
  - ○ Locations
    - − Hepatic bifurcation (Klatskin tumour)
    - − Distal CBD
    - − Intrahepatic (5-15%)
  - ○ MRI
    - − MRI "… is currently the imaging technique for cholangiocarcinoma" (Sleisenger and Fordtran's Gastrointestinal and Liver Disease. 9th Edition. Saunders/Elsevier, Philadelphia, 2010, page 1174).
    - − IDUS high frequency intraductal ultrasound
    - − CT/PET; sensitivity/specificity; intrahepatic, 93% and 80%, but extrahepatic, 53% and 33%, respectively.
    - − MRCP –
    - T1 –weighted, hypodense lesion
    - T2 –weighted, intense lesion
    - − Variable fibrosis and necrosis
    - − Atrophy
    - − Capsular retraction
    - − Biliary duct dilation
    - − Hypovascular (progressive, delayed hyperenhancement)

- ➢ Endoscopy
  - ○ ERCP + cytology
  - ○ Choledochoenteroscopy
  - ○ ERCP + choledoscopy (for dominant stricture; sensitivity 92%)

- ➢ Histopathology
  - ○ Few cells (paucicellular)
  - ○ Brush cytology
  - ○ FNA (fine-needle aspiration)
  - ○ Desmoplastic reaction
  - ○ FISH (fluorescence hybridization)
  - ○ Cytology
  - ○ Acinar or tubular structures
  - ○ Absent bile secretion
  - ○ Desmoplastic reaction
  - ○ Prominent colonization of stroma
  - ○ May be difficult to distinguish from metastatic adenocarcinoma

383

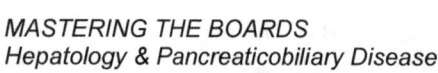

> Treatment
  - Liver
    - Transplantation
    - Resection

- Give the criteria for surgical resection of cholangiocarcinoma.
  - No extrahepatic metastases
  - No encasement or invasion of
  - No involvement of both segmental bile duct
  - No contralateral lobular atrophy

> Prognosis
  - When not a surgical candidate, survival rate
    - 1 year    28%
    - 5 year    5%
    - 5 year    29% to 36%
  - Liver transplantation combined with radiation, brachytherapy and chemosensitization
    - 5 year    82% survival rate

"The pain you feel today is the strength you feel tomorrow. For every challenge encountered there is opportunity for growth."

Unknown

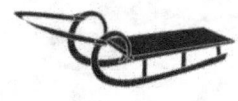

## LIVER TRANSPLANTATION (LT)

➢ Prognosis (survival rate [SR])

- o 92% 5 yr SR
- o 80% 10 yr SR

• Give the prognostic significance of a person requiring hemodialysis before LT.

- o "…return of adequate renal function is unlikely after transplantation of dialysis has been required for more than one month prior to liver transplantation" (Sleisenger and Fordtran's Gastrointestinal and Liver Disease. 9th Edition. Saunders/Elsevier 2010, page 1597); combined liver-kidney transplantation may need to be considered.

➢ Clinical

- o Causes of death Post-LT
  - "natural" causes ⎫ – 2x ↑ risk non-skin solid organ cancers
  - Malignancy 21% ⎭ – 30x ↑ lymphoproliferative disorders
  - Infection
  - Recurrent liver disease
  - "de-novo malignancy post-liver transplant (L-Tx)"

➢ Indications

• Give the indications for liver transplantation.

- o Acute liver failure (ALF; fulminant hepatic failure; King's College criteria)
- o Complications of cirrhosis
  - Ascites
  - Encephalopathy
  - ↓ synthetic dysfunction
  - Liver cancer (HCC)
  - Refractory variceal hemorrhage
  - By bleeding
    - Esophageal/gastric varices
    - Portal hypertensive gastropathy
  - Coagulopathy
  - $Na_s$ (serum sodium concentration)
  - Hepatopulmonary syndrome
  - Portopulmonary hypertension
  - DILI
  - Acute/chronic renal failure
  - ↑ MELD score
  - Hepatorenal syndrome
  - Vascular thrombosis, e.g., Budd-Chiari

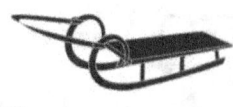

- Liver-based metabolic conditions causing systemic disease, and which may also cause liver disease
  - Primary oxaluria
  - Familial Amyloidosis
- Inherited liver diseases
  - $\alpha_1$-antitrypsin deficiency
  - Wilson disease
  - Urea cycle enzyme deficiencies
  - Glycogen storage disease
  - Tyrosemia

Adapted from: Lilly LB, Girgrah N, and Levy GA. *First Principles of Gastroenterology* 2005: pg. 634.

---

## SO YOU WANT TO BE A HEPATOLOGIST!

There are many indications for liver transplantation (LT) (Please see, Sleisenger and Fordtran's Gastrointestinal and Liver Disease. 9th Edition. Saunders/Elsevier 2010, Table 95.1, page 1594, Indications for Liver Transplantation). In adults,

- In adults, give the commonest diseases of the liver for which transplantation is performed include
  - HBC, 33%
  - Cholestatic disorders, 14%
  - ALD (alcoholic liver disease), 12%
  - NASH, 9%
  - HCC, 6%
  - HBV, 4%

Adapted from: Martin P, et al. *Sleisenger & Fordtran's gastrointestinal and liver disease: Pathophysiology/Diagnosis/Management* 2006: pg. 2037; and 2010, pg. 1594.

- Give the major indications for liver transplant (LT) in children.
  - Biliary atresia
  - Failed portoenterostomy (Kasai procedure) for biliary atresia.

---

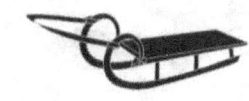

- ➢ Contraindications
    - ○ Definition of the word "Contraindications"
        - – Definition: Absolute contraindication – "…a clinical circumstance in which the likelihood of a successful outcome is so remove that liver transplantation should not be offered (Sleisenger and Fordtran's Gastrointestinal and Liver Disease. 9th Edition. *Saunders/Elsevier* 2010, page 1596),
        - – While there are many "absolute" contraindications to LT (please see (Sleisenger and Fordtran's Gastrointestinal and Liver Disease. 9th Edition. *Saunders/Elsevier* 2010, Table 95.2, page 1596 and Table 95.4, page 1600), there are many "shades of grey"

Please see, Feldman M., et al. Sleisenger and Fordtran's Gastrointestinal and Liver Disease. 9th Edition. Saunders/Elsevier 2010, Table 95.4, page 1600.

- • Give possible "relative" contraindications to liver transplantation.
    - ○ Patient
        - – Ongoing alcohol or drug abuse
        - – Non-adherence
        - – Lack of social support
        - – Serious underlying symptomatic illness
        - – Advanced cardio-pulmonary disease
        - – Sepsis
        - – Marked psychiatric impairment
        - – HIV/AIDS
        - – Diabetes mellitus
        - – Advanced age
        - – Obesity
        - – Multi-organ failure
        - – Increased intracranial pressure
        - – Jehovah Witness
        - – Non-adherence
    - ○ Anatomy
        - – Metastatic cancer
        - – Anatomical abnormalities
        - – PV thrombosis (large size)
        - – Outside Milan criteria for HCC (1 lesion <5 cm, 3 lesions <3 cm)
        - – Cholangiocarcinoma
    - ○ Liver
        - – Mild liver disease (Child <7, or MELD <9)

387

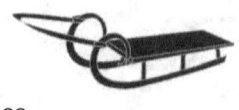

- o Co-morbidity
  - – Pulmonary hypertension
  - – Right heart dysfunction
  - – Extrahepatic cancer

Adapted from: Hay J. *Mayo Clinic Gastroenterology and Hepatology Board Review* 2008: pg. 433.

- Give medical methods introduced recently to **increase the availability** or to extend the fair allocation of livers for transplantation.
  - o MELD (Model for End-Stage Liver Disease)
    - – Equitable organ allocation
  - o MELD score and retransplantation
    - – The MELD score has helped to equitably allocate donor livers for transplantation, with the sick patients with higher MELD scores moving to "…the head of the line [waiting list]". When patients undergo retransplantation, then probability of survival is about 20% lower than their outcome expected following the initial transplantation.
    - – Maximal utility is achieved with MELD score for

      | HCV | 21 |
      |---|---|
      | Non-HCV | 24 |

  - o Modified MELD
    - – Hyponatremia (dilutional)
    - – HCC
    - – HPC (hepatopulmonary syndrome)
    - – Polycystic disease
  - o LDLT (liver-donor liver transplantation)
  - o Split decreased-donor grafts
  - o Marginal/extended criteria grafts

➢ Assessment

The **UNOS listing criteria** for status 1, 2A, 2B and 3 for liver transplantation.

❖ Status 1
  - o Fulminant hepatic failure. Onset within 8 weeks of initial symptoms and one of the following:
    - – Stage 2 encephalopathy
    - – Bilirubin > 15 mg/dl
    - – INR > 2.5
    - – Hypoglycemia (glucose level < 50 mg/dl)

388

- Primary non-function of graft transplanted within 7 days
- Hepatic artery thrombosis occurring within 7 days of transplantation
- Acute decompensated Wilson disease

❖ Status 2A

- Patient with chronic liver failure and a Child-Pugh score ≥10, in the critical care unit, with a life expectancy without a liver transplant of less than 7 days, with at least one of the following criteria:
  - Unresponsiveness active variceal hemorrhage with failure or contraindication of     surgical or transjugular intra-hepatic shunt
  - Hepatorenal syndrome
  - Refractory ascites/hepatorenal syndrome (hydrothorax)
  - Stage 3-4 encephalopathy unresponsive to therapy
- Contraindications to status 2A listing:
  - Extrahepatic sepsis unresponsive to antimicrobial therapy
  - Requirement for high dose or two or more pressor agents to maintain an adequate blood pressure
  - Severe, irreversible multi-organ failure

❖ Status 2B

- Patients with chronic liver disease and a Child-Pugh score ≥10, or ≥7 and one or more of the following clinical considerations:
  - Unresponsive variceal hemorrhage
  - Hepatorenal syndrome
  - Spontaneous bacterial peritonitis
  - Refractory ascites/hepatorenal syndrome (hydrothorax)
- Liver transplant candidates with hepatocellular carcinoma can be registered as status 2B if they meet the following criteria:
  - Thorough assessment has excluded metastatic disease
  - Recipient has one nodule ≤5 cm or three or fewer nodules all ≤3cm
  - Patient is not a resection candidate

❖ Status 3

- Patients with chronic liver disease and a Child-Pugh score ≥7

Adapted from: United Network Organ Sharing. *UNOS policy 3.6* June 23, 2009.

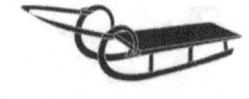

- Give the **protocol for evaluation** of potential living-related liver donors.

Stage 1
- o Complete history and physical examination
- o Laboratory blood tests: liver biochemical test, blood chemistry, hematology, coagulation profile, urinalysis, alpha-fetoprotein, carcinoembryonic antigen, and serologic tests for hepatitis A, B, and C, cytomegalorvirus, Epstein-Barr virus, and human immunodeficiency virus
- o Imaging studies: abdominal ultrasound examination, chest x-ray

Stage 2
- o Complete psychiatric and social evaluation
- o Imaging studies: computed tomography scan of the abdomen
- o Other studies: pulmonary function tests, echocardiography

Stage 3
- o Histology: liver biopsy
- o Imaging studies: celiac and superior mesenteric angiography with portal phase

Stage 4
- o Imaging studies: magnetic resonance cholangiogram Informed consent

Printed with permission: Ghobrial RM, et al. *Clin Liver Dis* 2000; 4: 553.

➤ Complications

- Give early and/or late non-pharmaceutical complications arising after liver transplantation.
  - o Surgery-related
    - – Non-specific
    - – Cannot get off of ventilator
    - – Dehiscence
    - – Ileus
    - – DVT (deep vein thrombosis)
    - – Atelectasis
  - o Metabolic
    - – Hypertension
    - – Hypercholesterolemia
    - – Diabetes mellitus
    - – Obesity
    - – Sexual dysfunction
  - o Abdominal bleeding
    - – Anastomoses (immediate)
    - – Site of implantation (immediate)

390

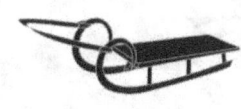

- Vascular complications
  - Suprahepatic/infrahepatic vena caval obstruction (immediate)
  - Hepatic artery thrombosis (early)
  - Portal vein thrombosis (early)
  - Hepatic artery stenosis (late)
- Biliary complications
  - T-tube insertion (early)
  - Anastomosis (early)
  - Stenosis of papilla vateri (early)
  - T-tube removal (late)
  - Anastomosis, extrahepatic (late)
  - Multiple strictures, intra-hepatic, abscesses
- Renal failure (adverse effects of treatment)
- Vascular
  - Coronary artery disease (dyslipoproteinemia)
  - Cerebrovascular
  - Peripheral vascular
- CNS/PNS
  - Depression
  - Neuropathy
  - Seizures
- Malignancy
  - Lymphoma
  - EBV-PTLD (Ebstein-Barr virus – post transplant lymphoproliferative disorder)
  - Pre-existing malignancies (within 5 years)
  - Acquired donor malignancy
  - Increased risk of all malignancies
    - Skin cancers (non melanoma)
    - Non-skin solid tumours
      - Head and neck
      - Esophagus
      - Kaposi sarcoma
      - Cervical (HPV)
      - Prostate
      - Lung
      - Breat
      - Colon

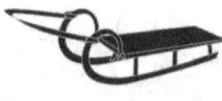

- o Infections
  - – Viral (HSV, CMV, EBV)
  - – Bacterial (lines, wound)
  - – Fungal (PCP, Candida - catheters)
- o Drug reactions
- o 1° graft failure
- o Rejection
- o Recurrence of disease
- o Death

Adapted from: Mueller AR, Platz KP, and Kremer B. *Best Practice & Research Clinical Gastroenterology* 2004;18(5): 882

## Non-GI adverse effects of immune suppression

- Give the most common adverse effects of immune-suppressive drugs frequently used after orthotopic liver transplantation.

| Adverse Effect | Cyclo-sporin | Tacro-limus | Gluco-Corticoids | Azathio-prine | Myco-phenolate Mofetil | mTOR Inhibitors |
|---|---|---|---|---|---|---|
| Alopecia | - | + | - | + | + | - |
| Arterial hypertension | +++ | ++ | +++ | - | - | + |
| Bone marrow suppression | + | + | - | +++ | +++ | ++ |
| Dermatitis | - | + (rash, pruritus) | + | - | - | ++ (oral ulcers, acne) |
| Gastrointestinal** Toxicity | + | + | + | + pancreatitis | +++ (gastritis and/or diarrhea) | ++ |
| Hirsutism and/or gingival hyperplasia | + | - | - | - | - | - |
| Hyperglycemia and diabetes mellitus | -(?) | + | +++ | - | - | - |
| Hyperlipidemia | ++ | + | ++ | - | - | +++ |
| Impaired wound healing | - | - | + | + | + | ++ |

392

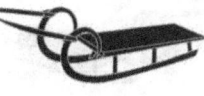

| Adverse Effect | Cyclo-sporin | Tacro-limus | Gluco-Corticoids | Azathio-prine | Myco-phenolate Mofetil | mTOR Inhibitors |
|---|---|---|---|---|---|---|
| Lymphoma malignancy | ++ | ++ | - | ? | ? | - |
| Myalgia arthralgia | - | - | + | + | - | ++ |
| Nephrotoxicity | +++ (K+, Mg²+) | +++ (K+, Mg²+) | - | - | - | + proteinuria |
| Neurotoxicity[a] | ++ | ++ | + psychiatric | - | + headache | - |
| Osteoporosis | + | + | +++ | - | - | - |
| Pneumonitis | - | - | - | - | - | + |

It should be noted that each agent has other specific adverse effects in addition to those listed in the table. [a]Neurotoxicity includes mainly peripheral neuropathy, headaches, tremor, convulsions, akinetic mutism, and insomnia.

? , Incidence unknown; - not reported; + rarely reported; ++ commonly reported; +++ very frequently reported adverse effect limiting usage of the drug.

Printed with permission:  Benten D, et al. *Nature Clinical Practice Gastroenterology and Hepatology* 2009;6:1:23-36.

**please see separate table of GI complications of immunosuppression associated with liver transplantation.

- Give gastrointestinal complications of transplant immunosuppression.
    - Infections
        - Viral: CMV (especially for MMF), HSV
        - Fungal: Candida albicans, candida tropicalis
        - Bacterial: versinia enterocolitica, Clostridium difficile
        - Parasites: microspordia, Strongyloides, *H. pylori* (70% in renal transplant recipients, and 60% in hemodialysis patients)
    - Mucosal injury and ulceration
        - Diarrhea, constipation dyspepsia (especially tacrolimus and MMF)
        - Ulcerations: stress/NSAID ulcers
            - Giant gastric ulcers (>3cm, lung transplant recipients)
        - Diverticular disease: complicated diverticulitis (perforation, abscess, Phlegmon, fistula); especially with polycystic kidney disease
        - Perforations: early, late (especially from diverticulitis or CMV colitis)

393

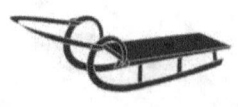

- o Biliary tract disease
  - Cholecystectomy (often as an emergency, high mortality [MR])
  - Cholelithiasis
- o Pancreatitis
  - 5% in liver, Tx, MR 64%
- o Liver
  - Acute cellular rejection
  - Acute early cellular rejection of graft occurs in the first few weeks after liver transplantation, especially for REC and AH
  - Chronic rejection occurs in 10% of liver transplant recipients, especially in HCV or AH
  - Recurrence of initial condition/retransplantation
  - Post liver transplantation steatosis
    - Steatosis occurs in as many as a third of persons following a liver transplantation (LT), with a histological diagnosis of NASH occurring in about 10% of these persons.
- o Post-transplant diabetes and cardiovascular disease
  - Early after liver transplantation, transient hyperglycemia occurs in 40% of patients, and 9-21% have persistent hyperglycemia (new onset diabetes)
  - Hyperlipidemia occurs in 20-50% of liver transplant patient, with a 2.6 fold higher risk of coronary artery disease (CAD) and 20% of deaths occurring 3 years after liver transplantation coming from CAD

Abbreviation: CAD, coronary artery disease

- Give factors which predict the risk for **post-LT steatosis.**
  - o Post-LT obesity
  - o Diabetes mellitus
  - o Hyperlipidemia
  - o Arterial hypertension
  - o Tacrolimus-based immunosuppression regimen
  - o Alcoholic cirrhosis as the primary indication for LT (Dumortier et al., AJG 2010; 105: 613-620).
  - o The more of these risk factors that are present, the higher their rate for steatosis: for example; 3 factors, 30% risk; 4-66%; 5-82%; 6 risk factors, 100% ped LT steatosis.

394

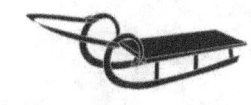

- Give the types of **hepatic rejection** after transplantation.
  - Hyperacute rejection
    - Hyperacute rejection (also known as massive hemorrhagic necrosis) seldom occurs, but when it does it results in rapid graft destruction with coagulative parenchymal necrosis owing to widespread endothelial dysfunction.
    - Endothelial cells are primarily targeted by a pre-existing anti-donor humoral immune response that leads to the deposition of antibodies, platelets, fibrin and erythrocytes within the portal venules and hepatic sinusoids.
    - Lymphocytes are usually absent and bile ducts unaffected.
    - This form of rejection is seen more commonly in recipients with ABO incompatible grafts.
  - Acute rejection
    - Acute rejection (also known as cellular rejection) is more common than hyperacute rejection, and usually occurs in the first 3 months post-transplantation.
    - It is characterized by portal tracts that are heavily infiltrated with lymphocytes, bile duct damage and venular inflammation.
    - Early acute rejection (within the first 3 months post-transplantation) generally responds well to increased doses of immunosuppressive agents, with resolution of biliary inflammation and stable long-term allograft function.
    - The degree of inflammation and graft damage does not correlate with either the response to increased immunosuppression or with long-term outcome.
    - By contrast, late acute rejection, recurrent rejection and steroid-resistant rejection are more likely to develop into chronic rejection.
  - Chronic rejection
    - Chronic rejection (also known as ductopenic rejection or vanishing bile duct syndrome) affects a small minority of liver allograft patients and may lead to graft loss.
    - A central late feature of chronic rejection is a loss of bile ducts (ductopenia), and pruning of the distal branches of the portal venous system owing to persistent inflammation and arterial foam cell infiltration and the presence of arterial foam cells.
    - Vanishing bile duct syndrome eventually ensues, with progressive cholestasis and liver dysfunction and, ultimately, graft failure.

Printed with permission: Eksteen and Neuberger. *Nature Clinical Practice Gastroenterology & Hepatology* April 2008;5(4): pg 210.

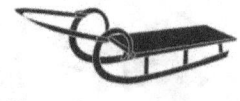

395

- o GI malignancy
  - – Lymphomas, Kaposi sarcomas, skin cancer
  - – Gastric MALT lymphomas; may be associated with *H. pylori*
  - – Colorectal cancer (liver Tx, RR, CRC 12.5)
  - – Colorectal Cancer (CRC) in UC (ulcerative colitis) plus primary sclerosing cholangitis (PSC)
    - ▪ In patients given a liver transplant for PSC in the settling of associated UC, the incidence of CRC is 1% per year, with a cumulative risk of colonic mucosal dysplasia of 15% at 5 years and 21% at 8 years
- o Post transplantation Lymphoproliferative disorder (PTLD) (10% of Tx pts; acute perforation, obstruction, bleeding; associated with EBV)

Printed with permission: Helderman JH, and Goral S. *J Am Soc Nephrol* 2002; 13: 277-287.

## Non-Skin Solid Organ Tumours

- o 10% per year
- o Squamous cell and basal cell skin cancer is 12-90 times more common in transplanted patient
- o Risk 2x > general population
  - – Head/neck Ca
  - – Esophageal Ca
  - – Karposi sarcoma
- o Non-melanoma skin cancer (NMSC)
  - – Alcohol L-Tx for ALD ↑ risk
  - – CRC
  - – IBD/PSC
    - ▪ 10% at 10 yrs
    - ▪ 22% at 20 yrs

## Post-Transplant Lymphoproliferative Disorder (PTLD)

- ➤ Demography
  - o There is a 10-fold increased risk of non-Hodgkins lymphoma (B-cell related to EBV) after liver transplantation, giving a relative risk of 3%
  - o Most commonly first 18 month post LT
  - o More immune suppression in heart Tx patients, so more PTLD.
  - o 5 year survival rate, 50%

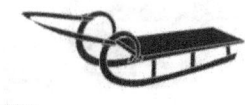

- ➢ Causes/associations
  - ○ EBV-associated latent infection in B-cells
  - ○ ↑ LDH, ↑ EBV viral load
- ➢ Pathology
  - ○ Extranodal, high grade, poor prognosis
  - ○ B cells originate from recipient, not from donor cells
  - ○ May occur in GI tract (e.g., colon)
- ➢ Treatment
  - ○ ↓ immune suppression (↓ by 25% to 50%)
  - ○ Short-term, 70% effective
  - ○ EBV treatment
  - ○ Multi-gent chemo (CHOP), radiation, surgery, rituximab
  - ○ Rituximab 50% remission rate (for CD20+ PTLD)

## Biliary Obstruction
- ○ Usually 1 month post L-Tx
- ○ Strictures of biliary tree occur in 20-35% of patients post liver transplantation, especially at the duct-to-duct anastamosis, or at the Roux-en-Y
- ○ Post transplant biliary strictures result from hepatic artery occlusion, chronic allograft rejection, or prolonged cold ischemia time
- ○ Common bile duct (CBD)
  - – Stone
  - – Stricture
  - – Bile duct injury and cholestasis in both post-LT HCV and with acute rejection cholestatic syndrome have a serious prognosis.
- ○ Ischemic stricture of CBD post L-Tx, above anastomosis
- ○ Chronic rejection
- ○ Post L-Tx, can see anastomosis on ERCP

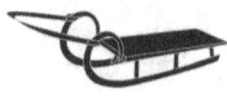

## Sexual Function and Pregnancy

- o ↓ libido in 25% of men and women after liver transplantation
- o Erectile dysfunction in 30% of men after liver transplantation
- o Post-transplant, pregnancy is associated with
  - ↑ fetal loss (18%)
  - ↓ birth weight (31%)
  - Premature delivery (39%)
  - Pre-eclampsia (21%)
  - The need for caesarian section (47%)
  - Allograft rejection occurs in 10-20% of women during pregnancy

## Recurrence of Liver Disease Leading to Need for Second Liver Transplantation

- Give the pathological features of acute cellular rejection after Liver Transplantation (LT).

  - o Portal tract — Inflammation, with lymphocytes eosinophils and plasma cell
    - Extension of inflammation into periportal area
  - o Bile ducts — Extension of inflammation into bile ducts
  - o Central vein — Lymphocytic infiltration around central vein, representing endothelitis

- Give examples of liver disorders which may recur in the liver following liver transplant (recurrence rates in brackets).

  - o Infection — HBV
    - HCV
  - o Inflammation — AIH
    - PBC
    - PSC
  - o Infiltration — HCC
    - NASH
    - Amyloid
  - o Toxins — ALD

Abbreviations: AIH, autoimmune hepatitis; ALD, alcoholic liver disease; HBV, hepatits B virus; HCC, hepatocellular cancer; HCV hepatitis C virus; NASH, non-alcoholic steatohepatitis; PBC, primary sclerosing cholangitis; PSC, primary sclerosing cholangitis

Adapted from: Lilly LB, Girgrah N, and Levy G.A. *First Principles of Gastroenterology* 2005: pg. 642.

398

# CASE SELF TEST STUDIES IN HEPATIC HISTOPATHOLOGY

## Alcoholic Liver Disease

**Case 1.** Clinical vignette: A 55-year-old sales executive presents for a physical examination pertaining to an insurance policy application. He has consumed 4 bottles of beer a day for 30 years. Past history, symptoms review, and physical examination is non-contributory. You suspect Alcoholic Liver Disease.

- Give the typical pathological features of Alcoholic Liver Disease.
  - Hepatocyte swelling and necrosis
  - Macrovesicular fatty change in centrilobular area
  - Mallory hyaline
  - Neutrophils, portal lymphocytes and macrophages
  - Sclerosing hyaline fibrosis

  Identify these features on the following slides.

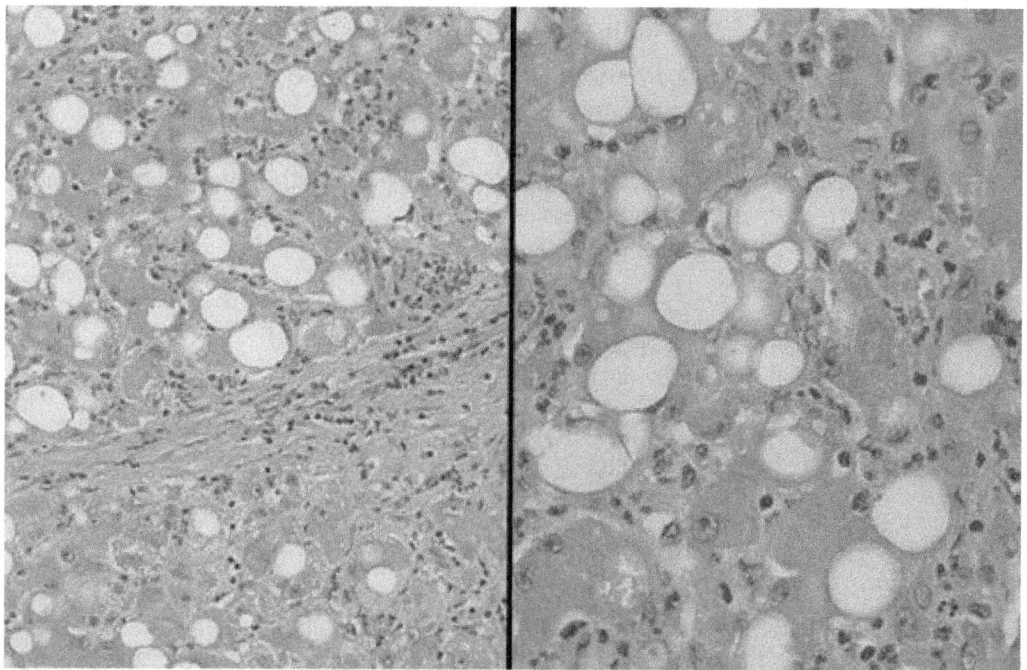

Reference: Colombat M, et al. Portal lymphocytic infiltrate in alcoholic liver disease. *Hum Pathol.* 2002;33;1170-4.

399

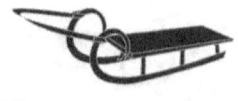

**Non-Alcoholic Steatohepatitis.**

**Case 2.** Clinical vignette: A 45-year-old type II diabetic with a BMI of 35 from Brandon, Manitoba presents with 2 x normal increased AST. There is no alcohol intake. This is a routine follow-up for mild hypertension, and she is otherwise well except for hypercholesterolemia. You suspect non-alcoholic steatohepatitis.

- Give the typical pathological features of non-alcoholic steatohepatitis.
  - o Micro- and macrovesicular steatosis, zone 3
  - o Lobular plasma cell and lymphocyte infiltrate
  - o Ballooning degeneration of hepatocytes
  - o "Chicken-wire" fibrosis

Identify these features on the following slide.

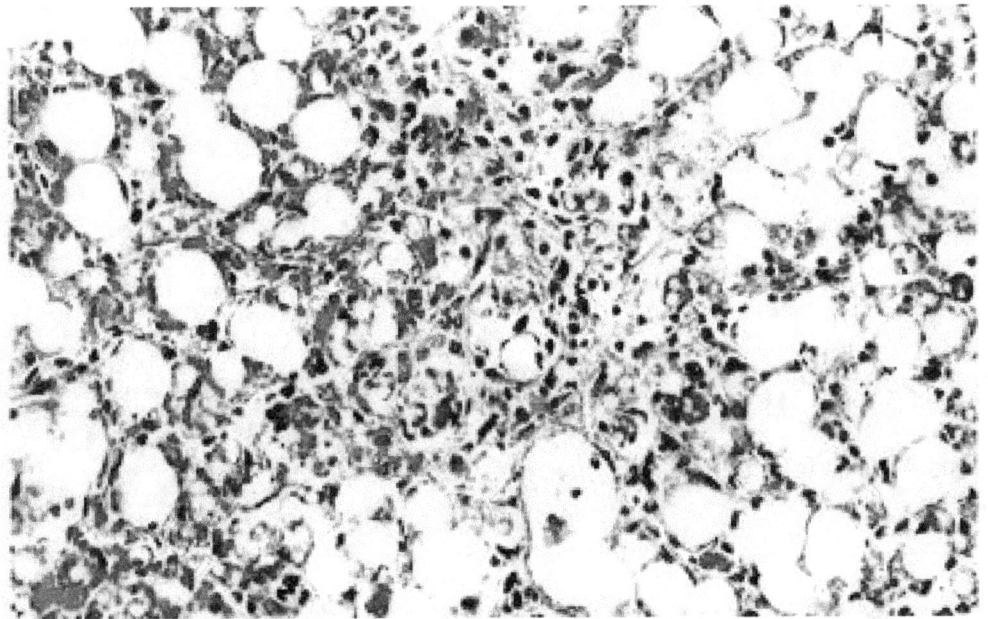

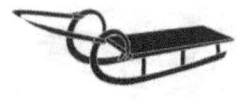

*MASTERING THE BOARDS*
*Hepatology & Pancreaticobiliary Disease*

A.B.R. Thomson

## Hepatitis A Virus Infection

**Case 3.** Clinical vignette: A 19-year-old young man from White Rock, BC, traveling in SE Asia presents with fatigue and jaundice. You suspect hepatitis A.

- Give the typical pathological features of Hepatitis A.
  - Portal and periportal inflammation
  - Ballooning degeneration
  - Relative sparing of centrilobular hepatocytes
  - Acidophil bodies or cytolysis (hydropic degeneration)
  - Bridging necrosis
  - Interface hepatitis

  Identify these features on the following slides.

Hepatitis A Virus Infection

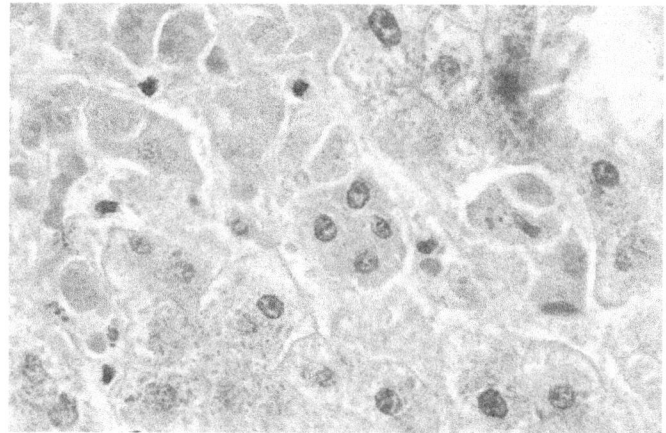

Hepatitis A Virus Infection

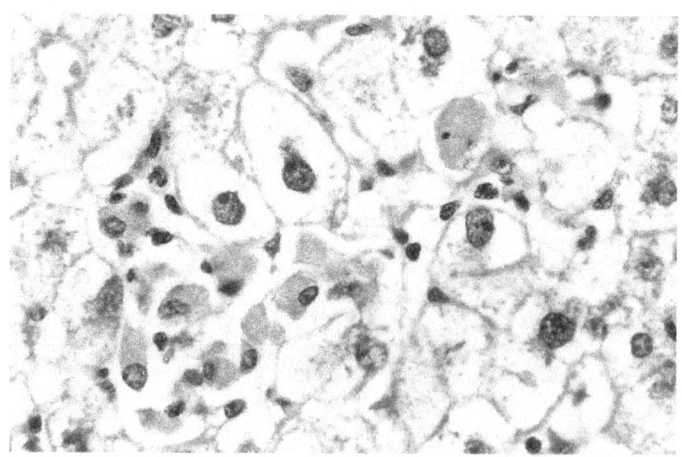

## Hepatitis B Virus Infection

**Case 4.** Clinical vignette: A 62-year-old businessman from Elk Point, AB, presents with recent onset of malaise and transaminitis. He denies alcohol intake. His younger brother died from HCC. You suspect Hepatitis B.

- Give the typical pathological features of Hepatitis B.

    o Piecemeal necrosis

    o Ground glass hepatocytes

Identify these features on the following slides.

Hepatitis B Virus Infection

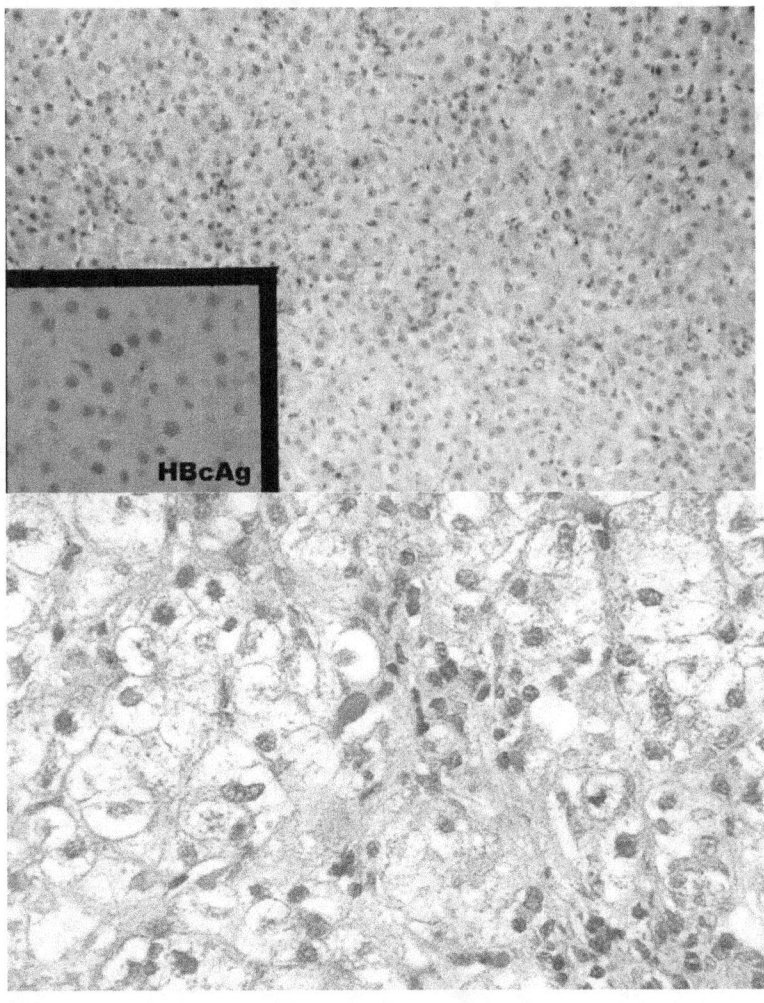

402

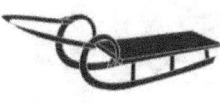

## Hepatitis C Virus Infection

**Case 5.** A 39-year-old hemophiliac physician from Brookville, ON, presents with fatigue and mild jaundice. You suspect Hepatitis C.

- Give the typical pathological features of Hepatitis C.
    - Sinusoidal lymphocytic infiltrate
    - Mallory hyaline
    - Macrovesicular steatosis
    - No/minimal plasma cells or eosinophils

Identify these features on the following slides.

Hepatitis C Virus Infection

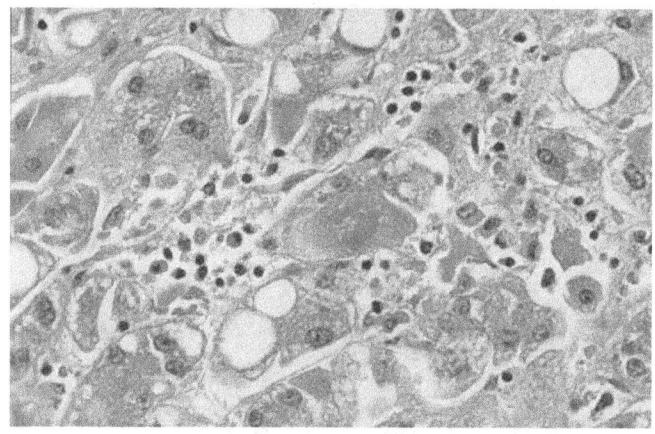

Hepatitis C Virus Infection

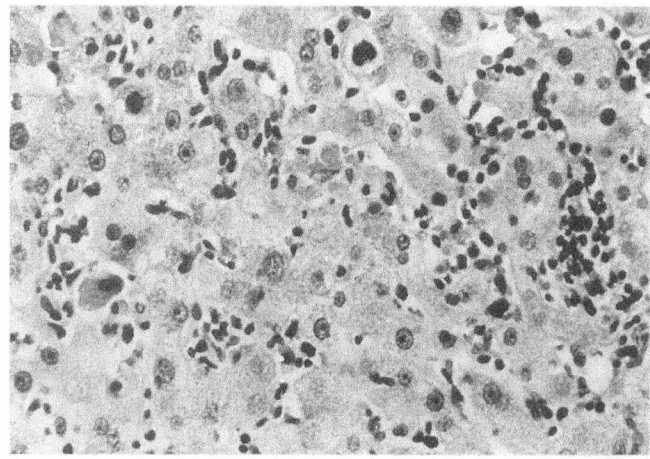

403

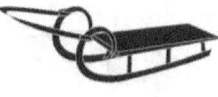

## Autoimmune Hepatitis

**Case 6.** Clinical vignette: A 45-year-old high school principal from Trois-Riviera, QC, with treated hypertension presents with a 6 month history of pruritus. The GGT and AP are increased twice normal. You suspect Autoimmune Hepatitis.

- Give the typical pathological features of Autoimmune Hepatitis.
    - Portal infiltrate with abundance of plasma cells
    - Bridging necrosis
    - Central necrosis with plasma cells

Identify these features on the following slide.

Autoimmune Hepatitis

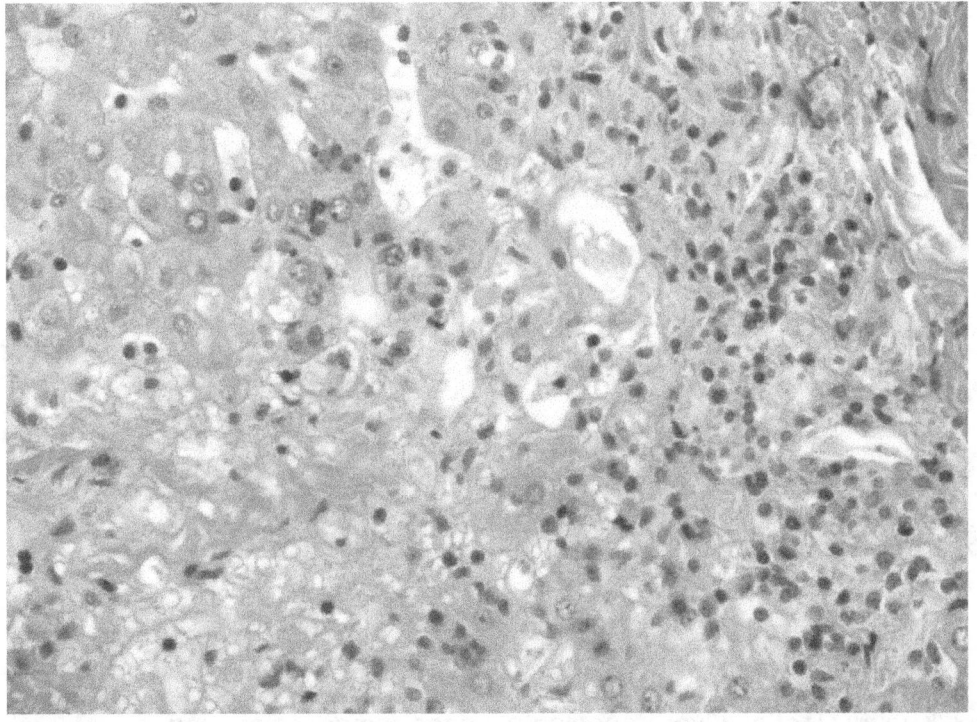

Reference: Khettry U, et al. Liver transplantation for primary sclerosing cholangitis: a long-term clinicopathologic study. *Hum Pathol.* 2003;34: 1127-36.

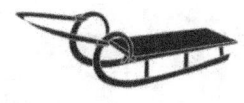

**Primary Sclerosing Cholangitis** (PSC)

**Case 7.** Clinical vignette: A 24-year-old male nurse from Red Earth, SK, with a 10 year history of ulcerative colitis presents with abnormal LFTs. You suspect Primary Sclerosing Cholangitis (PSC).

- Give the typical pathological features of PSC.

   o "Onion skin" fibrosis

Identify this feature on the following slide.

Primary Sclerosing Cholangitis (PSC)

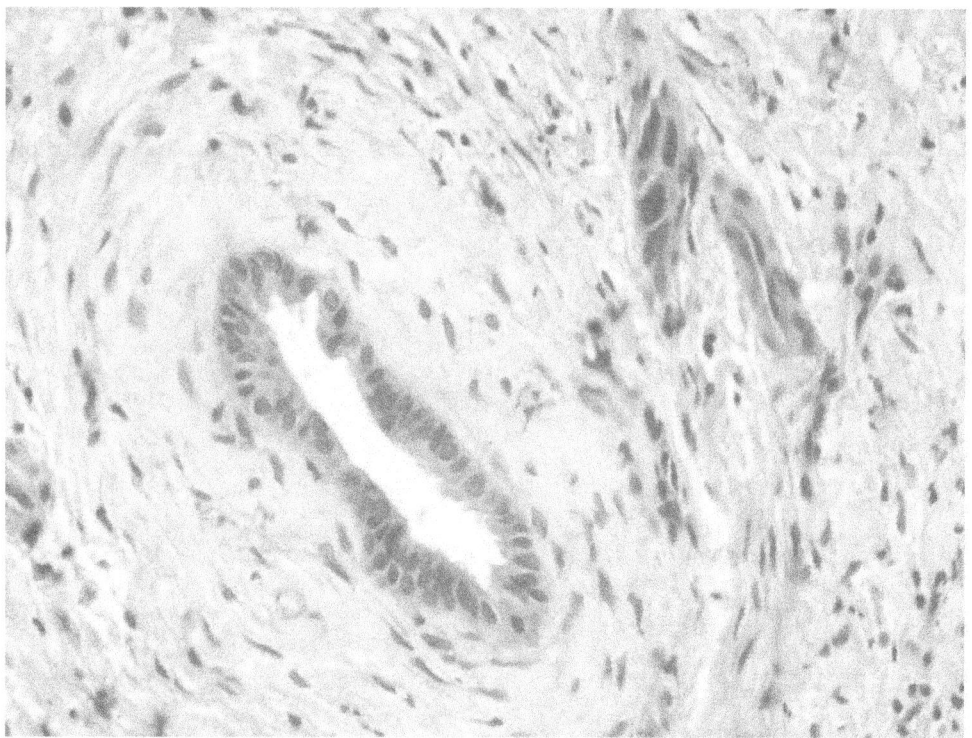

Reference: Khettry U, et al. Liver transplantation for primary sclerosing cholangitis: a long-term clinicopathologic study. *Hum Pathol.* 2003;34:1127-36.

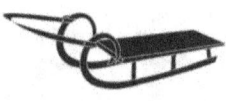

## Primary Biliary Cholangitis (PBC)

**Case 8.** Clinical vignette: A 50-year-old woman from Halifax, NS, presents with an asymptomatic elevation in her GGT and AP at the time of routine follow up of her dyslipoproteinemia. You suspect Primary Biliary Cholangitis (PBC).

- Give the typical pathological features of PBC.
  - Dense lymphocytic infiltrate in portal tracts
  - Minimal neutrophils
  - Granulomatous destruction and loss of medium-sized interlobular bile ducts
  - Destruction of bile ductules within the liver

Identify these features on the following slide.

Primary Biliary Cholangitis (PBC)

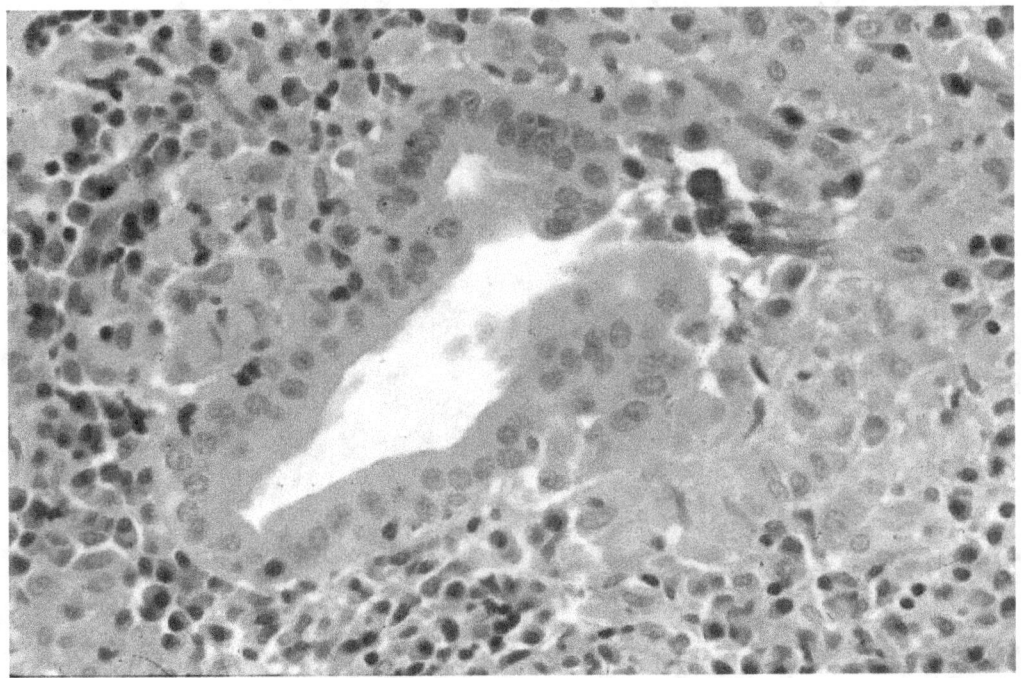

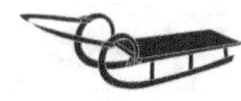

**Massive Hepatic Necrosis** (MHN)

**Case 9**. A distraught 19-year-old student from Mitchell, ON, consumed a bottle of unknown OTC pills, and presents to the ER with confusion and jaundice. You suspect Massive Hepatic Necrosis (MHN).

- Give the typical pathological features of MHN.
  - o Massive necrosis of hepatocytes in all zones
  - o Reticulin collapse
  - o Minimal inflammatory reaction

Identify these features on the following slide.

Massive Hepatic Necrosis (MHN)

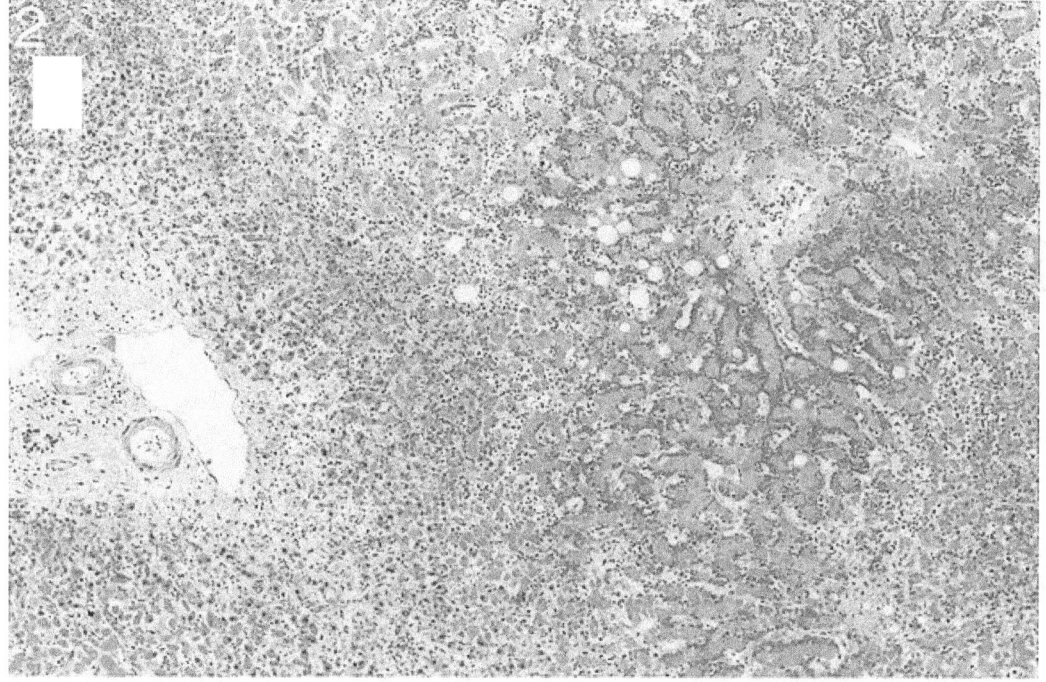

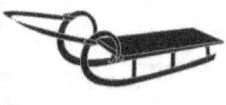

*MASTERING THE BOARDS*
*Hepatology & Pancreaticobiliary Disease*

A.B.R. Thomson

**Nodular Hyperplasia** (FNH)

**Case 10**. A 30 year old woman presents with abnormal liver enzymes. You suspect Focal Nodular Hyperplasia (FNH).

- Give the typical pathological features of FNH.
  - o Hepatocyte nodules surrounded by fibrous septa
  - o Foci of intense lymphocytic infiltrates

Identify these features on the following slide.

Nodular Hyperplasia (FNH)

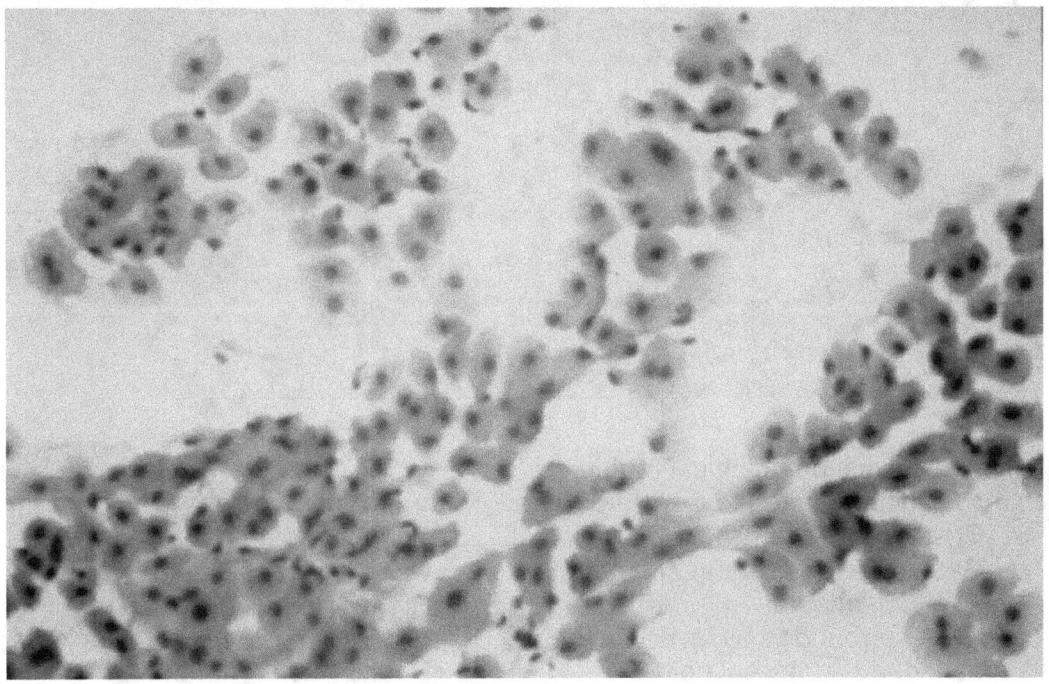

Reference: Gräntzdörffer I, et al.Angiotensin I-converting enzyme (CD143) is down-regulated in focal nodular hyperplasia of the liver. *Am J Surg Pathol* 2004;28(1):84-8; Wanless IR. Epithelioid hemangioendothelioma, multiple focal nodular hyperplasias, and cavernous hemangiomas of the liver. *Arch Pathol Lab Med* 2000;124(8):1105-7.

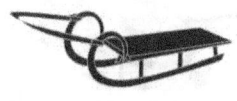

## Hepatocellular Carcinoma (HCC)

**Case 11.** Clinical vignette: A patient with known HIV and HBV from Calgary, AB, presents with worsening ascites and cachexia. You suspect hepatocellular carcinoma (HCC).

Hepatocellular carcinoma (HCC)

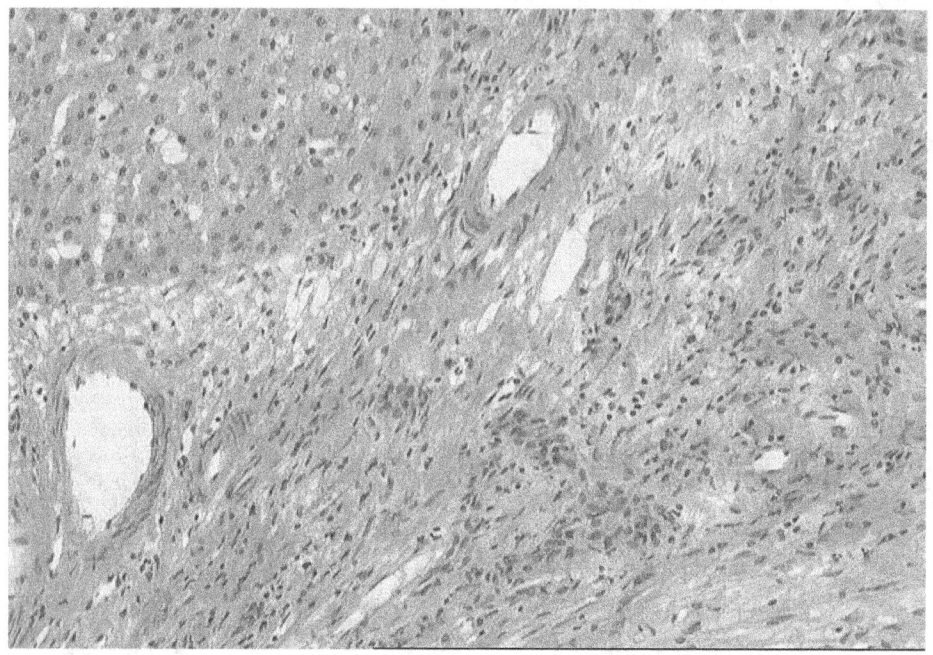

- Give the typical pathological features of HCC.
  - Well differentiated to bizarre pattern
  - Trabecular patterns
  - Sarcomatoid and clear cell patterns
  - Pseudoglandular
  - Cells surrounded by layer of flattened endothelial cells
  - Giant cells
  - Sinusoidal vessels surrounding tumour cells
  - Vascular invasion
  - Scanty stroma polygonal cells with distinct cell membranes
  - Higher N/C ratio
  - Granular eosinophilic cytoplasm
  - Round nuclei with coarse chromatin and thickened nuclear membrane

Reference: Fan Z, et al. Hep par 1 antibody stain for the differential diagnosis of hepatocellular carcinoma: 676 tumours tested using tissue microarrays and conventional tissue sections. *Mod Pathol* 2003;16:137-44; Itoh T, et al., Immunohistochemical detection of hepatocellular carcinoma in the setting of ongoing necrosis after radiofrequency ablation. *Mod Pathol* 2002;15:110-5. Identify these features on the following slides.

409

Hepatocellular Carcinoma (HCC)

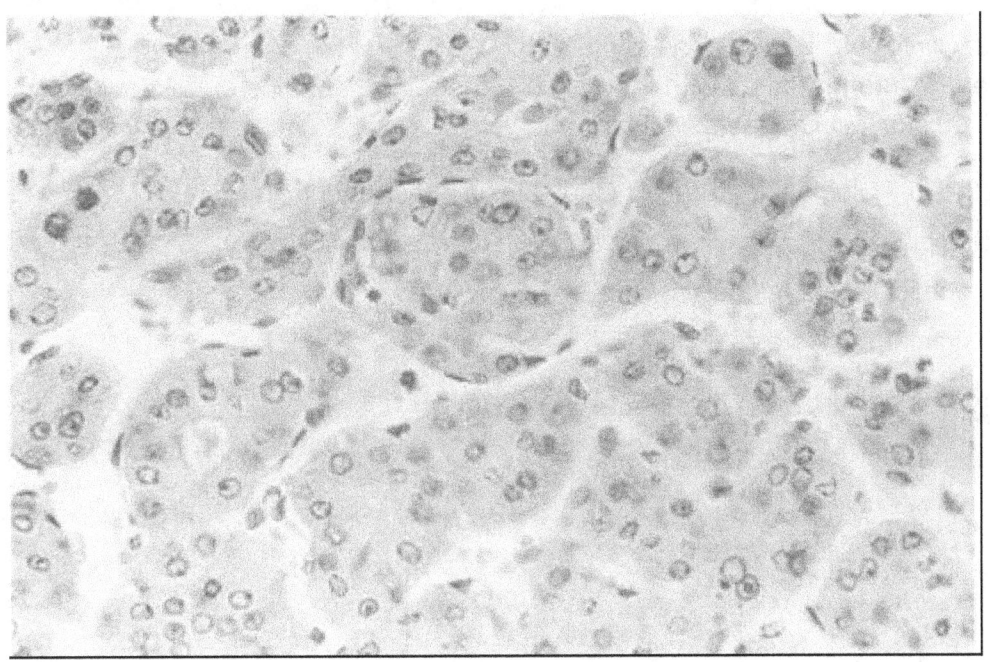

Hepatocellular Carcinoma (HCC)

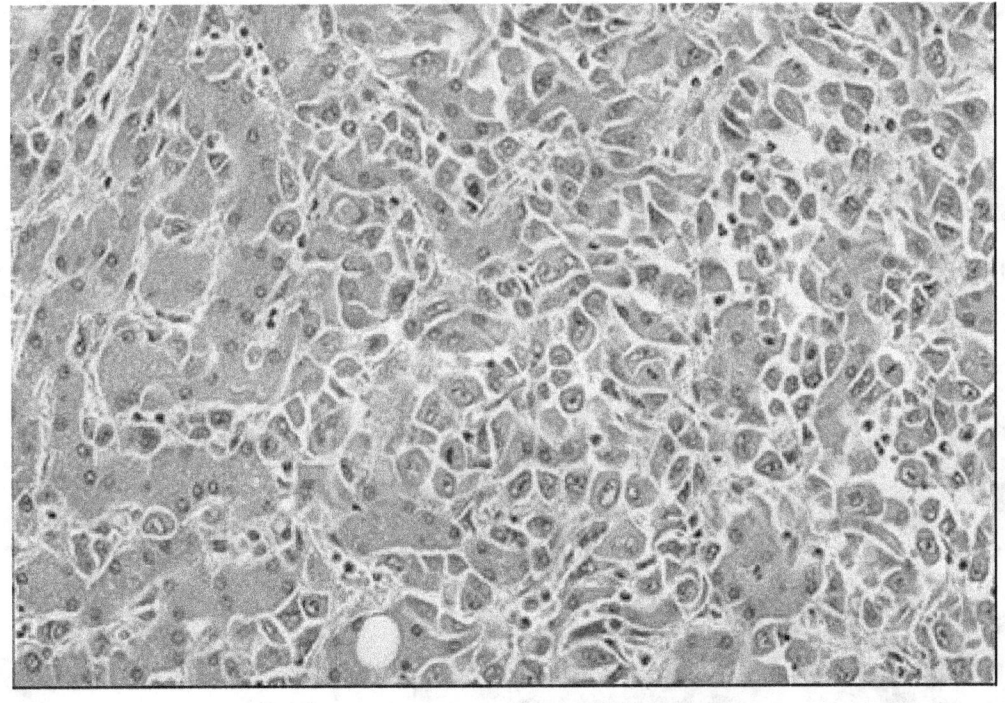

## Cholestasis Syndrome

**Case 12.** Clinical vignette: On a Royal College OSCE exam, this slide was presented for interpretation, with the only history being "jaundice of unknown origin." You suspect Cholestasis syndrome.

- Give the pathological features of Cholestasis syndrome include:
  - Bile plugs
  - Canalicular cholestasis
  - Ductular cholestasis
  - Cholangiolar proliferation

Identify these features on the following slides.

Cholestasis Syndrome

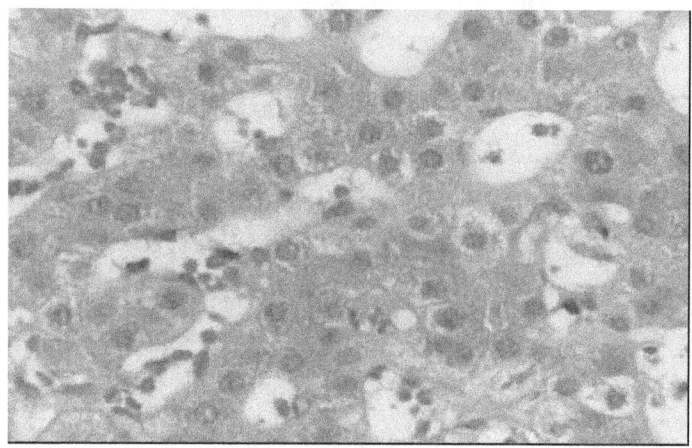

Cholestasis Syndrome

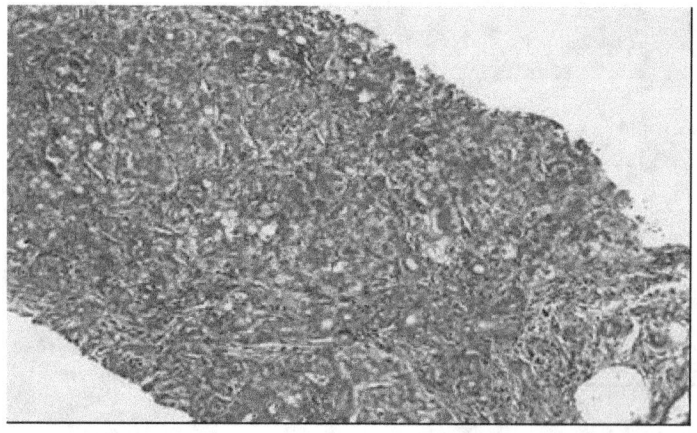

411

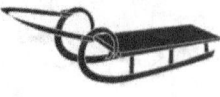

## Cirrhosis

**Case 13**. Clinical vignette: A 58-year-old man from P.E.I. with known alcoholic liver disease presents with resent onset abdominal distension and confusion. You suspect Cirrhosis.

- Give the typical pathological features of Cirrhosis include:
  - Disruption in architecture of entire liver
  - Bridging fibrous septa
  - Rounded parenchymal nodules of regenerating hepatocytes without central veins

Identify these features on the following slide.

Cirrhosis

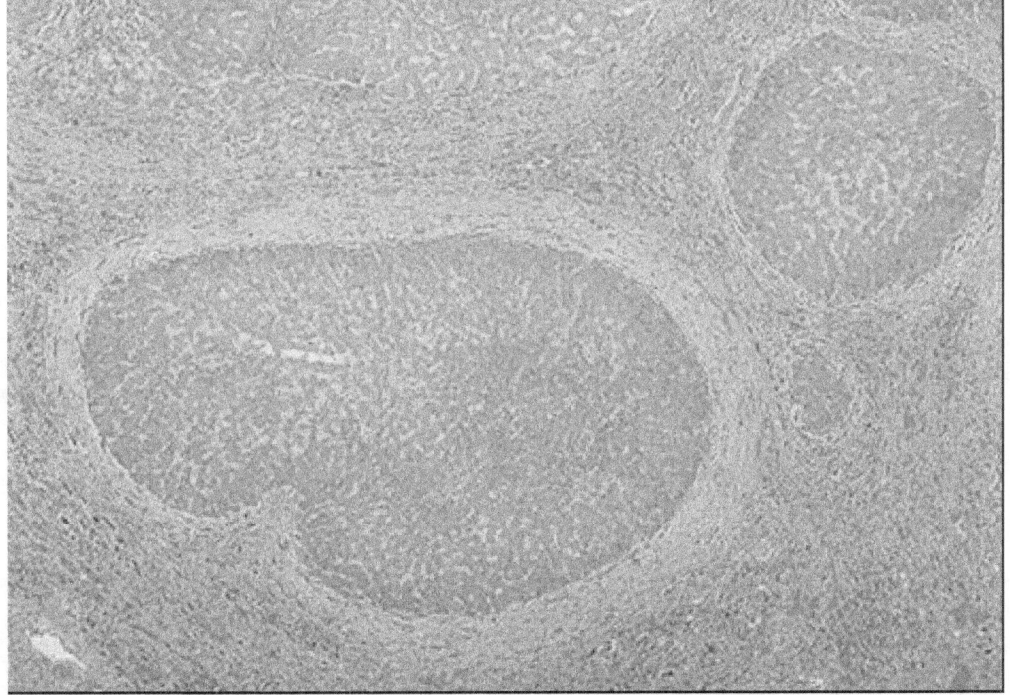

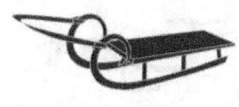

# BILIARY TREE AND GALLBLADDER

# TABLE OF CONTENTS

415

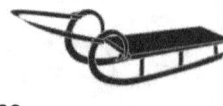

**ANATOMICAL OVERVIEW** of Bile ducts and Gallbladder (from small to large)

- o Canaliculus
- o Channels between hepatocytes
- o Terminal channels (aka canals of Hering)
- o Perilobular (aka intralobular) ducts
- o Zone 3 to zone 1
- o Interlobular ducts
- o Hepatic ducts (right and left)
- o Common hepatic duct
- o Cystic duct
- o Gallbladder
  - Neck
  - Infundibulum
  - Hartmann pouch
  - Body
  - Fundus
- o Common bile duct
- o Ampulla of Vater

- In the context of the anatomy of the gallbladder, give what is the **Hartmann pouch**, and what is its clinical significance?

  - o A. "Hartmann pouch is a bulging of the inferior surface of the infundibulum that lies close to the neck of the gallbladder" (Feldman M., et al. Sleisenger and Fordtran's Gastrointestinal and Liver Disease. 9th Edition. *Saunders/Elsevier*, Philadelphia, 2010, page 1049).

  - o Gallstones may become impacted in the Hartmann pouch, which blocks the cystic duct, and leads to cholecystitis.

"All our dreams can come true – if we have the

courage to pursue them."

Walt Disney

416

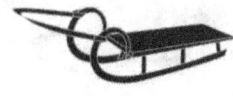

## CHOLELITHIASIS

- o Stones in the biliary tree usually arise from cholelithiasis.

- o However, multiple stones in the biliary tree, especially in the left hepatic system, suggests recurrent pyogenic cholangitis (RPC), aka "oriental cholangitis".
  - – RPC may be caused by infections, such as Clonorchis sinensis and Ascaris lumbricoides
  - – Because of the recurrent episodes of cholangitis, strictures may occur in biliary tract

After a liver biopsy a patient develops abdominal pain, hypertension and dropping hemoglobin concentration.

- • Give the findings on NG tube aspiration which may help to determine if the above scenario is likely due to acute bleeding from hemobilia.

| NG Tube Shows | Likelihood of Acute Bleeding |
|---|---|
| o No blood, but bile | < 5% |
| o No blood, no bile | < 15% |
| o Blood | > 95% |

- • Give causes of pneumobilia.

  - o Sphincterolomy

  - o Gallstone ileus

  - o Anaerobic infection of portal tract with Clostridium perfringens

"Harsh words are heavy and often fall with a big thud,
but a kind word will bounce on and on…"

Anonymous

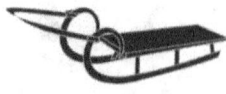

## STRICTURES AND STENTS

The commonest places for an injured biliary tree are the cystic duct and the duct of Luschka.

- Give the features in favour of using a plastic versus a metal stent for the management of a Hilar bile duct tumour.

| | Feature | | Plastic | Metal |
|---|---|---|---|---|
| o Stricture | – | Size | 3 mm | 10 mm |
| | – | Duration | < 6 mon (temporary) | 6 mon ("permanent") |
| o Stent | – | Cost | ~ $ 300 | ~ $ 1500 |
| | – | Covered | No | Yes |
| | – | Plastic stent can be inserted through a larger metal stent (3mm → 10 mm) | | |

- Give the anatomical sites which favour the use of covered versus uncovered metal stents.
  - o Covered
    - – Head of pancreas (HOP) (↑ risk of migration)
  - o Uncovered
    - – Intrahepatic duct

### Benign Biliary Strictures

➤ Types

- Give the **Bismuth** classification for benign biliary strictures.

| Classification | Location |
|---|---|
| I | > 2 cm distal to hepatic confluence |
| II | < 2 cm distal to hepatic confluence |
| III | Hilar stricture, hepatic confluence is preserved |
| IV | Involves the hepatic confluence, bile ducts are separated |

Source: Zepeda-Gomez S and Baron TH. Nat Rev Gastro Hep 2011; 8: 573-581.
➤ Causes/associations

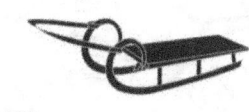

- Give causes of benign biliary strictures.

  - Conjugated
    - Choledochal cysts
    - Caroli disease
    - Caroli syndrome
    - Atresia

  - Biliary duct
    - Postsurgical
      - Cholecystectomy (open or laparoscopic)
      - Biliary anastomosis (orthetopic liver transplantation or biliary reconstruction
      - Biliary-enteric anastomosis
      - Trauma
      - Post-endoscopic biliary sphincterotomy
    - Post-ERCP
      - Primary sclerosing cholangitis
      - Post-radiation therapy
      - Infections (tuberculosis, histoplasmosis, viral, parasitic)
      - Choledochalithiasis
      - Autoimmune cholangiopathy
      - Inflammatory
      - Ischemia
        - Hypotension
        - Intrahepatic infusion of chemotherapy agents
        - Hepatic artery thrombosis

  - Sphincter of Oddi
    - Sphincter of Oddi dysfunction
    - Vasculitis

  - Pancreas
    - Chronic pancreatitis

Abbreviation: BBS, benign biliary strictures

Adapted from: Zepeda-Gomez S and Baron TH. Nat Rev Gastro Hep 2011; 8: 573-581, Box 1

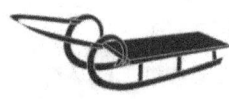

# SPHINCTER OF ODDI DYSFUNCTION (SOD)

➢ Subtypes

  o Stenosis

  o Dyskinesia

The Milwaukee Classification for biliary SOB is applied to biliary-type pain. However, SOD dysfunction may be a cause of recurrent idiopathic pancreatitis.

- Give the way in which the Milwaukee classification for possible pancreatic SOD differ from biliary SOD.

|  | Pancreatic SOD | Biliary SOD |
|---|---|---|
| Laboratory tests | ↑ Lipase or amylase | ↑ ALT, AST, AP |
| Duct diameter | Bile duct > 10 mm | Pancreatic duct > 6 mm in the head, 5 mm in the body of pancreas |

➢ Causes/associations

  o SOD is usually suspected in the setting of biliary-like pain with or without a gallbladder (without stones), or idiopathic recurrent pancreatitis.

  o The cause of SOD is unknown.

- Give conditions associated with SOD.

  o Post liver transplantation

  o Hyperlipidemia

  o AIDS (acquired immunodeficiency syndrome)

  o Chronic use of opium

➢ Clinical

  o Biliary-type pain after cholecystectomy

  o Biliary-type pain with intact gallbladder and no stones

  o Recurrent idiopathic pancreatitis (↑ ALT, ↑ AP, CBD > 10 mm)

➢ Diagnosis

  o Scintigraphy

  o Fatty meal ultrasonography

  o Morphine + neostigmine low sensitivity/specificity (Nardi test)

  o SOM (sphincter of Oddi manometry) may show ↑ SOD (sphincter of Oddi) (> 35 to 40 mmHg)

420

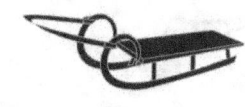

- ➢ Sphincter of Oddi Manometry (SOM)
  - ○ SOM - specific, not sensitive
  - ○ SOM, done at time of ERCP
  - ○ The insertion of the manometry of catheter may cause spasm
  - ○ SOD patients have a high complication rate
    - - Post-ERCP
    - - Post-ERCP placement of the stent

- • Give non-invasive tests for biliary or pancreatic SOD, as well as their performance characteristics.
  - ○ Biliary scintigraphy (ultrasound) after
    - – Fatty meal (stimulated ultrasound testing of diameter of biliary duct)
    - – CCK injection (for biliary SOD)
    - – Secretin injection (for pancreatic SOD)

|  | For Biliary SOD | For pancreatic SOD |
|---|---|---|
|  | Fatty meal | Secretin |
| ▪ Sensitivity | 21% | 88% |
| ▪ Specificity | 97% | 82% |

- ➢ Classification

- • Give the modified **Milwaukee Classification** for Biliary Sphincter of Oddi Dysfunction (SOD).

| Type | Biliary-type Pain | ↑ LEs | DBD (> 10 mm) | ↑ SO Pressure |
|---|---|---|---|---|
| I | + | + | + | 65% to 85% |
| II | + | Either ↑ LEs or DBD | +/- | 55% |
| III | + | - | - | 28% |

Abbreviations: DBD, dilated bile duct; LE, liver enzymes (ALT, AST, AP [alkaline phosphatase])

Adapted from: Sleisenger and Fordtran's Gastrointestinal and Liver Disease. 10th Edition. *Saunders/Elsevier* 2016, Table 63.1, page 1078.

421

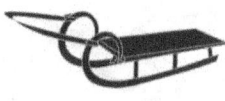

> Treatment
>> o When sphincter pressure > 40 mmHg, response to sphincterotomy, 91% (vs 25% with sham sphincterotomy)
>> o When sphincter pressure < 40 mmHg, response to sphincterotomy is only 42% (sham, 33%)

|  | Relief (%) | |
| --- | --- | --- |
| Success of Sphincterotomy | ABN SOM | N-SOM |
| I | 90-95 | 90-95 |
| II | 85 | 35-42 |
| III | 55-60 | < 10% high risk of complication |

>> o Because of the technical difficulties with SOM and its sometimes unreliable results, the test is not always done to diagnose SOD.
>> o However, with type II or III disease, if the SOM is normal, the response to ERCP plus sphincterotomy is much lower (see below), and it could be argued that in type II or III patients, SOM should be obtained.
>> o SOD are diagnosed with the modified Milwaukee criteria rather than an abnormal SOM (i.e., SOD which is not manometrically proven).

- Give possible causes for failure to achieve pain relief after biliary sphincterotomy for presumed sphincter of Oddi dysfunction (SOD).

  o Sphincter
    - Inadequate initial sphincterotomy (remaining ↑ SOD pressure)
    - Restenosis

  o Pancreatitis
    - Chronic pancreatitis with a normal pancreatogram
    - Nonpancreaticobiliary pain (beware functional gastrointestinal disease)

Source: Elta, Grace H. *Sleisenger & Fordtran's gastrointestinal and liver disease: Pathophysiology/Diagnosis/Management* 2006: pg. 1365.

---

! Caution Alert!

  o For reasons which are unclear, the risk of post-ERCP pancreatitis is ↑ 3x (>25%) when the indication for the ERCP is SOD.
    - For this reason a stent may be placed after ERCP to ↓ risk of post-ERCP pancreatitis in persons who turn to have SOD.
  o When SOD is diagnosed, and the patient is not post-liver transplant, does not have hyperlipidemia, does not have HIV/AIDs or is not a chronic opium user (conditions associated with ↑ SOM and thereby SOD), watch out for a possible intra-ampullary neoplasm mimicking SOD.

---

422

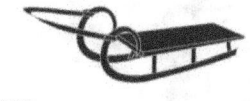

# CHOLELITHIASIS

- ➤ Types of gallstones
    - ○ Composition
        - – Cholesterol
            - ▪ Crystals of cholesterol monohydrate
            - ▪ Calcium bilirubinate
            - ▪ Calcium carbonate/phosphate
        - – Pigment
            - ▪ Calcium bilirubinate
        - – Mixed
        - – Rare
            - ▪ Calcium carbonate
            - ▪ Calcium-fatty acids
    - ○ Site
        - – Intrahepatic
            - ▪ Brown pigment
        - – Gallbladder
            - ▪ Cholesterol >> black pigment
        - – Bile duct
            - ▪ Mixed
    - ○ Physical state of cholesterol
        - – Low concentrations
            - ▪ Monomers of bile acids (BA)
        - – CMC (critical micellar concentration)
            - ▪ Simple micelles are spontaneously formed with BA monomers
                - – Small (~ 3 nm diameter)
                - – Disk-like macromolecular aggregates
                - – Solubilize and incorporate
            - ▪ Cholesterol
            - ▪ Phospholipids
            (mostly lecithin, with some phosphatidylethanolamines and sphingomyelin) to form mixed micelles (~ 4-8 nm diameter)
        - – Biliary vesicles
            - ▪ Secreted by hepatocytes
            - ▪ Composed of cholesterol monohydrate crystals and phospholipids
            - ▪ Large (40-100 nm diameter)
            - ▪ Multilamellar spherical structures
            - ▪ As the gallbladder (GB) absorbs $H_2O$, the GB bile becomes concentrated
            - ▪ The stability of the biliary vesicles determines the stability of bile molecular rearrangements such that
            - ▪ In high concentrations of BA, there are the biliary vesicles may transform into mixed micelles

423

- Phase diagram and triangular co-ordinates
  - The maximal solubility of cholesterol is determined by the relative molar percentages of cholesterol, phospholipids and bile acids
  - This allows for the quantification of the degree of saturation of bile with cholesterol
  - This quantification of cholesterol saturation is the CSI (cholesterol saturation index), aka the lithogenic index
  - Examples of CSI
    - < 1 unsaturated
    - 1 saturated
    - > 1 supersaturated (↑ risk of forming gallstones)

Pigmental gallstones are seen in patients with chronic hemolytic anemia, liver disease, and with TPN.

SO YOU HAVE NOW GIVEN UP – ON BEING A (PEDIATRIC) GASTROENTEROLOGIST!

Congenital abnormalities of the biliary tree include choledochal cysts, Caroli disease and Caroli syndrome.

- Give why biliary atresia is sometimes not included in this list of congenital abnormalities of the biliary tree.

  - Injury to biliary tract occurs after birth
  - There is some evidence for an in utero infection (e.g., HSV, retrovirus, Rhesus rotavirus).

"Happiness cannot come from without. It must come from within."

Helen Keller

424

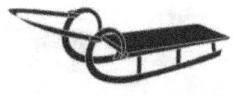

- Give differences, (besides their colour) between black versus brown pigmented stones.

| Characteristics | Black | Brown |
|---|---|---|
| o Site | GP | GB, HBT |
| o Infected bile | No | Yes |
| o Association with chronic hemolytic anemia | Yes | Yes |
| o Composition of stones | Polymers of calcium bilirubinate | Monomers of calcium bilirubinate plus cholesterol, fatty acids, bile salts, phospholipids |
| o B-glucuronidase forming unconjugated bilirubin glucuronide | Endogenous | Exogenous (E. Coli, roundworms, Clonorchis sinensis) |
| o Reduced acidification of bile | Yes | - |
| o Gallbladder dysfunction | No | No |

Abbreviations: GB, gallbladder; HBT, hepatobiliary tree

➤ Genetics

- o Testing
  - ABC B4 gene (PC transporter)
  - ABC B11 gene (bile salt export pump)
  - CYP7AI (cholesterol 7α-hydroxylase)
  - FXR farnesoid x
  - E4 allele of APOE (apolipoprotein E)
  - NTCP (Na+ dependent taurocholate cotransporting peptide)
  - TNF receptor 2
  - SHP (small heterodimer partner)

There are over a dozen genes and gene predicts that have been identified (please refer to Sleisenger and Fordtran's Gastrointestinal and Liver Disease. 9th Edition. Saunders/Elsevier, Philadelphia, 2016, Table 65.1, page 1115.

- Give cinical observations which suggest that there may be genetic factors leading to the formation of gallstones ↑ risk of gallstones.

  - o ↑ risk of gallstone
    - Siblings
    - Monozygotic twins
    - Relatives of index person with gallstones

425

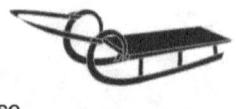

➤ Pathophysiology

"Phase Diaphragm"

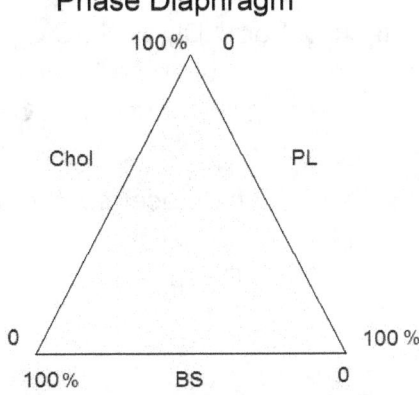

- o If cholesterol saturation index (CSI) > 1, bile is saturated, and cholesterol can precipitate and form crystals
- o Note: This figure is also refrred to as "triangular co-ordinates"

Abbreviations: BS, bile salts; chol, cholesterol; PL, phospholipids

- o The lithogenicity of bile is finally determined by the molar % of cholesterol (CH), phospholipids and bile acids.
- o The amount of CH available for transport across the CM of the hepatocyte is determined by a balance between
  - – Entry of CH across the sinusoidal membrane (SM), exit across the SM
  - – Metabolism in hepatocyte cytosol
  - – Exit across the canalicular membrane (CM)
- o Gallbladder
  - – ↓ cholesterol nucleation and crystallization
  - – ↓ gallbladder motility
- o Intestine
  - – Intestinal factors

- After an episode of cholecystitis, give circumstances when it is appropriate to perform early laparoscopic cholecystectomy.
  - o Pregnancy
  - o Severe acute cholecystitis
  - o Gallstone pancreatitis
  - o Intractable pancreatitis

426

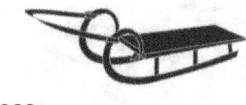

❖ Liver

- Give the role of the hepatocyte in the **metabolism** of cholesterol (CH).

    o CH uptake across the SM from LDL, HDL, CMR secretion of
        - CH across SM in VLDL back into portal blood
        - As CH in N-HDL (nascent HDL), using ABCA1

    o Metabolism
        - De Novo synthesis of CH from acetate, through HMG-CoAR
        - Esterification of CH to CE (cholesterol ester) by way of ACAT
        - 7α-hydroxylation of CH to BA (bile acids) by
            ▪ CYP7A1
            ▪ CYP27A1

    o ↑ hepatic secretion of cholesterol
        - ↑ hepatic uptake of HDL-C → CETP (cholesterol ester transfer protein)
        - ↑ intestinal CH absorption and ↑ hepatic VLDL synthesis → Apolipoprotein (APO) E and APOB genes polymorphisms
        - 7α-hydroxylase (CYP7A1) gene variant → ↓ conversion of CH (cholesterol) to BA (bile acids) in the "neural" pathway
        - ↓ PL secretion
            ▪ ABC B4 (aka MDR3 [multidrug resistant gene 3]) missense mutation of phosphatidylcholine (PC) transporter in hepatocyte CM
            ▪ ↓ CYP7A1
            ▪ ↑ HMG-CoA reductase
            ▪ ↓ bile PC
            ▪ ↑ bile CH

    o Transfer of CH across CM by ABCG5/-G8

    o If cholesterol saturation index (CSI) is > 1, bile is saturated, and cholesterol precipitates and form crystals

Abbreviations: ACAT, acyl-coenzyme A: cholesterol acyltransferase; CM, canalicular membrane of hepatocytes; CMR, chylomicron remnants; CYP27A, 27-hydroxylase ("acidic" pathway); CYP7A1, cholesterol 7α-hydroxylase ("neutral" pathway); HDL-L, high-density lipoprotein; HMG CoAR, 3-hydroxyl-3-methy glutaryl-coenzyme A reductase; LDL, low-density lipoprotein; SM, sinusoidal membrane of hepatocytes; VLDL, very-low-density lipoprotein

427

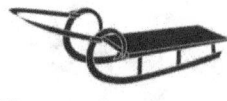

- ❖ Gallbladder
    - o Fasting period
        - – 7α-hydroxylation of CH to BA (bile acids) by
        - – ↑ volume of bile
        - – ↑cholesterol absorption ("loss of capacity for selective absorption of biliary cholesterol and phospholipids") by GB
            - → ↑ stiff sarcoplasmic membranes
            - → ↓ activation of G-proteins in muscularis propria
            - → ↑ storage of cholesterol esters (CE)
            - → ↓ motility of gallbladder
            - → ↑ inflammation and proliferation
    - o Postprandial
        - – ↓ binding of CCK to CCK-1 receptors
        - – Aberrant splicing of CCK-IR (cholecystokinin-1 receptor)
            - ▪ ↓ gallbladder motility
        - – ↓ emptying continued BG bile supersaturation
        - – ↑ post-emptying (residual) volume
    - o Interdigestive period
        - – ↓ filling
        - – ↑ lithogenic hepatic bile enters duodenum
        - – ↓ cholesterol solubilisation
    - o ↑ mucin glycoproteins
        - – Binds cholesterol (CH), phospholipids (PL), bile acids (BA)
        - – ↑ nucleation factors
        - – ↓ antinucleation factors
        - – ↑ vesicles fusion/aggregation
        - – ↑ mucin in lithogenic bile
    - o ↓ motility
        - – Contraction of gallbladder (GB)
            - ▪ ↑ parasympathetic
            - ▪ ↓ sympathetic
        - – ↑ fasting residual GB volumes
        - – ↓ response to CKK
        - – Likely important in CF, pancreatic insufficiency

428

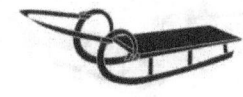

- o GB sludge   – Cholesterol monohydrate crystals, Ca bilirubinate, mucin
  - Radiolucent cholesterol stones
  - – Black stones – hypersecretion of bilirubin conjugates into bile
    - Hemolysis
    - Cirrhosis
  - – Pigmental gallstones are seen in patients with chronic hemolytic anemia, liver disease, and with TPN.

---

Useful Quotes

- o Early operation [for acute cholecystitis] is preferable because
  - – ↓ total length of hospitalization
  - – ↓ costs
  - – ↓ morbility
  - – Deaths related to progressive acute cholecystectomy are prevented"

Sleisenger and Fordtran's Gastrointestinal and Liver Disease. 9th Edition. *Saunders/Elsevier* 2010, page 1130.

---

❖ Small intestine

- Give small intestinal factors contributing to the formation of gallstones.
  - o ↑ intake of CH
  - o ↑ cholesterol absorption
    - – $1°$ ↑ inefficiency of uptake
    - – $2°$ ↑ dietary intake
  - o ↓ transit
    - – ↑ gram + anaerobic bacteria → ↑ $7α$-dehydroxylase activity
    - – ↑ conversion of $1°$ cholic acid to $2°$ deoxycholic acid
    - – ↑ deoxycholic → ↑ lithogenicity of bile
  - o Dysfunction/resection of the terminal ileum → ↓ bile acid absorption → if hepatic synthetic reserve is associated from ileal loss → supersaturation of bile → stone formation

429

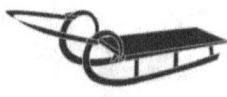

*MASTERING THE BOARDS*
*Hepatology & Pancreaticobiliary Disease*

A.B.R. Thomson

➢ Causes/associations

• Give clinical risk factors for the development of gallstones.

- o Hereditary
- o Classical "4 Fs"
  - – Female
  - – Fertile
  - – Forty
  - – "fat" (obesity)
- o Diet
  - – ↑ calories
  - – ↑ carbohydrates (refined)
  - – ↑ saturated fats
- o Origin
  - – Sweden
  - – Chile
- o Gastric bypass surgery
  - – TPN
  - – Cholelithiasis
  - – Acalculous cholecystitis
- o Dyslipidemias
  - – ↓ HDL-cholesterol
  - – ↑ triglycerides
- o Drugs
  - – Estrogen/OCP (oral contraceptive pill)
  - – Clofibrate
  - – Octreotide
  - – Ceftriazone
- o Diabetes
- o Loss of ileal function
- o Spinal cord injuries

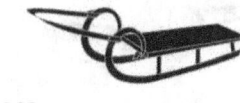

- Give the mechanisms by which some classes of drugs lead to ↑ risk of cholelithiasis.
  - Conjugated estrogens and contraceptive steroids
    - Cholesterol synthesis
      - Estrogens activate the hepatic estrogen receptor α
      - The activated hepatic estrogen receptor α stimulate SREBP-2-responsive genes
      - Activated SREBP-2-responsive genes leads to
        - ↑ cholesterol synthesis and secretion into bile
        - Supersaturation of bile with cholesterol
    - Lipoproteins
      - Estrogens cause ↑ expression of hepatic LDL receptor
      - ↑ hepatic LDL receptor leads to ↑ clearance of LDL
      - ↑ clearance of LDL causes
        - ↓ plasma LDL
        - ↑ plasma HDL
        - ↑ liver LDL
    - ↑ uptake of LDL into the liver causes
      - ↑ cholesterol synthesis
      - ↑ secretion into bile
    - Smooth muscle
      - Estrogens slow smooth muscle motility, leading to gallbladder stasis
  - Clofibrate
    - Clofibrate cause ↓ activity of 7α-hydroxylase
    - ↓ 7α-hydroxylase leads to
      - ↓ synthesis and secretion of bile acids from cholesterol
      - ↓ cholesterol solubility in bile
  - Octreotide cause
    - ↓ gallbladder emptying
    - ↓ small intestine transit
    - ↑ "dwell" time for cholic acid to be dehydroxylated into the 2 bile acid, deoxycholic acid
    - ↑ deoxycholic acid absorption in EHC and return to the liver
    - ↑ deoxycholic acid secretion into bile canaliculus
    - ↓ solubilisation of cholic and chenic acids
  - Ceftriaxone

When the saturation of ceftriaxone in bile is exceeded, ceftriaxone
  - Forms insoluble salts with calcium → biliary sludge

431

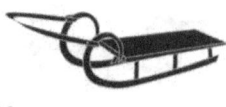

> Clinical

- Give the natural history of asymptomatic stones biliary pain, and acute cholecystitis.
  - o Asymptomatic stones   – Risk of symptoms developing, 1.5% per year

  - o Biliary pain          – Recurrence pain after 1 episode, 6% per year (~70%)
                            – Severe complications, 1% to 2% per year

  - o Acute cholelithiasis  – Resolves, 50%
                            – Duct stones, 15%
                            – Gangrenous gallbladder, 7%
                            – Empyema, 6%
                            – Perforation, 3%
                            – Empty edematous cholecystitis, 1%

  - o Recurrent choledocholithiasis after sphincterotomy, 12%

---

Tricks of the Art: Palpation of gallbladder

  - o Gallbladder (GB) may often be enlarged without a palpable liver; you can better feel the GB with the patient on her/his left side.

  - o Obstructive jaundice plus palpable GB-unlikely to be due to stones (unless stones in cystic duct or Hartmann pouch).
    - – Impossible to insert a finger between kidney and erector spinae muscle; there is a band of resonance anteriorly over an enlarged kidney
    - – Pancreatic cysts may be palpable, but tumours rarely
    - – Ovarian tumours may be palpated in the midline, including at the umbilicus
    - – Distended bladder is symmetrical, unless a diverticulum is present

---

- In the context of cholelithiasis, give the meaning of **Mirizzi syndrome**.
  - o Acute cholecystitis complicated by jaundice due to
    - – Type I
      - ▪ Stones in cystic duct at neck of gallbladder compresses hepatic duct causing CD (cystic duct) / Hartmann pouch obstruction, or causes stricture in the extrahepatic bile duct
    - – Type II
      - ▪ Stone erodes into the hepatic duct, forming a cholecystocholedochal fistula

432

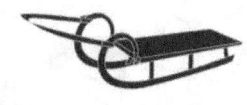

## SO YOU WANT TO BE A GASTROENTEROLOGIST!

- Give the mechanism of the pain experienced in acute cholecystitis.
    - Stones irritate the gallbladder (GB) mucosa
    - The irritated GB mucosa releases phospholipase A
    - Phospholipase A converts lecithin to lysolecithin
    - Lysolecithin stimulates prostaglandin synthetase
    - ↑ prostaglandin synthetase leads to the production of ↑ prostaglandin in the GB wall
    - ↑ prostaglandins cause pain from cholelithiasis

The selection criteria for the use of oral ursodeoxycholic acid (UDCA) dissolution of gallstones relate to the characteristics of the stones, biliary pain without complications, and a functionaing gallbladder. Please see Sleisenger and Fordtran's Gastrointestinal and Liver Disease. 9th Edition. *Saunders/Elsevier* 2010, Table 66.1, page 1122 for details.

## SO YOU WANT TO BE A GASTROENTEROLOGIST!

- Give the anatomical reason why the gallbladder is at high risk for the development of necrosis.
    - The gallbladder is at high risk of developing necrosis because the blood supply to the gallbladder is the cystic artery, an end artery, thereby placing the gallbladder at risk of ischemic necrosis if the blood flow through the cystic artery becomes impaired.

- Give risk factors are associated with an ↑ risk of the patient with gallstones developing gangrenous or emphysematous cholecystitis.

Risk factors for the development complicated acute cholecystitis:

- Diabetic
- Cardiovascular disease
- Male gender
- WBC > 150,000 / mm$^3$

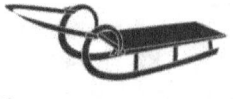

*MASTERING THE BOARDS*
*Hepatology & Pancreaticobiliary Disease*

A.B.R. Thomson

➢ Complications

• Give the complications of gallstone disease.
  o Emphysematous cholecystitis
    – Multiple air pockets in wall of gallbladder in patient with acute cholelithiasis
    – Air pockets formed from Cl. Welchii, E. Coli, anaerobic streptococci (gas-forming organisms)
    – May occur in diabetics or the elderly (atherosclerosis of cystic artery)
  o Cholecystoenteric fistula
    – Gallstone erodes through the wall of the neck of gallbladder into the duodenum stones larger than 25 mm may obstruct
      ▪ Terminal ileum (gallstone ileus)
        – Mortality rate, 20%
      ▪ Gastric outlet (Bonvert syndrome)
    – Three signs on plain abdominal film which are pathognomic of gallstone ileus
      ▪ Pneumobilia suggesting cholecystoenteric fistula (duodenum or jejunum, stomach or hepatic flexure)
      ▪ Small bowel dilation
      ▪ Gallstone in RLQ (right lower quadrant, site stone obstructing the terminal ileum
  o Mirizzi syndrome
  o Porcelain gallbladder
    – Focal or diffusion
    – Intramural calcification of the pancreas
    – With focal calcification, risk of gallbladder adenocarcinoma is 20%

➢ Diagnostic imaging

| Abdominal Ultrasound for Stones | Sensitivity |
| --- | --- |
| o In GB | 95-98% |
| o In CBD | 50% |

  o It has been suggested that an abdominal ultrasound is the best test to exclude other intra-abdominal conditions which may give similar clinical findings of RUQ pain, fever, leucocytosis, hyperamylasemia (or elevated serum lipase concentration.

434

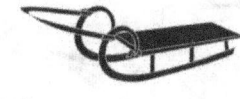

- However, this approach can be challenged based on the performance characteristics of abdominal ultrasound, CT scan, and hepatobiliary scanning.

- ERCP "gallstone pancreatitis" (GSP) – only 10% have stone in CBD
  - When to be suspected GSP
    - Jaundice          } ERCP + Stone removal
    - LE's increasing   }

---

**SO YOU WANT TO BE A GASTROENTEROLOGIST!**

Cholescintigraphy (aka hepatobiliary scintigraphy) has a sensitivity of about 95% and a specificity of about 90% for acute cholecystitis, and a normal scan excludes acute cholecystitis.

- Give the names of the chemicals used for hepatobiliary scintigraphy.

  - HIDA      o  99 m Tc – labelled hydroxyl iminodiacetic acid
  - DISIDA    (diisopropyl iminodiacetic acid)

- In the context of an abdominal ultrasound performed for cholelithiasis, give the meaning of the wall-echo shadow sign (aka "double-arc shadow")

  - The wall-echo shadow sign is the presence of Echogenic stones and acoustic shadowing in a contracted gallbladder filled with stones.

---

Please see Sleisenger and Fordtran's Gastrointestinal and Liver Disease. 9th Edition. *Saunders/Elsevier* 2010, Table 67.2, for details of the diagnostic criteria for acute
acalculous cholecystitis.

"In order to succeed, your desire for success
should be greater than your fear of failure."

Bill Cosby

435

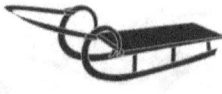

# ACUTE CHOLANGITIS

➢ Diagnostic imaging

• Give the pros and cons of imaging tests for the diagnosis of acute cholangitis.

| Parameter | Abdominal Ultrasonography | CT | MRCP | EUS | ERCP |
|---|---|---|---|---|---|
| o Availability | Widely available | Helical CT is rare | Available | Limited | Available |
| o Portability | Portable | No | No | Limited | Limited |
| o Invasiveness | Non-invasive | Non-invasive | Non-invasive | Invasive | Invasive |
| o Need for sedation | No | No | Some patients | Yes | Yes |
| o Sensitivity for detection of stones | Low | High (best for helical CT) | High | As good as, if not better than ERCP | Gold standard in most studies |
| o Sensitivity for detection of strictures | Low | Fair | Best non-invasive method | Good | Excellent |
| o Sensitivity for detection of tumours | Low | Good | Good | Excellent | Fair |
| o Advantages | Widely available and non invasive | Widely available and accurate | Accurate without radiation exposure | Excellent for small stones, can be done at same time as ERCP | Therapeutic capability |
| o Disadvantage | Low sensitivity | Effects on renal function, poor detection of small stones, not portable | Not compatible in patients with implanted metal devices, poor detection of small stones, not portable | Invasive, poor imaging of intrahepatic ducts | Invasive, possible worsening of condition owing to contrast injection |

Abbreviations: ERCP, endoscopic retrograde cholangiopancreatography; EUS, endoscopic ultrasonography; MRCP, magnetic resonance cholangiopancreatography

Printed with permission: John G. Lee. *Nature Reviews Gastroenterology and Hepatology* 2009;6:533-541, page 535.

436

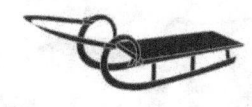

# COMMON BILE DUCT DISEASE

➢ Diagnostic imaging

• Give the advantages and limitations imaging modalities for detecting stones in the common bile duct.

| Imaging Modality | Description | Advantages | Limitations |
|---|---|---|---|
| ○ Transabdominal ultrasonography | – Non-invasive procedure whereby high-frequency sound waves are converted into images | ▪ First-line imaging modality<br>▪ Noninvasive<br>▪ Widely available and inexpensive<br>▪ Sensitivity 22%–65%*<br>▪ Specificity 70%–98%* | Artifacts may be caused by pneumobilia, surgical clips, biliary stents, duodenal diverticula, and calcifying pancreatitis |
| ○ Endoscopic ultrasonography | – Use of a duodenoscope with an ultrasound transducer at its tip; images are more accurate and detailed than ones obtained by traditional ultrasonography because of the proximity of the transducer to the organs of interest | ▪ More cost-effective than ERCP as a diagnostic tool<br>▪ Sensitivity 85%–97%*<br>▪ Specificity 90%–95%* | Not widely available; operator dependent; artifacts may be caused by pneumobilia, surgical clips, biliary stents, duodenal diverticula and calcifying pancreatitis |
| ○ Intraductal ultrasonography | – Imaging of the biliary tree with an ultrasound transducer mounted at the tip of a catheter inserted through duodenoscope | ▪ Sensitivity 97%–100%* | Probes have limited durability; stones, sludge and air bubbles may be indistinguishable |

437

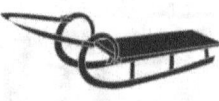

| Imaging Modality | Description | Advantages | Limitations |
|---|---|---|---|
| o Laparoscopic intraoperative ultrasonography | – Intraoperative use of a specialized laparoscopic probe with an ultrasound transducer at the tip that is positioned to visualize the biliary system | ▪ Sensitivity 80%–83%*<br>▪ Specificity 99%–100%* | Technically difficult to perform, especially in obese individuals; operator dependent; suboptimal visualization of the intrapancreatic portion of the common bile duct; artifacts may be caused by pneumobilia; detects sludge and small stones that are of limited clinical significance |
| o ERCP | – Injection of a contrast agent directly into the common bile duct and imaging at duodenoscopy; considered the "gold standard" against which other imaging modalities are compared | ▪ Sensitivity 89%–90%*<br>▪ Specificity 98%–100%* | Operator dependent; overall complication rate 4%–6%; mortality associated with procedure 0.1%–0.5% |
| o Intraoperative cholangiography | – Insertion of a catheter through the cystic duct at the time of surgery, followed by injection of a contrast agent into the common bile duct and fluoroscopic imaging | ▪ Sensitivity 75%–100%*<br>▪ Specificity 97%–100%* | Prolongs the duration of the surgical procedure; fluoroscopy use in the operating room |

438

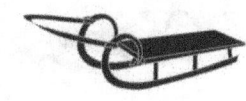

| Imaging Modality | Description | Advantages | Limitations |
|---|---|---|---|
| o Helical computed tomography cholangiography | – Computed tomography of the biliary system following intravenous administration of a contrast agent | ▪ Sensitivity 71%–85%* <br> ▪ Specificity 88%–97%* | Similar drawbacks to those with intravenous cholangiography |
| o Intravenous cholangiography | – Injection of a contrast agent intravenously, followed by radiographic imaging of the biliary system | ▪ Relatively non-invasive; provides information on the biliary ductal system <br> ▪ Sensitivity 48%–50%* <br> ▪ Specificity 95%–97%* | Risk of reaction to contrast agent (1%) or renal impairment <br> Limited value in patients with elevated bilirubin level because of decreased excretion of dye into the biliary system |
| o Magnetic resonance cholangiopan-creatography | – Magnetic resonance imaging whereby the hepatobiliary and pancreatic system are visualized using a specialized sequence | ▪ Can be used when endoscopic ultrasonography and ERCP is not possible (e.g.,, after Roux-en-Y gastric or biliary procedures); diagnostic accuracy decreased if stones < 5 mm or common bile duct >10 mm <br> ▪ Sensitivity 85%–100%* <br> ▪ Specificity 91%–97%* | Hard for patients with claustrophobia to tolerate <br> May cause dysfunction of certain pacemakers or implantable cardiac defibrillators, or may dislodge of metallic prostheses |

Abbreviation: ERCP, endoscopic retrograde cholangiopancreatography.

*Using different reference standards across multiple studies.

Printed with permission: Almadi MA, et al. Management of suspected stones in the common bile duct. CMAJ. 2012;184(8):884-92. Table 2.

439

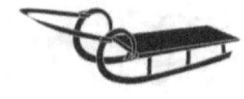

**SO YOU WANT TO BE A GASTROENTEROLOGIST!**

- Give the differential diagnosis for the situation where abdominal ultrasound shows dilated intrahepatic duct, normal extrahepatic duct and small (contracted gallbladder) filled with stones.

  o These three features on abdominal ultrasound suggest compression of the common hepatic duct, such as from
    - Tumour (Klatskin tumour at bifurcation of R. & L. intrahepatic ducts with the hepatic duct)
    - Stone in neck of gallbladder or cystic duct (Mirizzi syndrome, Type I)

- Give the approximate values for the performance characteristics for diagnostic imaging studies of the biliary tree.

| | Cholelithiasis (> 2 mm) | | Acute cholelithiasis | | Choledochalithiasis | |
|---|---|---|---|---|---|---|
| | Sens | Spec | Sens | Spec | Sens | Spec |
| o Abdominal ultrasound with acoustic shadow | > 95% | > 95% | Murphy sign, PPV, > 90% (if cholelithiasis is present) | | < 50% for stones ~ 75% for diameter > 6 mm (dilation) | |
| o Oral cholecystography | > 90% | > 90% | - | - | - | - |
| o Hepatobiliary scintigraphy | - | - | 95% | 90% | - | - |
| o ERCP | 80% | - | - | - | 95% | 95% |
| o EUS | - | - | - | - | 95% | 97% |
| | | | | | PPV, 99% NPV, 98% | |
| o MRCP | - | - | - | - | 93% | 94% |

Abbreviations: NPV, negative predictive value; PPV, positive predictive value; sens, sensitivity; spec, specificity

440

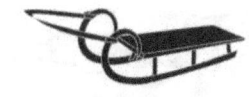

## SO YOU WANT TO BE A GASTROENTEROLOGIST!

- In the context of suspected gallbladder disease, give the meaning of the **Couvoisier sign.**

  - o Painless jaundice plus a palpable gallbladdddr suggests a cancer obstructing the bile duct, such as cancer of the head of the pancreas.

## SO YOU WANT TO BE A GASTROENTEROLOGIST!

- Time for a trick question! Is cholecystectomy associated with an increased risk of colorectal cancer?

  - o "Yes, but…….."; the risk is statistically significant, but the relative risk is low, < 2.0.

- ➢ Prevention
  - o UDCA (ursodeoxycholic acid) to prevent stone formation
    - – Gallstones and symptoms are frequent after bariatric surgery, when the patient is on a very low calorie diet.
    - – As a result, there is
      - ▪ ↑ liver synthesis of cholesterol
      - ▪ ↑ gallbladder (GB) mucin
      - ▪ ↓ GB motility
    - – Giving UDCA prophylactically reduces gallstones from 28% to 3%

441

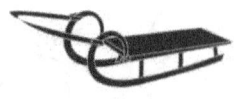

- Criteria for use of UDCA
  - Functioning gallbladder on HiDA scan
  - Radiolucent stones
  - Patent cystic duct
  - 20% to 70% dissolution rates
  - Current indication
    - Prevention of development of cholelithiasis in high risk persons (e.g., bariatric surgery, short bowel syndrome)

---

**SO YOU WANT TO BE A GASTROENTEROLOGIST!**

- Give the success rate for UDCA for the dissolution of gallstones, when appropriately used.

  - ↓ risk of biliary pain and acute cholecystitis, even without dissolution of stones

  - Dissolution rates of stones

    | Size, mm | Rates |
    | --- | --- |
    | < 5 | 70% |
    | < 10 | 49% |
    | >10 | 29% |

  - Recurrence of stones when stopping UDCA after initial successful dissolution, 50% in 5 years

---

- ESWL – extracorporeal shock-wave lithotripsy
  - For large impacted stones, not amenable to endoscopic removal
  - Complications
  - Hemobilia (10%)
  - Biliary sepsis (4%)

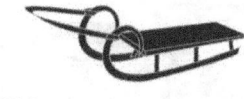

# SO YOU WANT TO BE A GASTROENTEROLOGIST!

Recommended selection criteria are available for **extracorporeal shock-wave lithotripsy** (ESWL) (Please see Sleisenger and Fordtran's Gastrointestinal and Liver Disease. 9th Edition. *Saunders/Elsevier* 2010, Table 66.2, page 1123; and 10th Edition, 2016, page 1137). These are identical for UDCA, except that diameter of the single or multiple stones is optimally < 6 mm (and 6-10 mm acceptably) for ESWL.

- Give the success rate for ESWL when appropriately used.

  | o Free of stones | Months | Proportion |
  | --- | --- | --- |
  | | 6 | 47% to 77% |
  | | 12 | 68% to 84% |

  | o Recurrence (cumulative) | Years | Proportion |
  | --- | --- | --- |
  | | 3 | 27% |
  | | 5 | 41% |
  | | 10 | 54% |

- Give factors which predict a poor response to ESWL.

  - Stones that are
    - Multiple
    - Large (> 16 mm diameter)
    - Dense (CT density > 84 Hounsfield unit)
  - Failure of dissolution or recurrence
  - Biliary pain, 33%
  - Petechiae, 8%
  - Obstruction of cystic duct, 5%
  - Hematurin, 4%
  - Gallstone pancreatitis, 2%
  - Hepatic hematomas, < 1%

443

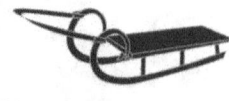

- o Surgery
  - – Open cholecystectomy
  - – MR > 65  0.03%
    -      < 65  0.5%
  - – Laparoscopic cholecystectomy
    - ▪ MR    0.15%
    - ▪ Intra-operative conversion to open procedure    2-8%
    - ▪ Bile duct injury (same as for open cholecystectomy 0.14-0.5%
  - – Nasocystic drain
    - ▪ Use a nasocystic drain of a "hot" gallbladder (cholecystitis) in high risk patients
    - ▪ For EUS, the probe must be < 1 cm from GI tract
    - ▪ Treatments with EUS
      - – Make a fistula
      - – Insert a stent
      - – Drain. debride cavity

---

### SO YOU WANT TO BE A GASTROENTEROLOGIST!

- Give the risks of laparoscopic cholecystectomy.
  - o Major morbidity, 5%
  - o Need to convert from lap "chole" to open cholecystectomy, 3%
  - o Bile duct injury, 0.5% (depends on surgeon's experience)
  - o Mortality, 60/ $10^5$ (0.06%)
  - o Stricture
  - o Choledocholthiasis

---

Abbreviations: CHD, common hepatic duct; CBD, common bile duct; SOD, sphincter of Oddi; IBS, irritable bowel syndrome.

Adapted from: Glasgow RE. and Mulvihill SJ. Treatment of Gallstone Disease. *Sleisenger & Fordtran's Gastrointestinal and Liver Disease: Pathophysiology/Diagnosis/Management* 2006; pg. 1424-1436.

➢ High risk patient

- o Percutaneous cholecystectomy, followed by lap'chole'
- o Early surgery preferred for acute cholecystitis

Sleisenger and Fordtran's Gastrointestinal and Liver Disease. 9th Edition. *Saunders/Elsevier* 2010, page 1105 and 1130.

444

Useful Quotes

"...... the natural history of gallstones in diabetic patients follows the same pattern observed in non-diabetic patients.
Prophylactic cholecystectomy is generally not recommended in patients with insulin-resistant diabetes mellitus and asymptomatic gallstones".

* Note:
- When diabetic patients develop biliary pain, early cholecystectomy should be performed because these patients have an increased risk of developing gangrenous cholecystitis.

Useful Quotes

"...... cholecystectomy may be undertaken during pregnancy with minimal fetal and maternal morbidity but only when necessary".
If cholecystectomy necessary, attempt to perform in T2, second trimester
- Cholecystectomy necessary, attempt to perform in T2, second trimester

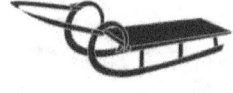

## ASGE Guidelines on Competence in Performing ERCP

- o 200 cases performed by trainee with expert supervision
- o 80-90% cannulation rate
- o Continued completion of 50 sphincterotomies / year

Useful Trivia

".... It is unlikely that the ampulla [of Vater] is obstructed [by impaction of a stone within the common channel of the ampulla of Vater] in the presence of a normal serum bilirubin [i.e., the absence of hyperbilirubinemia]....."

(Sleisenger and Fordtran's Gastrointestinal and Liver Disease. 9th Edition. *Saunders/Elsevier*, Philadelphia, 2010, page 1035).

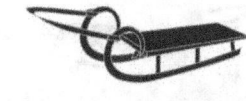

# ACALCULOUS GALLBLADDER DISEASE

➢ Risk factors

➢ Diagnostic imaging

- Give the findings on abdominal ultrasound, CT scanning and hepatobiliary scanning which suggest the diagnosis of acalculous cholecystitis.

o Abdominal ultrasound (US)
  - Gallbladder (GB) wall > 4 mm*

  - Positive US Murphy sign
  - Collection of pericholecystic fluid

o CT scan
  - GB wall > 4 mm
  - Sloughed GB mucosa

  - Pericholecystic fluid
  - Intramular air

o Hepatobiliary scan
  - Lack of "hot spot"** (failure of filling of GB, with passage of radionucleotide into duodenum)

* in absence of ascites or hyoalbuminemia
** false negatives with fasting or ICU illness

447

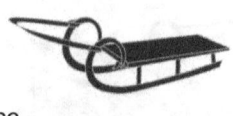

*MASTERING THE BOARDS*
*Hepatology & Pancreaticobiliary Disease*

A.B.R. Thomson

- Give the performance characteristics of 3 diagnostic imaging tests for acalculous cholecystitis.

| Diagnostic Imaging Test | Sensitivity | Specificity |
| --- | --- | --- |
| o Abdominal ultrasound | 67% to 92% | 90% |
| o CT scan | > 95% | > 95% |
| o Hepatobiliary scan[1] | > 90% | 90% |

[1] The morphine-augmented cholescintigraphy increases specificity to about 95%

---

## SO YOU WANT TO BE A GASTROENTEROLOGIST!

- In the context of acalculous biliary pain and in the setting of apparently an idiopathic post-cholecystectomy syndrome, give the meaning of the **Meltzer-Lyon** test.

  o The Meltzer-Lyon test is the collection and staining of the stool to establish the presence of microlithiasis as a possible cause of post-cholecystectomy syndrome.

- Give the microscopic appearance of the substance examined in the Meltzer-Lyon test.

  o The Meltzer-Lyon test involves collecting and examining the stools for microlithiasis in the setting of the post-cholecystectomy syndrome.

  o Microscopic examination may show rhomboidal cholesterol crystals or granules of calcium bilirulonate.

---

> Treatment

---

Useful Quotes

"Cholecystectomy has not typically been recommended for patients with acalculous pain and a normal GBEF [gallbladder ejection fraction > 35% on hepatobiliary scanning after the slow IV infusion of CCK]."

---

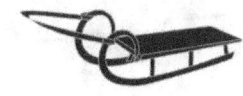

A Follow-up Useful Quote

".....although the GBEF [gallbladder ejection fraction on hepatobiliary scanning] is used commonly to evaluate patients with acalculous biliary-type pain, it is not a reliable predictor of the response to cholecystectomy."

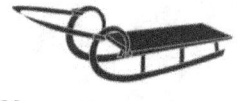

# CONGENITAL ABNORMALITIES OF THE BILIARY TRACT

## Biliary Atresia

➢ Definition

   o "biliary atresia is characterized by the complete obstruction of bile flow as a result of the destruction or absence of all or a portion of the extrahepatic bile ducts" (Sleisenger and Fordtran's Gastrointestinal and Liver Disease. 10th Edition. *Saunders/Elsevier*, Philadelphia, 2016, page 1062).

➢ Pathology

   o Bile duct proliferation

   o Bile stasis in canaliadae and cells

   o Bile plugs in portal treads

   o Edema

   o Fibrosis

➢ Surgical treatment

   o Kasai hepatoportoenterostomy

   o Liver transplantation (for failure of portoenterostomy)

## Choledochal Cyst

➢ Definition

   o Choledochal cysts are congenital anomalies of the biliary tract that are manifested by cystic dilation of the extrahepatic and intrahepatic bile ducts" (Sleisenger and Fordtran's Gastrointestinal and Liver Disease. 10th Edition. *Saunders/Elsevier*, Philadelphia, 2016, page 1067).

➢ Types

   o CBD (common bile duct)

     – Diffuse, fusiform dilations        I

     – Diverticula        II

     – Dilation of intraduodenal portion of CBD    III

       (aka choledochal cyst)

   o Intra- and extrahepatic bile duct cysts    IV

   o Intrahepatic cysts (Caroli disease)    V

450

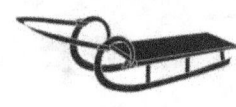

- ➢ Clinical
  - ○ Abdominal pain
  - ○ Jaundice
  - ○ Palpable mass (cyst)

- ➢ Complications of choledochal cysts
  - ○ Biliary tree
    - – Cholangitis
    - – Strictures
    - – Cholangiocarcinoma (occurs in 30%, especially type I and II)
  - ○ Pancreas
    - – Recurrent pancreatitis

## Caroli Disease

- ➢ Definition
  - ○ Segmental, saccular, congenital dilation of intrahepatic ducts, without obstruction

- ➢ Pathology
  - ○ Intrauterine malformation of ductal plate
    - – Dilated ducts associated with
      - ▪ Congenital hepatic fibrosis
      - ▪ Medullary sponge kidney
      - ▪ Choledochal cysts, type V
    - – Stones form in dilated ducts
      - ▪ Cholangitis (~33%)
      - ▪ Cholangiocarcinoma (10%)

- ➢ Causes/associations
  - ○ Intrahepatic duct stones
  - ○ Bacterial cholangitis
  - ○ Renal tubular ectasia
  - ○ ARPKD (autosomal recessive polycystic kidney disease)

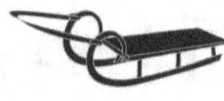

**Caroli Syndrome**

➢ Definition: Same as caroli disease, plus

  o Heart failure (HF)

  o Choledochal cysts

---

Trivia alert: Note subtle differences between Caroli disease and Caroli syndrome

---

Please see Sleisenger and Fordtran's Gastrointestinal and Liver Disease. 9th Edition. *Saunders/Elsevier* 2010, Figure 94.10, for Algorithm's to use to Approach the Patient with a Hepatic Mass Lesion without or with associated cirrhosis

**Alagille Syndrome** (Familial Intrahepatic Cholestasis [FIC])

➢ Definition

  o Autosomal dominant familial intrahepatic cholestasis due to a decrease in the number of interlobular portal bile ducts (ratio of interlobular portal bile ducts to portal bile ducts to portal tracts < 0.4) due to mutations in the jagged 1 ($JAG_1$) gene, leading to periportal fibrosis and cirrhosis.

➢ Genetic

  o 94% of Alagille syndrome patients have mutations in the $JAG_1$ gene, and the remainder have mutations in the gene coding for the $NOTCH_2$ receptor.

➢ Clinical

  o Face
    − Wide forehead
    − Deeply set and widely spaced eyes
    − Small chin
    − Triangular face

  o Ears
    − Big

  o Spine
    − Short
    − Butterfly vertebrae

  o Heart
    − Murmurs (commonly pulmonary stenosis)

452

# GALLBLADDER CANCER

➢ Demography
  o 1/10$^5$, with global incidence rates of GB-Ca parallel to incidence rates of cholelithiasis.

➢ Causes/associations

• Give conditions associated with ↑ risk of development of GB-Ca.
  o Calcification of gallbladder
    – GB-Ca 80% have cholelithiasis (all types of stones, especially > 10 mm)
    – Porcelain gallbladder (selective mucosal calcification, type II / III)
  o Polyps > 2 cm
    – Adenomyomatosis
    – Very small risk
    – Forget symptoms → laparoscopic cholecystectomy (LC), any size of polyp
    – No symptoms
      ▪ ≥ 1 cm polyp → LC
      ▪ < 1 cm plus stones → LC
      ▪ < 1 cm, no stones → US q 6 to 12 months
    – Symptoms → LC, regardless
  o Bile duct
    – Choledochal cysts
    – Caroli disease
    – Pancreatic duct draining into bile duct
    – Cholangiocarcinoma [cholelithiasis, 2% develop GB-Ca]
    – Au PBD (anomalous union of the pancreatic and bile ducts outside the duodenal wall in a long common channel)
    – Consider prophylactic cholecystectomy
  o Primary sclerosing cholangitis (PSC)
    – 20% develop GB-Ca
    – 50% of masses in GB of PSC patient are cancer
  o Biliary dysplasia
    – Toxins e.g., 2° bile acids, mustard oil
  o Infection
    – Chronic Salmonella Typhi/paratyphi carrier state
    – E. Coli
    – H. pylori
  o Family history, first degree relative

453

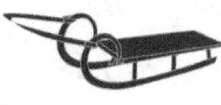

# CHOLESTEROLOSIS

➤ Definition

- o "Macrophages in the wall of the gallbladder" appearing foamy from accumulation of cholesterol esters plus triglyceride.

➤ Types

- o Diffuse collections of cholesterol in GB wall, ending at cystic duct
- o Focal collections of cholesterol
- o Polyps (2 to 10 mm)
- o Combined diffuse plus polypoid accumulations

➤ Microscopy

- o Foamy macrophages of variable distribution (please see above)
- o Hyperplasia of the mucosa
- o Hyperplasia may be villous in appearance

# ADENOMYOMATOSIS

➤ Definition

- o "An acquired, hyperplastic lesion [of the gallbladder] characterized by excessive proliferation of surface epithelium with imaginations into the thickened muscularis (Rokitansky-Aschoff sinus) or even more deeply" to produce tiny diverticulae (Sleisenger and Fordtran's Gastrointestinal and Liver Disease. 10th Edition. Saunders/Elsevier, Philadelphia, 2016, page 1159).

- • In the context of adenomyomatosis of the gallbladder give the characteristics of the Rokitansky-Aschoff sinuses.

- o Deep
- o Branched
- o Hyperplasia of the muscle layer

➤ Type

- o Generalized
- o Fundic
- o Segmental (may produce a narrowing of the lumen of the gallbladder)
- o "segmental adenomyomatosis should be considered a potentially premalignant lesion"

454

# ABBREVIATIONS

| | |
|---|---|
| $^{99m}$Tc-MAA | Perfusion body scan with $^{99m}$ Technetium-labeled macroaggregated albumin |
| $AaPO_2$ | Alveolar-arterial pressure gradient for oxygen |
| AFLP | Acute fatty liver of pregnancy |
| AFP | Alpha- fetoprotein |
| AH | Autoimmune hepatitis |
| ALD | Alcoholic liver disease |
| ALF | Acute liver failure |
| ALP | Alkaline phosphatase |
| ALT | Alanine aminotransferase |
| AMA | Antimitochondrial antibodies |
| ANA | Antinuclear antibodies |
| ARBs | Angiotensin receptor blockers |
| ASA | Anti-smooth muscle antibody |
| AST | Aspartate aminotransferase |
| ATN | Acute tubular necrosis |
| BID | Twice a day |
| BMI | Body mass index |
| BNP | Brain natriuretic peptide |
| BPM | Beats per minute |
| BUN | Blood urea nitrogen |
| CAD | Coronary artery disease |
| CAT | Computerized axial tomography |
| CBD | Common bile duct |
| CEE | Contrast enhanced echocardiography |

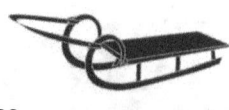

| | |
|---|---|
| CHD | Common hepatic duct |
| CLT | Cadaveric liver transplatation |
| CT | Computerized tomography |
| CTP | Child Turcotte Pugh |
| E | Hepatitis B e antigen |
| E/A ratio | Ratio of early to late (arterial) phases of ventricular filling |
| ECG | Electrocardiogram |
| EGD | Esophagogastroduodenoscopy |
| ELISA | Enzyme linked immunosorbent assay |
| ERCP | Endoscopic retrograde cholangiopancreatography |
| ESLD | End-stage liver disease |
| EUS | Endoscopic ultrasonography |
| EVBL | Endoscopic variceal band ligation |
| EVL | Endoscopic variceal ligation |
| EVR | Early virologic response |
| FH | Family history |
| FNH | Focal nodular hyperplasia |
| GAVE | Gastric antral vascular ectasia |
| GGT | Gamma-glutamyltransferase |
| GI | Gastrointestinal |
| H | Hemalysis |
| HBV | Hepatitis B virus |
| HCC | Hepatocellular carcinoma |
| HCV | Hepatitis C virus |
| HE | Hepatic encephalopathy |

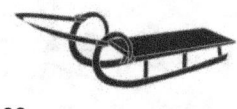

| | |
|---|---|
| HH | Hereditary hemochromatosis |
| HOMA | Homeostatic model assessment |
| HRS | Hepatorenal syndrome |
| HRT | Hormone replacement therapy |
| HSC | Hepatic stellatecells |
| HVPG | Hepatic venous pressure gradient |
| IBS | Irritable bowel syndrome |
| ICP | Intracranial pressure |
| ICP | Intrahepatic cholestasis of pregnancy |
| INR | International normalized ratio |
| IV | intravenous |
| IVC | Inferior vena cava |
| IVDU | IV drug use |
| LCHAD | Long chain 3-hydroxyacyl-CoA-dehydrogenase |
| LDLT | Live donor liver transplantation |
| LP | Thrombocytopenia |
| MAP | Mean arterial pressure |
| MCV | Mean corpuscular volume |
| MDA | Malondialdehyde |
| MELD | Model for end stage liver disease |
| MPAOP | Mean pulmonary artery occlusion pressure |
| MRCP | Magnetic resonance cholangiopancreatography |
| MRI | Magnetic resonance imaging |
| MTOR | Mammalian target of rapamycin |
| NA | Not available |
| NAS | NASH activity score |

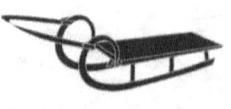

| | |
|---|---|
| NASH | Non alcoholic steatohepatitis |
| NNFL | Non-NASH fatty liver |
| NP | Not applicable |
| NRH | Nodular regenerative hyperplasia |
| NVR | No virologic response |
| OGIS | Oral glucose insulin sensitivity index |
| OLT | Orthotopic liver transplantation |
| OR | Odds ratio |
| PA | Pulmonary artery |
| $PaO_2$ | Partial pressure gradient for oxygen |
| PBC | Primary biliary cholangitis |
| PCLD | Polycystic liver disease |
| PCR | Polymerase chain reaction |
| PEI | Percutaneous ethanol injection |
| PFT | Pulmonary function testing |
| PHG | Portal hypertensive gastropathy |
| PHT | Portal hypertension |
| PMN | Polymorphonuclear (neutrophil) cell count |
| PNH | Paroxysmal nocturnal hemoglobulinuria |
| PO | Orally |
| PPH | Portopulmonary hypertension |
| PS | Performance status |
| PSC | Primary sclerosing cholangitis |
| PT | Prothrombin time |
| PV | Pulmonary vein |
| PVR | Pulmonary vascular resistance |

458

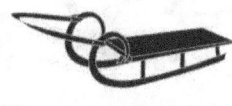

| | |
|---|---|
| QD | Once daily |
| QUICKI | Quantitative insulin-sensitivity check index |
| RBBB | Right bundle branch block |
| RBC | Red blood cell count |
| RFA | Radiofrequency ablation |
| RIBA | Recombinant immunoblot assay |
| RV | Right ventricular |
| RVR | Rapid viral response |
| SAAG | Serum ascites albumin gradient |
| SBP | Spontaneous bacterial peritonitis |
| SC | Subcutaneously |
| SMA | Smooth muscle antibodies |
| SMR | Standard mortality ratio |
| SOD | Sphincter of Oddi |
| SS | Simple steatosis |
| SVR | Sustained viral response |
| TACE | Transarterial chemoembolization |
| TAE | Transarterial embolization |
| TID | Thrice a day |
| TIPS | Transjugular intrahepatic portosystemic shunt |
| TMP-SMX | Trimethoprim sulfamethoxazole |
| UDCA | Ursodeoxycholic aid |
| ULN | Upper limit of normal |
| US | Ultrasound |
| VR | Viral response |

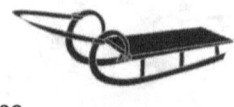

# PANCREAS

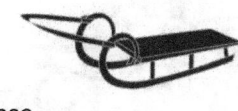

# TABLE OF CONTENTS

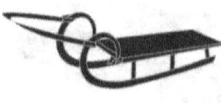

*MASTERING THE BOARDS*
*Hepatology & Pancreaticobiliary Disease*

A.B.R. Thomson

# PANCREATITIS

- ➢ Definitions
    - ○ **Acute pancreatitis** is "......an event triggered by sudden pancreatic injury that is followed by sequential inflammatory responses" (Sleisenger and Fordtran's Gastrointestinal and Liver Disease. 9th Edition. Saunders/Elsevier, Philadelphia, 2010, page 901).
        - – Alternate definitions:....an acute inflammatory process of the pancreas with variable involvement of other regional tissue or remote organ systems" (Sleisenger and Fordtran's Gastrointestinal and Liver Disease. 9th Edition. Saunders/Elsevier, Philadelphia, 2010, page 931).
        - – "...best defined clinically by a patient with [or all of the following criteria: (1) symptoms such as epigastric pain, consistent with the disease; (2) a serum amylase or lipase greater than three times a year limit of normal; or (3) radiologic imaging consistent with the diagnosis, usually using computed tomography (CT) or magnetic resonance imaging (MRI) (Sleisenger and Fordtran's Gastrointestinal and Liver Disease. 9th Edition. Saunders/Elsevier, Philadelphia, 2010, page 960).
    - ○ Acute pancreatitis is..... an event triggered by sudden pancreatic injury that is followed by sequential inflammatory responses (Sleisenger and Fordtran's Gastrointestinal and Liver Disease. 9th Edition. Saunders/Elsevier, Philadelphia, 2010, page 901).
    - ○ **Chronic pancreatitis** ".....is a process that usually begins with recurrent pancreatitis and ends with immune-related destruction of the pancreas and widespread glandular fibrosis" (Sleisenger and Fordtran's Gastrointestinal and Liver Disease. 9th Edition. Saunders/Elsevier, Philadelphia, 2010, page 931).
    - ○ **Hereditary pancreatitis** is "......recurrent acute or chronic pancreatitis in an individual from a family in which the pancreatitis phenotype appears to be inherited through a disease-causing gene mutation expressed in an autosomal dominant pattern."
        - – Caused by mutations in $PRSS_1$ (cationic trypsinogen) gene
        - – Clinical phenotype: recurrent acute pancreatitis
        - – Penetrance of genotype to phenotype 80%
    - ○ **Familial pancreatitis** is "....pancreatitis from any cause that occurs in a family with an incidence [of pancreatitis] that is greater than would be expected by chance alone, given the size of the family and incidence of pancreatitis within a defined population" (familial may or may not be caused by a genetic defect).
        - – Usually caused by
            - ▪ SPINK1 mutations, or
            - ▪ CFTR – SPINK1 genotypes atypical (homozygous or atypical compound heterozygous.

462

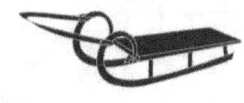

- o **Tropical pancreatitis** is "......a form of early age-onset, non-alcoholic chronic pancreatitis occurring in tropical regions what is often clustered among family members, and that has a complex genetic basis."
  - SPINK1 N34S mutations are common

- ➢ Demography
  - o Wide variation in quoted incidence ~ $25/10^5$
  - o Incidence depends on causes
  - o Most common causes are alcohol excess and cholelithiasis

- ➢ Causes/associations

- • Give causes of acute pancreatitis.
  - o Idiopathic
    - Pancreas divisum
    - Choledochocele

  - o Inherited
    - CFTR, SPINK 1 & 2, CT gene and other mutations

  - o Infection
    - Viral (mumps, Coxsackie, CMV, HSV, HIV)
    - Bacterial (Mycoplasma, Legionella, Leptospira, Salmonella)
    - Fungal (Aspergillus)
    - Parasitic (toxoplasma, cryptosporidium, Ascaris)

  - o Inflammation
    - Penetrating gastroduodenal ulcer
    - Crohn disease

  - o Ischemic
    - Ischemia
    - Vascular bypass surgery
    - Vasculitis

  - o Immune
    - Idiopathic autoimmune pancreatitis

  - o Obstruction
    - Gallstones
    - Biliary sludge
    - ERCP
    - Juxta-ampullary diverticulum
    - Ampullary neoplasms
    - Pancreatic neoplasms
    - Ampullary stenosis
    - Sphincter of Oddi dysfunction (SOD)

463

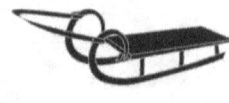

o Trauma      – Blunt trauma

                         – Penetrating trauma

                         – Post ERCP

o Metabolic      – Hypertriglyceridemia

                         – Hypercalcemia

o Medications/      – Ethanol
  toxin

                         – Methanol

                         – Scorpion venom

                         – Drugs: immunosuppressant, pentamadine, DDI, furosemide, thiazides, sulfasalazine, 5-ASA, salicylates, L-asparaginase, azathioprine, valproate, estrogen, sulindac, and others (see next question please)

---

xxxxxxxxxxxxxxxxxxxxxxxxxxxxxxxxxxxxxxxxxxxxxxxxxxxxxxxxxxxxxxxxxxx

SO YOU WANT TO BE A GASTROENTEROLOGIST!

•   Give systemic diseases associated with pancreatitis.

     o Endocrine           – Diabetes (ketoacidosis)

                               – Hypercalcemia

                               – Hypertriglyceridemia

     o Hematology        – HUS (hemolytic uremic syndrome)

     o MSK                      – SLE (systemic lupus erythematosus)

     o Transplantation     – The surgery itself

                               – Immune suppressant drugs

*Note: These conditions may of course be included in the answer to the previous question.

xxxxxxxxxxxxxxxxxxxxxxxxxxxxxxxxxxxxxxxxxxxxxxxxxxxxxxxxxxxxxxxxxxx

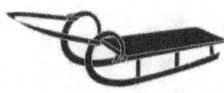

➢ Genetics

Acute pancreatitis may be caused by or associated with genetic defects which disrupt mechanisms which normally protects the process from trypsin associated injury, and therapy increases the susceptibility of the pancreas.

- Give examples of major susceptibility genes which cause or predispose to pancreatic disease.
  - Cationic trypsinogen ($PRSS_1$) [protease serine 1]) gene mutations. There are 3 forms of trypsinogen
    - $PRSS_1$
      - Cationic trypsinogen (65%)
      - Protease serine 1 gene
    - $PRSS_2$
      - Anionic trypsinogen (30%)
    - $PRSS_3$
      - Mesotrypsin
  - $PST_1$ (aka $SPINK_1$ [serine protease inhibitors Kazal type 1])
  - Cystic fibrosis conductance regulator gene
  - SBDS (Schwachman-Bodian-Diamond Syndrome) gene
  - CASR (Calcium-sensing receptor) gene polymorphism
    - Trypsin
      - TAP (trypsinogen activation peptide) =

$$\text{Trypsinogen} \xrightarrow{\text{enterokinase}} \text{trypsin + TAP}$$
$$\text{Trypsin (autoactivation)}$$

➢ Pathophysiology
  - Inadvertent activation of trypsin in the pancreas is prevented by several protective mechanisms to prevent autodigestion

- Give major factors involved in the pathophysiology of acute pancreatitis.
  - Failure of the normal mechanisms of protecting pancreas from autodigestion by trypsin and the pancreatic proenzymes activated by trypsin.
  - Activation of complement and Kinin systems
  - Associated genetic abnormalities
    - $SPINK_1$ (aka PSTI, pancreatic secretory trypsin inhibitor) mutations, resulting in loss of the normal effect of inactivating 20% of trypsin activity.
    - $PRSS_1$ (cationic trypsinogen gene)

465

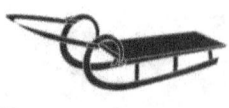

- o Associated metabolic abnormalities e.g.,
  - ↑ serum triglyceride
  - ↑ serum $Ca^{2+}$
  - Acidosis
- o Disassociation
  - Between continued synthesis but blocked secretion of pancreatic enzymes
  - Enzymes accumulate in acini, causing damage
  - Possible colocalization of pancreatic enzymes in the lysosomes
- o Disruption of tight junctions
  - Pancreas: loss of paracellular barrier of acinar cells and intralobular pancreatic duct cells
  - GI tract: ↑ translocation of gut bacteria
- o Microcirculatory changes
  - Vasoconstriction
  - Release of VCAM-1 (an endothelial adhesion molecule)
    - PGs (prostaglandins)
    - PAF (platelet activating factor)
    - Leukotrienes
  - Ischemia
  - AV shunting in gut (plus ischemia → GI bleeding)
  - Possible reperfusion injury
- o Immune changes
  - Activation of complement and release of C5a
  - Recruitments of PMNs and macrophages
  - ↑ proinflammatory cytokines
  - ↑ mediators of inflammation
    - Arachidonic acid metabolites
    - NO (nitric oxide)
    - Reactive oxygen metabolites
- o Failure of anti-autodigestion mechanisms

- Give the mechanisms that prevent autodigestion.
  - o Separation of zymogen granules and lysosomes within the acinar cell
  - o Trypsin inhibitors (SPINK) within the acinar cells and the pancreatic duct
  - o The digestive enzymes secreted as precursors
  - o Activation of trypsin actually occurs OUTSIDE the pancreas by duodenally secreted enterokinases (pepsinogen activated kinase)

Adapted from: Hirota M, et al. *J Gastroenterol* 2006;41(9):832-6.

466

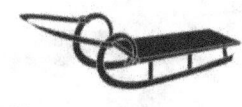

- Give the mechanisms by which the activity of trypsin is switched on and off.
  - Activation of trypsin
    - TAP (trypsinogen activation peptide)
    - The trypsin plus TAP peptides form the inactive trypsinogen enzyme.
    - The TAP is cleared from trypsinogen to form the active trypsin.
    - The activation of the cleavage of TAP results from enterocyte brush border membrane enterokinase, or by other molecules of trypsin.
    - This activation of trypsin by trypsin is called "autoactivation".
    - Trypsin is activated by $\uparrow Ca^{2+}$ ($\uparrow Ca^{2+}$ blocks trypsin degradation), and is inactivated (degraded) in the acinar cell by $\downarrow Ca^{2+}$ ($\downarrow Ca^{2+}$ blocks activation).
    - Degradation of trypsin also results from CTRC (chymotrypsin-C)
  - Dereactivation (autolysis) of trypsin
    - Trypsin may autolyse itself ("trypsin-mediated autolysis") by acting at its own connecting chain.
    - CTRC (chymotrypsin C, aka enzyme Y) degrades the connecting chain calcium
    - Calcium binding pockets ("switch" sites)
      - The local concentration of $Ca^{2+}$ will either modify trypsin by exposing or blocking the separate sites for exposing of the activation site ($\uparrow$ activation), or the autolysis ($\uparrow$ deactivation site).
  - Calcium
    - The local concentration of $Ca^{2+}$ will activate or deactivate trypsin, either by exposing the activation site or the blocking site (autolysis).
    - The intra-acinar (autoreaction) concentration of $Ca^{2+}$ is detected ("sensed") by the G-protein coupled receptor CASR (calcium-sensing receptor).
    - Low $Ca^{2+}$ favours autolysis, and high $Ca^{2+}$ favours autoreaction.
    - Intra acinar cell $Ca^{2+}$ concentrations may increase as a result of numerous factors:
      - $\uparrow$ extracellular $Ca^{2+}$
      - $\uparrow Ca^{2+}$ entry
        - Opening of $Ca^{2+}$
          - Channels
          - Tunnels
          - Bile reflux

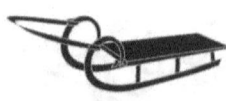

> Types

- Give the types of acute pancreatitis.
  - o Interstitial (edematous) pancreatitis
    - Mild disease on CT/MRI
    - No extrahepatic organ dysfunction
  - o Severe (necrotizing) pancreatitis
    - Atlanta criteria
      - Pseudocyst
    - Organ failure
      - SBP < 90 mmHg
      - Pa $O_2$ ≤ 60 mmHg
      - Serum creatinine > 2 mg/dL
      - GIB > 500 mL/24 hr
    - Local complications (sterile or infected)
      - Abscess (not all guidelines use this term; infected pancreatic necrosis)
      - Peripancreatic necrosis
    - Adverse early prognostic signs
      - Ranson signs (3 or more criteria for non-gallstone pancreatitis)
      - APACHE – II (> 8 points)

Abbreviations: GIB, gastrointestinal bleeding; SBP, systolic blood pressure

> Clinical

- Perform a focused physical examination for acute pancreatitis.

  - o Abdomen
    - – Pigment
      - Centre (periumbilical), Cullen sign
      - 1 or both flanks Grey Turner sign
  - o Lung
    - – Tachypnea
    - – Shallow breathing signs of effusions, atelectasis
  - o CNS
    - – Confusion
    - – Agitation
    - – Hallucinations
    - – Coma
  - o Eyes
    - – Jaundice
    - – Band keratopathy
    - – Lipemia retinalis
    - – Purtsher retinopathy

468

- ○ Salivary glands     – Parotid glands large and tender
- ○ Skin     – Subcutaneous fat necrosis
  - Tender, red nodules
  - Distal extremities
  - Scalp, trunk, buttocks
  - Eruptive xanthomas
  - Thrombophlebitis
- ○ MSK     – Polyarteritis

---

**SO YOU WANT TO BE A GASTROENTEROLOGIST!**

- In the context of acute pancreatitis, give the meaning of Purtsher Retinopathy.

  - ○ In the patient with acute pancreatitis, there may be micro-embolization to the choroidal and retinal arteries.

  - ○ This arterial embolization causes
    - Flame-shaped retinal hemorrhage, with cotton spots
    - Sudden blindness in the affected eye

  - ○ Purtsher retinopathy is the development of sudden blindness in the persons with pancreatitis due to microembolization to the choroidal and retinal arteries, causing hemorrhages and cotton spots.

---

➢ Complications

- Give complications of acute pancreatitis.

  - ○ Local
    - Sterile necrosis
    - Infected necrosis
    - Abscess
    - Pseudocyst
    - Gastrointestinal bleeding

  - ○ Pancreatitis-related:
    - Splenic artery rupture or splenic artery pseudoaneurysm rupture
    - Splenic vein rupture
    - Portal vein rupture
    - Splenic/portal vein thrombosis, leading to gastroesophageal varices with rupture
    - Pseudocyst or abscess hemorrhage
    - Postnecrosectomy bleeding

- o Non-pancreatitis-related:
  - Mallory-Weiss tear
  - Alcoholic gastropathy
  - Stress-related mucosal gastropathy
- o Splenic injury
  - Infarction
  - Rupture
  - Hematoma
- o Fistulization to or obstruction of small or large bowel
- o Right-sided hydronephrosis
- o Systemic (systemic cytokine response, aka "cytokine" storm)
  - CNS
    - Retinopathy
    - Psychosis
  - Heart
    - Shock (circulatory failure)
    - Death
  - Lung
    - Respiratory failure
  - GI
    - Bleeding
    - Pseudocyst
    - Abscess (infected pancreatic necrosis)
  - Endocrine
    - Hyperglycemia
    - Hypoglycemia
    - Hypocalcemia
    - Hypomagnesemia
    - Subcutaneous nodules due to fat necrosis
  - Nutrition
    - Malnutrition
  - Blood
    - Disseminated intravascular coagulation (DIC)
  - Kidney
    - Acute renal failure

Adapted from: Keller J, et al. *Best Practice & Research Clinical Gastroenterology* 2007; 21(3): pg. 524.

470

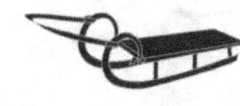

➢ Causes/associations

SO YOU WANT TO BE A GASTROENTEROLOGIST!

A patient with acute pancreatitis develops **upper GI bleeding** (UGIB).

- Give causes of the UGIB which are related to the underlying acute pancreatitis.
  - Portal vein — - Rupture
  - Splenic artery — - Rupture
  - Splenic vein — - Rupture; - Gastric varices +/- esophageal varices
  - Pseudocysts — - Pseudoaneurysms; - Rupture of pseudoaneurysm (mortality rate, 40%); - Bleeding from wall of pseudocyst
  - Surgery, drainage — - Necrotizing pancreatitis; - Walled-off pancreatic necrosis (WOPN); - Pseudocyst

- Give the anatomical basis for the development of gastric varices arising from splenic vein thrombosis.
  - Obstruction of splenic vein → ↑ flow in short gastric veins → coronary vein → development of variceal channels in gastric cardia/fundus.

- Give the factors associated with severe pancreatitis.
  - Patients
    - "4 Os"
    - Older > 55 yr
    - Obese (BMI > 30 kg/m$^2$)
    - Orientation
      - Altered mental status
    - Organs
      - Comorbidities
    - Systemic inflammatory response syndrome (SIRS)
  - Laboratory
    - Hematocrit (Hct) > 44%, and rising
    - Blood urea nitrogen (BUN) > 20 mg/dL, and rising
    - ↑ $Cr_s$ (serum creatinine)

- o Diagnostic imaging
  - – Lungs
    - Infiltrations
    - Effusion(s)
  - – Pancreas
    - Extrapancreatic fluid collection
      - –Large
      - –Many

Adapted from: Sleisenger and Fordtran's Gastrointestinal and Liver Disease. 10th Edition. Saunders/Elsevier, Philadelphia, 2016, Box 58.2, page 971.

Atlanta Classification of Severity of Acute Pancreatitis

| Endpoints | Mild | Moderately Severe | Severe |
|---|---|---|---|
| o Organ failure | - | < 48 hr | > 48 hr |
| o Complications local/systemic | - | + | + |

- o Local complications
  - – Pancreas
    - Necrosis
    - Walled-off necrosis
    - Pseudocyst
  - – Peripancreatic
    - Fluid
    - Necrosis

- Give the **performance characteristics** of predictors of severity of acute pancreatitis.

| | Sensitivity | Specificity | PPV | NPV |
|---|---|---|---|---|
| o Ranson (cut off, 3 signs) | | | | |
| – At 48 hours | 40% to 88% | 43% to 90% | 50% | 90% |
| o Apache-II (< 9, survive; >13, usually die) | | | | |
| – At admission | 34% to 70% | 76% to 98% | | |
| – At 48 hr | < 50% | 90% to 100% | | |
| o SIRS (≥ 2 organs failing on same day) | | | | |
| o Hematocrit > 44%, detecting organ failure) | | | | |
| – At admission | 72% | | | |
| – At 24 hr | 94% | | | 96% |
| o BUN – ↑ MR 2.2x for every ↑ 5 mg/dL in first 24 hr | | | | |
| o C-reactive protein | 60% to 100% | 75% to 100% | | |
| o Fluid on peritoneal lavage | 36% to 72% | 80% to 100% | | |
| o Procalcitonin | 86% | 95% | | |

472

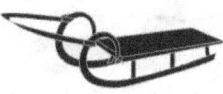

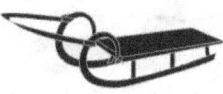

Abbreviations: NPV, negative predictive value; PPV, positive predictive value; SIRS, systemic inflammatory response system

Note: it is the NPV of Ranson criteria and hematocrit which are most helpful clinically, in terms of predicting who will not have severe acute pancreatitis

---

MCQ Alert

- o In a patient with acute pancreatitis, suspect severe pancreatitis (necrosis), if the stem provides
    - – History / signs
        - ▪ Mention of cytokines / leukotrienes
        - ▪ Fever, hypotension, tachycardia, dyspnea, oliguria
        - ▪ Abdominal guarding, rebound tenderness, ileus
        - ▪ Hemorrhage
        - ▪ Persisting /non-responsive pain
        - ▪ Organ failure
    - – Abnormal blood tests
    - – Abnormal CT scan (e.g., hematocrit or WBC, but not the level of the elevation of an
    - – Non-enhancing areas of large portions (> 50%) of pancreas

- o The patient has experienced repeated episodes of severe abdominal pain radiating to the back, in associating with high levels of alcohol ingestion. On the occasion she/ he had similar pain and alcohol abuse, and the serum amylase or lipase is normal. You are offered several plausible MCQ choices, as well as acute pancreatitis. Chronic pancreatitis is the answer
    - – Caution: normal serum amylase or lipase do not R/O chronic pancreatitis.

- o In the patient with acute pancreatitis, suspect biliary tract gallstones if
    - – Bilirubin > 4 mg/dL
    - – ALT, AST > 1000 U/mL

- o If the patient with acute pancreatitis has also been drinking alcohol recently, the ALT, AST may be > 1000 U/mL, and the bilirubin may be increased (true, often > 15 mg/dL). But, alcoholics have an ↑ risk of having gallstones, so beware of gallstone pancreatitis in the alcoholic.

---

473

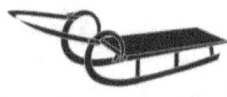

- Give the specific predictions made from **scoring systems** of acute pancreatitis.

| System | Prediction | |
|---|---|---|
| ❖ Scoring system | | |
|   o Ranson score | – Pancreatic necrosis<br>– Infected necrosis<br>– Systemic complications<br>– Death | ▪ Late (48 hr) identification<br>▪ Low sensitivity and specificity<br>▪ Best use is to exclude severe disease |
|   o Apache-II score | – Severity<br>– Death | ▪ Best use to exclude severe disease |
|   o Multisystem organ failure (MOF) | | |
|   o CT grading scores | – Local complications (pseudocyst, abscess) | |
|   o BISAP | – Complications<br>– Death | ▪ Early identification |
| ❖ Blood unit tests | | |
|   o BUN | – Pancreatic necrosis<br>– Organ failure | |
|   o C-reactive protein | – Severity of pancreatitis | |
|   o Peritoneal lavage | – Death | |
|   o Procalcitonin | – Organ failure<br>– Urinary trypsinogen activation peptide severity | |

Abbreviation: BISAP, Bedside Index for Severity of Acute Pancreatitis; BUN, blood urea nitrogen

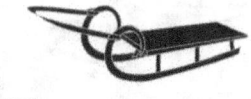

- Give the components which comprise the **Marshall scoring system** for the diagnosis of Multisystem Organ Failure (MOF).
  - – 2 or more falling on same day
  - – Mortality rate ~ 50%
  - o Heart
    - – Myocardial infarction
    - – Dysrhythmias
    - – Pericardial effusions
  - o Lung
    - – Pleural effusion
    - – Pneumonia
    - – Atelectasis
    - – Elevated diaphragm
    - – ARDS
  - o Kidney
    - – Hypovolemia
    - – Hypotension
    - – Acute tubular necrosis
    - – Shock
  - o CT Grading System (Balthazar) and CT Severity Index
    - – Extent of fluid collection and necrosis

- ➤ Laboratory
  - o Pancreatitis-associated protein (PAP) and Pancreatic-specific protein (PSP)
    - – Same accuracy as serum amylase for diagnosing acute pancreatitis
  - o The most laboratory tests used to predict the severity of acute pancreatitis are surrogate markers of local inflammation.
  - o Urinary TAP (trypsinogen activation peptide) is a marker for
    - – Pancreatic necrosis
    - – Systemic inflammatory response (sepsis)
  - o The extent of elevation of serum amylase or lipase do not correlate with the severity of pancreatitis.
  - o Elevated serum amylase or lipase concentrations are only ~85% sensitive, and their specificity, especially for values of < 3x ULN, is only ~50%.
  - o Recurrent attacks of acute pancreatitis may be caused by alcohol abuse or by gallstones. In the patient with both alcohol use and known gallstones, the finding of an ↑ ALT (> 3x ULN) is often used clinically as a reliable indicator of biliary pancreatitis.

475

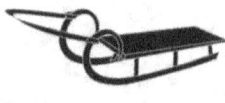

- Give causes of an elevated serum amylase/lipase.
  - Salivary glands
    - Salivary gland disease, e.g., mumps
  - Stomach
    - Peptic ulcer disease with penetration
  - Small bowel
    - Intestinal ischemia
    - Small bowel obstruction
    - Bowel perforation
    - Celiac disease
  - Pancreas
    - Pancreatitis
    - Pancreatic cancer
  - Colon, appendix
    - Appendicitis
  - Biliary tree
    - Cholecystitis

- Give the reason why serial serum ionized $Ca^{2+}$ must be measured in the patient with acute pancreatitis.
  - Hypocalcemia may occur in acute pancreatitis.
  - Correct any associated hypomagnesemia
  - Cautious use of IV calcium gluconate to prevent dysrhythmia (IV $Ca^{2+}$ increases binding of $Ca^{2+}$ to myocardial receptors; ↑ $Ca^{2+}$ on myocardial receptors displaces $K^+$ from the myocardial receptors, leading to dysrhythmia)

Please see Sleisenger and Fordtran's Gastrointestinal and Liver Disease. 9th Edition. Saunders/Elsevier 2010, Table 58.8, for Table of Complications of Acute Pancreatitis

- Give causes of falsely negative serum amylase in acute pancreatitis.
  - Blood sampled too late after onset of symptoms (T1/2, 10 hrs)
  - Not correlated with severity of pancreatitis (may be normal with fatal disease, or with mild disease)
  - Acute on chronic pancreatitis
  - Hypertriglyceridemia-associated pancreatitis (↑ triglyceride in serum may produce an inhibitor of amylase, resulting in falsely low serum amylase concentrations)

476

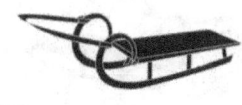

- Give causes of **falsely** positive serum amylase.
  - Macroamylasemia (amylase binds to immunoglobulin in serum, and is not filtered/excreted by kidney)
  - Disease of
    - Salivary glands
    - Fallopian tubes
    - Ovary
      - Cyst
      - Cystadenoma
  - Kidney
    - Renal failure - ↓ clearance of amylase
    - Hemodialysis (> peritoneal dialysis)
  - Psychiatric disorders
    - Munchausen syndrome

---

### SO YOU WANT TO BE A GASTROENTEROLOGIST!

- In the context of an elevated serum amylase, give the rational for measuring **UACR** (a urinary amylase-to-creatinine ratio), and **urinary salivary amylase**.

  - ↓ UACR — In macroamylasemia, where amylase is bound to immunoglobulin and persists in the blood because of lack of renal excretion, the UACR may be low
    - UACR may also be low with renal insufficiency
    - UACR may be high when contaminated with salivary amylase

  - ↑ urinary salivary amylase — Saliva contains amylase, and if the patient spits into the urine collection, the total amylase level will be increased, and the UACR will also rise.
    - Persons with Munchausen Syndrome may spit into urine sample, so that the urine total amylase and UACR are increased.

- Give the advantage of measuring serum lipase rather than amylase to diagnose acute pancreatitis.

  - Serum lipase concentrations are not elevated in disorders of salivary glands, fallopian tubes or ovary with Munchausen syndrome or macroamylasemia.

  - Measurement of the serum lipase concentration has greater sensitivity, and especially better specificity.

---

477

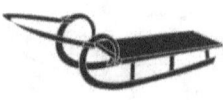

➢   Diagnostic imaging

The **abdominal plain film** (APF) is useful to support the diagnosis of acute pancreatitis.

- Give findings on the APF (abdominal plain film) which suggest acute pancreatitis, and distinguish between the "sentinel loop" and the "colon cut-off" signs.

    - Stomach          – Anterior displacement
                       – Separation of the contours of the stomach and transverse colon

    - Duodenum         – Descending portion displaced and stretched by head of enlarged pancreas

    - Jejunum/Ileum    – "sentinel loop" (localized dilated segment of small bowel)
                       – Ileus

    - Colon            – "colon cut-off" sign
                           ▪ Spasm of colon with
                               – Proximal dilation
                               – Distal lack of gas
                       – Irregular haustral pattern

    - Gallbladder      – Calcified stones

    - Pancreas         – Stones
                       – Calcification
                       – Ascites
                       – Retroperitoneal air (abscess)
                           ▪ Gas-forming organism
                           ▪ Microperforation of gut
                           ▪ Adjacent pseudocyst

    - **Abdominal ultrasound** may be hypoechoic in acute pancreatitis, but its usefulness may be limited by

        – Overlying bowel gas (in ~ 1/3),

        – ↓ sensitivity to detect CBD stones

        – The challenge to differentiate hypoechoic areas from acute versus chronic pancreatitis, a malignancy

        – Not sensitive to detect cholelithiasis/choledochalithiasis in acute pancreatitis; use MRI or EUS

    - Sensitivity of detecting CBD stones EUS = ERCP = MRCP > US or CT

    - In the patient with suspected necrotizing pancreatitis, EUS is superior to ERCP because of the lack of risk of introducing infection.

478

- Give the way to distinguish on diagnostic imaging the possibilities of alcoholic pancreatitis versus biliary tract stones.
  - Abdominal ultrasound
    - Not sensitive for bile duct (BD) stones
    - May show indirect evidence of
      - Stones
        - Dilated BD or cystic duct
      - Cholecystitis
        - Gallbladder wall > 4 mm
        - ↑ pericholecystic fluid

- Treatment
  - Risk stratification for necrotizing pancreatitis
  - Pain control
  - Evaluate for cause
    - Alcohol
    - Gallstones
    - Drugs
    - ↑ TG (> 1000 mg/dL)
    - ↑ $Ca^{2+}$
    - Post ERCP
  - IV fluids, approximately 250 cc/hr (3 cc/kg per hr) for 24 hr, then reassess for rate/volume depending upon clinical status.
  - NG/NJ tube feeding (no difference in outcome, NG = NJ feeding)
  - Antibiotics
    - Only if infected necrosis suspected (usually after day 10)
    - Do not give prophylactically since only 1/3 of patients with necrosis develop infected necrosis
  - Early ERCP for
    - Gallstone pancreatitis (ALT 3XULN, PPV- 95%; ↑bilirubin on day
    - Sphincterotomy and stone extraction
  - CT-guided FNA for culture
  - Debridement (necrosectomy)
    - By surgery, endoscopy, radiology
  - Treatment complications

Abbreviation: EUS, endoscopic ultrasound; FNA, fine needle aspiration; NG/NJ, nasogastric/nasojejunal; ULN, upper limit of normal; US, ultrasound

Adapted from: Forsmark CE and Baillie J. *Gastroenterology* 2007;132(5):2022-44.

479

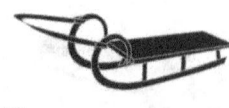

# TYPES OF ACUTE PANCREATITIS

## Alcoholic Pancreatitis

➤ Pathology

- ○ "About 60% of ......persons who present with their first attack of acute alcoholic pancreatitis have already developed histologic chronic pancreatitis" (Feldman M., et al. Sleisenger and Fordtran's Gastrointestinal and Liver Disease. 9th Edition. *Saunders/Elsevier*, Philadelphia, 2010, page 989).

- ○ In persons with acute alcoholic pancreatitis who have not yet developed obvious chronic pancreatitis, stopping alcohol.
  - – ↓ rate of progression to chronic pancreatic insufficiency
  - – Does not alter the frequency of recurrent attacks of acute pancreatitis

➤ Pathophysiology

- Give the pathophysiology of acute pancreatitis due to alcohol abuse.

  - ○ Direct effect of alcohol and its "toxic" metabolites on pancreatic acinar cells.

  - ○ ↑ lithogenicity of pancreatic fluid (alcohol-related ↑ secretion and viscosity of pancreatic juice → precipitation of protein (such as GP-2) → formation of pancreatic stones (crystals of calcium carbonate, polysaccharides, fibrillar proteins, and a gel-like matrix)

  - ○ Acute and sometimes subclinical pancreatitis → scaring of preductular area → stasis of ductules → progression to fibrosis

  - ○ Acute pancreatitis activates trypsin → ↑ inflammation → ↑ cytokines → activates pancreatic stellate cells → fibrosis

- Give the pathophysiology of alcoholic pancreatitis.

  - ○ Direct injury by alcohol or a metabolite
    - – Liver
      - ▪ Acetaldehyde
    - – Pancreas
      - ▪ FAEs (fatty acid esters) → ↑ $Ca_i^{2+}$

  - ○ Oxidative stress
    - – Production of free radicals
    - – ↑ peroxidation of membrane lipids

480

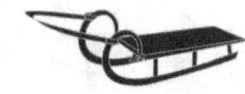

- CCK
  - Alcohol-associated ↑ sensitivity of acinar cells to CCK
  - Redirection of CCK-mediation zymogen granule exocytosis from apical to basolateral membrane of acinar cell.

- Genes/enzymes
  - Alcohol-associated
    - Altered expression of genes responsive to physiologic stress
  - Over
    - ↑ expression/activity of necrosis/apoptosis

- Stellate cells
  - ↑ activity of pancreatic acinar cells associated stellate (myofibroblastic) cells
    - ↑ extracellular matrix → ↑ fibrosis → ischemia
    - ↑ proliferation
    - Phagocytosis
  - Alcohol / alcohol metabolites
  - Cytokines (from necrosis of cells)
  - Growth factors (PDGF, TGF-B1)
  - Transcription factors
  - Angiotensin II
  - Autocrine factors

- Protein precipitation (plugs)
  - Alcohol stimulates pancreatic secretion of fluid with ↑ protein, ↓ volume and $HCO_3^-$

- Gain of function gene mutation, leading to SAPE
  - CFTR (cystic fibrosis transmembrane conductance regulator gene)
  - PRSS1 (cationic trypsinogen gene)
  - SPINK1 (a trypsin inhibitor)
  - These genetic mutations are hypothesized to lead to repeated episodes of acute pancreatitis, which set in motion a process that leads to chronic pancreatitis (SAPE, sentinel acute pancreatitis event)

Abbreviations: $Ca_i^{2+}$, intracellular $Ca^{2+}$; CCK, cholecystokinin; PDGF, platelet-derived growth factor; SAPE, sentinel acute pancreatic event; TGF, transforming growth factor

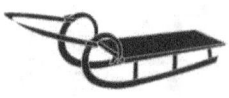

## Infuence of Obesity on Acute Pancreatitis

## ERCP-Associated Acute Pancreatitis

- ➤ Definition
  - Pain + > 3x ↑ amylase within 24 hours requiring admission > 48 hrs
  - Use prophylactic stents in high risk patients

- ➤ Causes/associations
- Give risk factors associated with the development of post-ERCP pancreatitis.
  - Operator related
    - Lower ERCP volume
  - Patient related
    - Younger age
    - Female sex (possibly)
    - Suspected sphincter of Oddi dysfunction (SOD)
    - Normal bilirubin
    - History of pancreatitis, recurrent of post-ERCP pancreatitis

482

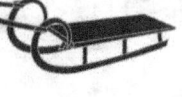

- o Procedure-related factors
  - – Prior episode of post-ERCP pancreatitis
  - – Trainee participation in procedure
  - – Difficult or multiple cannulation attempts
  - – Multiple pancreatic contrast injections
  - – Pancreatic acinerization
  - – Precut sphincterotomy
  - – Endoscopic papillary balloon dilation
  - – Sphincter of Oddi manometry
  - – Distal common bile duct diameter ≤ 10 mm
  - – Procedures not involving stone removal
  - – Recent biliary sphincterotomy
  - – Ampullectomy
  - – Sphincter of Oddi dysfunction

Abbreviation: CCK, cholecystokinin; ERCP, endoscopic retrograde cholangiopancreatography

Printed with permission: Blero D, et al. Nat Rev Gastroenterol Hepatol. 2012;9(3):162-72; and adapted from: Elta GH. *Gastrointest Endosc* 2008;67(2):262-64.; and Freeman ML, et al. *Gastrointest Endosc* 2001;54(4):425-434.

## Pancreatic Necrosis

➢ Definition

- o "Necrotizing pancreatitis is defined, in the absence of laparotomy or autopsy, by the presence of greater than 30% of non-enhancement of the pancreas on a contrast-enhanced CT scan", or MRI (Feldman M., et al. Sleisenger and Fordtran's Gastrointestinal and Liver Disease. 9th Edition. *Saunders/Elsevier* 2010, page 981).

➢ Clinical

- o Persons with pancreatic necrosis resulting from an episode of acute pancreatitis may progress to developing chronic pancreatitis associated with exocrine (exo) or endocrine (endo) insufficiency.
  - – Overtime, WOPN (walled-off pancreatic necrosis) develops, and if symptomatic may be safely drained with
    - ▪ Short stature
    - ▪ Surgery
    - ▪ Percutaneous drainage
    - ▪ Endoscopic drainage

483

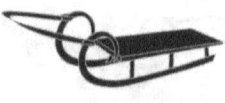

## SO YOU WANT TO BE A GASTROENTEROLOGIST!

- Give the pathophysiology of the multiple failure organ failure in necrotizing pancreatitis.

  - Heart
    - SIRS (systemic inflammatory response syndrome)
      - Activation of
        - Trypsin
        - Phospholipase
        - Elastase
      - Release into portal circulation of TNF, PAS
        - Activation of hepatic Kupffer cells
        - ↑ CRP (C-reactive protein)
        - ↑ IL-6

  - Lung
    - ARDS (acute respiratory distress syndrome)
      - Breakdown of surface from
        - ↑ activity of phospholipase A

  - Kidney
    - ↓ SBP (hypotension) ↓ blood volume (hypovolemia)

  - GI tract
    - Microcirculatory changes e.g., vasoconstriction → ischemia, AV shunting in gut

- In the context of the patient with chronic pancreatitis and upper GI bleeding, give what is "hemosuccus pancreaticus".

  - Hemosuccus pancreaticus is bleeding from the wall of the pseudocyst into the pancreatic duct.

> Investigation
  - CT-FNA helps to establish if necrosis is infected

> Pathology
  - Necrosis of pancreatic tissue, often with associated peripancreatic fat necrosis, and accompanied by disruptions in pancreatic ducts.
  - Necrotizing pancreatitis may be infected (1/3) or non-infected (2/3)

484

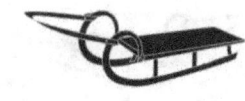

- Walled-off pancreatic necrosis (WOPN)
  - Several weeks after pancreatic necrosis and duct disruption, the cystic area contains liquid as well as solid material (non-enhancing pancreatic parenchyma on contrast-enhanced CT scan).
- Pancreatic abscess
  - ".....infected pseudocyst or infected liquefied collections without significant solid debris (pancreatic necrosis" (Sleisenger and Fordtran's Gastrointestinal and Liver Disease. 9th Edition. *Saunders/Elsevier*, Philadelphia, 2010, page 1038).
  - Strictly speaking, a pancreatic pseudocyst is not a cyst, because although there may be cystic spaces filled with pancreatic secretion fluid from a duct which has been disrupted by obstruction or inflammation, the cystic space does not have an epithelial lining, and so is actually not a true cyst.
  - Cytology of fluid in pseudocysts may show histocytes.
  - ERCP/MRCP – shows communication with pancreatic duct

➢ Treatment
- Avoid using routine prophylactic antibiotics in necrotizing pancreatitis (i.e., to attempt to prevent non-infected necrosis from becoming infected).
- For infected necrosis or abscess
  - Use IV antibiotics which act against gram-negative aerobic or anaerobic species, and which penetrate the pancreas (e.g., imipenem, fluoroquinolones, metronidazole)
  - These antibiotics the mortality from infected pancreatic necrosis
- Avoid early debridement (necrosectomy)
  - Mortality rate 15% to 73%
  - Wait 4 weeks before considering surgical drainage

| Development of Insufficiency | No Necrosectomy | Necrosectomy |
| --- | --- | --- |
| Endocrine | 26% | 75% |
| Exocrine | 13% | 58% |

- Up to two-thirds of patients having a surgical resection for pain from chronic pancreatitis develop steatorrhea.

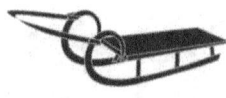

# Gallstone Pancreatitis

- ➤ Definition
    - o "...... an outcome following ERCP and sphincterotomy in gallstone pancreatitis [which] results from reduced biliary sepsis rather than impairment in pancreatitis".

- ➤ Clinical
    - o Abdominal pain, ↑ serum lipase, ↑ ALT > 150 IU/L (2-3x > ULN): PPV (positive predictive value) 0.95 (95% likelihood of gallstone pancreatitis)

- ➤ Laboratory
    - o Serum lipase: amylase > 2.0 suggests alcoholic pancreatitis, not gallstone pancreatitis (sensitivity, 91%; specificity 76%).
    - o An almost normal AP and/or total bilirubin do occur with obstruction of the CBD (common bile duct).

- • Give a comment on the use of an elevated serum ALT as a test to support the **diagnosis of gallstone pancreatitis** by giving its performance characteristics.
    - o An elevated (> 3x ULN) is often serum ALT to differentiate biliary pancreatitis from alcoholic pancreatitis, has a specificity of 96%, but a sensitivity of only 48%, yielding a positive predictive value of 95%.
    - o Thus, a normal ALT does not exclude gallstone pancreatitis, but an ↑ ALT does suggest gallstone pancreatitis.

- ➤ Diagnostic imaging
    - o In this setting of ↑ suspicion of gallstone pancreatitis, don't be side-tracked if abdominal ultrasound is normal (pancreatitis → ileus → bowel air may obscure pancreas).

- ➤ Treatment
    - o It is these patients with acute cholangitis who are helped by ERCP plus sphincterotomy in mild-to-moderate gallstone pancreatitis.
    - o The ERCP and sphincterotomy must be done within 28 hours.

- ➤ Prevention
    - o "ERCP in patients with severe gallstone acute pancreatitis is best reserved for patients with suspected biliary obstruction....." (Feldman M., et al. Sleisenger and Fordtran's Gastrointestinal and Liver Disease. 9th Edition. *Saunders/Elsevier*, Philadelphia, 2010, page 1035).

486

# Drug-Associated Pancreatitis

➢ Classification

- Give a classification of drugs associated with induction of acute pancreatitis.

  - Class I: implicated in > 20 reports, at least one documented case following re-exposure
    - Asparaginase
    - Azathioprine
    - Cytarabine
    - Didanosine
    - Estrogen preparations
    - Furosemide
    - Mercaptopurine
    - Mesalamine
    - Opiates
    - Pentamidine
    - Pentavalent antimonials
    - Steroids
    - Sulfasalazine
    - Sulindac
    - Tetracycline
    - Trimethoprim/sulfamethoxazole
    - Valproic acid

  - Class II: implicated in > 10 reports
    - Acetaminophen
    - Carbamazepine
    - Cisplatin
    - Cyclopenthiazide
    - Enalapril
    - Erythromycin
    - Hydrochlorothiazide
    - Interferon Alfa-2b
    - Lamivudine
    - Octreotide
    - Phenformin
    - Rifampicin

Note that the list represents only a sample of drugs which have been reported to be associated with hyperamylasemia +/- clinical pancreatitis

Printed with permission: Keller J, et al. *Best Pract Res Clin Gastroenterol* 2007;21(3):519-33.

487

## Acute Recurrent Pancreatitis

- ➤ Less common causes of acute pancreatitis
  - ○ Pancreas divisum
    - – Symptoms may develop in those with acute recurrent pancreatitis arising from relative destructions to the flow of pancreatic juice through the minor papilla.
    - – The presence of pancreas divisum is associated with a high risk of post-ERCP pancreatitis
  - ○ Sphincter of Oddi dysfunction (SOD)
    - – Postulated to be the cause of acute recurrent pancreatitis when the basal presence in the pancreatic sphincter is > 40 mmHg
  - ○ IBD and drugs
    - – The ↑ rate of acute pancreatitis in persons with inflammatory bowel disease (IBD, risk is ↑ 4x in Crohn disease and 1.5x in Ulcerative Colitis) may be due to drugs used to treat the conditions, such as 5-ASA/ sulfasalazine or azathioprine / 6-mercaptopurine.
  - ○ Celiac disease
  - ○ Severe burns
  - ○ Smoking (possibly making the effects of alcohol worse)
  - ○ AIP (autoimmune pancreatitis)
    - – ↑ IgG4
    - – May be associated with
      - ▪ Acute pancreatitis
      - ▪ Chronic pancreatic insufficiency
      - ▪ Stricture of main pancreatic ducts
      - ▪ Diabetes

"There is never a better measure of what a person is than what he does when he's absolutely free to choose."

William M Bulger

488

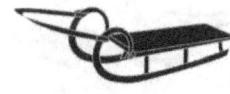

## CHRONIC PANCREATITIS

➢ Definition

    o There are numerous definitions of chronic pancreatitis
- Pancreatitis is a spectrum
- Acute pancreatitis is an identifiable event, whereas
- Chronic pancreatitis is an ongoing process of

    o There may be typical symptoms and changes on diagnostic imaging, as well as the above changes in histology.

➢ Demography

    o The incidence of chronic pancreatitis is approximately $8/10^5$ per year, and the prevalence is $27/10^5$.

    o 10 year survival rate is 70%

    o The standardized mortality ratio (SMR) is 3.6:1, with higher mortality rates associated with
- Advanced age
- Alcohol etiology
- Continued alcohol use (↑ SMR by 60%)
- Smoking (especially in alcoholics)

➢ Causes/associations

• Give causes of chronic pancreatitis.

❖ Hereditary

    o CT (cationic trypsinogen) gene

    o Autosomal dominant
- Hereditary pancreatitis (PRSS1 mutations)

    o Autosomal recessive or modifier genes
- CFTR mutations
- SPINK1 mutations
- IgG4 associated

    o PSTI (pancreatic secretory trypsin inhibitor) aka **SPINK₁** (serine protease inhibitor, Kazal type 1)

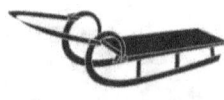

489

- o SPINK$_1$
  - – Colocalized in zymogen granules in the pancreatic acinar cells.
  - – Secreted with trypsinogen.
  - – Presents the premature activation of trypsinogen in the pancreatic acinar cells.
  - – Mutations, or polygenic mutation of CFTR- SPINK$_1$ are associated with familial pancreatitis.

Useful additional material : Feldman M., et al. Sleisenger and Fordtran's Gastrointestinal and Liver Disease. 9th Edition. Saunders/Elsevier, Philadelphia, 2010, Table 57-4 (Clinical manifestation of cystic fibrosis) and Table 57-5 (Frequency of gastrointestinal manifestations in cystic fibrosis), page 941).

- o SPINK$_1$ N34S is the most common SPINK$_1$ mutation
- o SPINK$_1$ mutations lead to less trypsin inhibition.
- o These loss-of-function polymorphisms are important
  - – When acute pancreatitis occurs.
  - – When there is recurrent premature activation of trypsin (e.g., CFTR or PRSS, mutation).
- o An acute phase reactant
  - – ↑ SPINK$_1$ with inflammation of pancreas
- o "SPINK$_1$ acts as the first line defense against prematurely activated trypsinogen" (Feldman M., et al. Sleisenger and Fordtran's Gastrointestinal and Liver Disease. 9th Edition. Saunders/Elsevier, Philadelphia, 2010, page 937).
- o SPINK$_1$ mutations such as with CFTR or PRSS$_1$ increase the risk of fibrosis.

- ❖ Acquired
  - o Benign pancreatic duct obstruction
    - – Traumatic stricture
    - – Stricture after severe acute pancreatitis
    - – Duodenal wall cyst
    - – Pancreas divisum
  - o Malignant pancreatic duct stricture
    - – Ampullary or duodenal carcinoma
    - – Pancreatic adenocarcinoma
    - – Intraductal papillary mucinous neoplasm

490

- o Autoimmune
  - Associated with autoimmune diseases (e.g., Sjögren's syndrome, primary biliary cholangitis, primary sclerosing cholangitis)
- o Tropical
  - Tropical calcific pancreatitis
  - Fibrocalculous pancreatic diabetes
- o Metabolic
  - Diabetes
  - Alcohol
  - Hypercalcemia
  - Hyperlipidemia
  - Hypertriglyceridemia
  - Lipoprotein lipase deficiency
  - Apolipoprotein C-II deficiency
- o Postnecrotic chronic pancreatitis
- o Idiopathic
  - Early-onset
  - Late-onset
- o Asymptomatic pancreatic fibrosis
  - Chronic alcoholism
  - Old age
  - Chronic renal failure
  - Radiotherapy

Adapted from: Chari ST. *Mayo Clinic Gastroenterology and Hepatology Board Review:* pg 470; and 2010: pg. 988; and Keller J, and Layer P. *Best Practice & Research Clinical Gastroenterology* 2008; 22(1): pg. 106.

There are numerous gene mutations in $PRSS_1$.

- • Give the mutations which are $Ca^{2+}$-dependent or $Ca^{2+}$-independent mutations in PRSS1.
- ❖ $Ca^{2+}$ dependent
  - o The main genetic mutations in $PRSS_1$ are $R_{122}H$ and $N_{29}I$ mutations.
  - o $PRSS_1$ gene mutation is associated with hereditary pancreatitis.
  - o The $R_{122}H$ is a "conversion mutation" which alters the high fidelity regulatory mechanism of $PRSS_1$.
  - o The switch on/off represents a process to enhance trypsin activity ("gain-of-function").

491

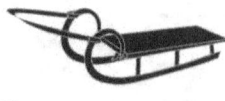

- o The $R_{122}H$ and $N_{29}I$ mutations of $PRSS_1$ result in
  - – ↑ activation, or
  - – ↓ inactivation

❖ $Ca^{2+}$-independent-mutation
  - o Process related to maintenance of intracellular pH.

➢ Clinical

Abdominal pain is common in persons with pancreatitis. It is now questioned whether the pain is due to increased pressure in the duct or parenchyma of the pancreas, resulting in tissue ischemia.

- • Give evidence for alternate theories relating to neuroimmune interaction, for the **pain** of chronic pancreatitis.
  - o Nerves
    - – ↑ number and diameter of nerves in the pancreas
    - – ↑ inflammation around these nerves and ganglia
    - – Axons release pain mediators, such as
      - ▪ Substance P
      - ▪ CERP
      - ▪ Glutamate
  - o GAP-43 (growth-associated protein 43)
    - – ↑ NGF (nerve growth factor) and TrkA (NGF receptor)
    - – ↑ endogenous proteases
  - o CCK
    - – ↑ sensitivity of pancreas to stimulation by CCK
    - – ↑ duct pressure
    - – Redirecting pancreas enzymes to basolateral rather than apical portion of acinar cells

➢ Complications

- • Give the factors responsible for the development of **diabetes mellitus** in chronic pancreatitis.

| | |
|---|---|
| o Loss of Islet cells | – From chronic pancreatitis disease-associated destructive process |
| | – From resection of pancreas |
| | – ↑ amylase → ↑ insulin resistance |
| o Hepatic insulin receptors | – ↓ number |
| | – ↓ function |

492

- Give the median times for the development of complications of chronic pancreatitis.

| Complication | Etiology of pancreatic disease | Approximate median time (yr) to onset of complication |
|---|---|---|
| o Pancreatic insufficiency | o Alcohol | 13 |
| | o Idiopathic | |
| |    – Early onset | 26 |
| |    – Late onset | 17 |
| o Diabetes | o Alcohol | 20 |
| | o Idiopathic | |
| |    – Early onset | 26 |
| |    – Late onset | 12 |

➢ Laboratory

Diagnostic tests of chronic pancreatitis

- o There is no "gold standard" for diagnostic form (structure) and function.

- o The tests are for altered pancreatic form (structure) and function.

- o The performance characteristics improve as the disease becomes more severe; why is this?

Because "...... 30% to 50% damage to the [pancreatic] gland is necessary before direct pancreatic function tests yield reliable results (Sleisenger and Fordtran's Gastrointestinal and Liver Disease. 10th Edition. *Saunders/Elsevier*, Philadelphia, 2016, page 1009).

- o It is in the persons with mild-to-moderate disease that you wish to be able to make an early diagnosis.

- Give the effect of disease severity on the performance characteristics of the combined **secretin-CCK test** for chronic pancreatitis.

| | Sensitivity | Specificity |
|---|---|---|
| Overall | 67% | 90% |
| Moderate-severe | 79% | |

- o Pancreatic function testing may be abnormal even in the absence of structural changes.

- o However, persons with abnormal pancreatic structure as shown on ERCP may have hormonal stimulation test results.

493

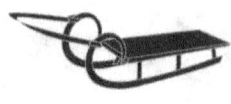

- Give tests of exocrine pancreatic functions.
  - o Direct invasive intubation tests
    - - CCK/secretin stimulation
    - - Lundh meal
    - - ERCP and pancreatic aspiration
  - o Indirect non-invasive tests
    - - Stool fats and nitrogen
    - - Stool trypsin, chymotrypsin, and elastase
    - - Breath tests
    - - Oral function tests (bentiromide test and pancreolauryl test)
  - o Blood determinations
    - - Trypsinogen
    - - Lipase
    - - Pancreatic amylase

Adapted from: Sleisenger and Fordtran's Gastrointestinal and Liver Disease. 10th Edition. Saunders/Elsevier, Philadelphia, 2016, Table 59.3, page 1010.

- For laboratory tests to detect and to differentiate big vs small duct disease in chronic pancreatitis.

| Test | Possible Findings in 'Big Duct' Disease | Findings in 'Small Duct' Disease |
|---|---|---|
| o Fecal elastase | – Usually low (<100/g of stool) | – Usually normal |
| o Serum trypsin | – Usually low (< 20 ng/mL) | – Usually normal |

➤ Diagnostic imaging
  - o Accuracy of detection on abdominal ultrasound: gallstones, > 90%; dilated CBD, 55-91%; CBD stones, 20-75%
  - o Contract enhanced CT useful to grade pancreatitis, and to detect necrosis as well as neoplasm; equivalent to gadolinium-enhanced dynamic MRCP (but contrast-enhanced MRCP is superior to contrast enhanced CT to detect CBD stones) (Arvanitakis M, et al. *Gastroenterology* 2005:715-23.
  - o **Microlithiasis** occurs in 37-89% of persons with idiopathic acute pancreatitis, and some experts recommend cholecystectomy for associated symptoms

494

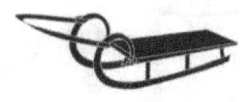

- Definitions
  - Microlithiasis, stones < 3 mm
  - Biliary sludge, a suspension of crystals, mucin, glycoproteins, cellular debris, and protein across material
  - Biliary crystals, crystals of calcium bilirubinate, calcium carbonate, or cholesterol monohydrate; the use of duodenal drainage to assess the presence of biliary crystals has a sensitivity of 65%, and a specificity of 94-100%
  - The risk of pancreatitis following ERCP is high in persons with IAP (ideopathic acute pancreatitis), sphincter of Oddi dysfunction (SOD), or a post history of pancreatitis (12.5% risk)

In situations where the results of pancreatic structure vary from the functional tests, it is suggested that ".....hormonal stimulation testing appears to be somewhat more sensitive and specific than ERCP" (Feldman M., et al. Sleisenger and Fordtran's Gastrointestinal and Liver Disease. 9th Edition. *Saunders/Elsevier*, Philadelphia, 2010, page 999).

- Give the performance characteristics for **diagnostic imaging** tests chronic pancreatitis.

| Diagnostic Imaging Test | Sensitivity | Specificity |
|---|---|---|
| o   Abdominal ultrasound | 50% to 80% | 80% to 90% |
| o   CT | 75% to 90% | > 85% |
| o   Multidetector CT | > 80% | ~100% |
| o   ERCP | 70% to 90% | 80% to 100% |
| o   EUS | | |
| > 3 diagnostic criteria | 83% | 57% |
| Advanced disease | 73% | 81% |
| > 4 criteria | 90% | 86% |

  - MRCP agrees with ERCP in about 90% of patients, with lower values for changes that are
    - Subtle
    - In pancreatic tail
    - Side branches of pancreatic duct

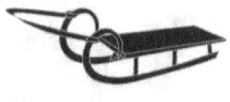

A caution about EUS:

- o   Certain patient- and disease-related factors can mimic the EUS changes of pancreatitis, and lead to a false diagnosis.

| Patient-related | Disease-related |
|---|---|
| o   Age | o   Diabetes mellitus |
| o   Tobacco | o   Chronic renal disease |
| o   Alcohol | |

- For laboratory and/or diagnostic imaging tests to detect and to differentiate big versus small duct disease in chronic pancreatitis.

| Diagnostic Test | Possible Findings in 'Big Duct' Disease | Findings in 'Small Duct' Disease |
|---|---|---|
| o   Abdominal ultrasonography | – Pancreatic atrophy<br>– Pancreatic duct dilation<br>– Pancreatic calcifications<br>– Pseudocyst | – Usually normal |
| o   Computerized tomography | – Pancreatic atrophy<br>– Pancreatic duct dilation<br>– Pancreatic calcifications<br>– Pseudocyst | – Usually normal or equivocal |
| o   MRCP | – Pancreatic atrophy<br>– Pancreatic duct dilation<br>– Irregularity or stricture<br>– Pancreatic calcifications<br>– Pseudocyst | – Usually normal or equivocal |
| o   Endoscopic ultrasonography | – Abnormal (> 4 features of chronic pancreatitis | – May be abnormal |
| o   ERCP | – Abnormal | – Normal of minimally abnormal |
| o   Direct hormonal stimulations test (e.g., secretin test) | – Abnormal | – Usually abnormal |

Abbreviations: MRI, magnetic resonance imaging, MRCP, magnetic resonance cholangiopancreatography.

Source: Lieb JG II, and Forsmark CE. *Journal Compilation* 2009;29:713.

496

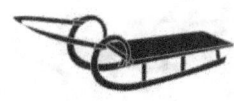

Ampulla of Vater

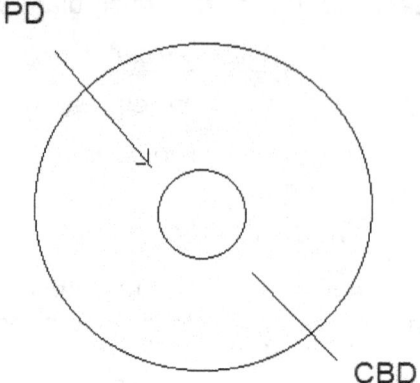

CBD, common bile duct; PD, pancreatic duct
Scope 11 mm: CBD size −compare to scope

- o Diameter of CBD
    - – Age
        - ▪ < 50    6 mm
        - ▪ > 50    ↑ mm / 10 yrs
    - – After cholecystectomy – 11 mm

- ➢ Pathology
    - o Acute inflammation
        - – Lymphocytes
        - – Plasma
        - – Metaplasia
    - o Chronic self-sustaining inflammation
    - o Acute inflammation (lymphocytes, plasma cells, macrophages),
    - o Fibrosis within and between lobules
    - o Duct metaplasia
    - o Eosinophilic protein plugs in duct, as well as
    - o Destruction of acinar cells and islets of Langerhans.
    - o The similar histological changes of chronic pancreatitis may be seen in
        - – Advanced ages
        - – Diabetes
        - – Chronic kidney disease

- Within the context of chronic pancreatitis, distinguish the histological features of ACP (autoimmune chronic pancreatitis) from IDCCP (idiopathic duct centric chronic pancreatitis)

|  | ACP | IDCCP |
| --- | --- | --- |
| o Cells | – ↑ lymphocytes<br>– ↑ plasma cells<br>– IgG4 positive | – Neutrophils, as well as lymphocytes and plasma cells |
| o Veins | – Obstructive phlebitis | |
| o Fibrosis | – "Wharled" (aka LPSP [lymphoplastic sclerosing pancreatitis] | |

- Give the pathology of obstructive chronic pancreatitis.

  o Obstructive chronic pancreatitis is
    - A distinct disease entity
    - Caused by a single dominant narrowing or stricture of the pancreatic duct
    - Caused by diffuse interlobular and intralobular fibrosis"
    - This fibrosis is ".....usually equally and symmetrically distributed in the affected area."

(Feldman M., et al. Sleisenger and Fordtran's Gastrointestinal and Liver Disease. 9th Edition. *Saunders/Elsevier*, Philadelphia, 2010, page 993).

➢ Treatment

- Give current approaches to the management of pain in the patient with chronic pancreatitis.
  o General measures
    - Manage associated/causative factors
    - Cessation of alcohol intake, smoking
    - Analgesics
    - Gabapentin
    - SSRIs, TCAs

- o Neural interruption
  - Percutaneous or endoscopic (EUS) celiac axis nerve blocks
  - Surgical (thorascopic) splanchic nerve resection
    - Pain relief at 1 yr~ 50-75% (lower rates with longer follow-up)
- o Reduction of intrapancreatic pressure
  - Pharmaceological
    - Anticholinergics, PPI, somatostatin, pancreatic enzyme replacement
  - Endoscopic (decompression techniques)

| | |
|---|---|
| • Sphincterotomy, endoscopic dilation and stenting<br>• Stone removal (endoscopic or ESWL) | Useful for "big-duct" chronic pancreatitis (dilation of main pancreatic duct seen on diagnostic imaging, in contrast to small duct disease (aka minimal [structural] change chronic pancreatitis). |

- o ESWL (extracorporeal shock-wave lithotripsy) provides 2-year pain improvement in ~62%.
- o Surgery
  - Surgical drainage, if pancreatic duct dilated (Puestow)
  - Organ resection
    - Partial, complete, with/without pancreatic islet cell transplant

➢ Prognosis
  - o The 80% immediate reduction of pancreatic pain using pancreatics jejunostomy or the modified Pueston operation falls with the duration of follow-up.

Adapted from: Forsmark CE. *Sleisenger & Fordtran's gastrointestinal and liver disease: Pathophysiology/Diagnosis/Management* 2006: pg 1288-1294.

- • Give causes for failure to achieve pain relief after biliary sphincterotomy for pancreatic pain.
  - o Sphincter
    - Inadequate initial sphincterotomy
    - Ductal edema post sphincterotomy
    - Restenosis
    - Residual sphincter of Oddi dysfunction (SOD)
    - Failure of sphincterotomy in SOD types II, or III
  - o Pancreatic
    - Subtle chronic pancreatitis with a normal pancreatogram (small duct disease)
  - o Non-pancreatic
    - Nonpancreaticobiliary pain, especially functional gastrointestinal disease

499

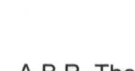

- Give the rational for the use of non-enteric rather than enteric coated pancreatic enzyme replacement products to reduce the pain of pancreatitis.
  - Normally
    - When fat and protein enter the duodenum and proximal jejunum, CCK is released from I cells, and stimulates the release of pancreatic digestive enzymes (proteases, but not fluid or $HCO_3^-$).
    - Pancreatic serine proteases secreted into the duodenum destroy an intestinal CCK-releasing factor.
    - With ↓ CCK-releasing factor, there is ↓ CCK release and ↓ continued secretion of pancreatic enzymes.
  - Pancreatic enzymes and feedback control of secretion of pancreatic enzymes
    - Taking replacement pancreatic enzymes by mouth destroys the intestinal CCK-releasing factor.
    - With ↓ intestinal CCF-releasing factor, there is ↓ CCK, ↓ secretion of pancreatic enzymes, and less pancreatic pain.
  - Why non-enteric rather than enteric coated pancreatic replacement enzymes.
    - Non-enteric coated pancreatic replacement enzymes are delivered to the feedback-sensitive duodenum and proximal jejunum, from which CCK-releasing factor is released and destroyed.
    - Enteric coated enzymes will partially bypass the duodenum and proximal jejunum, so that there is less destruction of CCK-releasing factor, and this results in more CCK being released.

- Please see Harrison's Internal Medicine, 17th Edition, 2008, page 2016, for the protease and the lipase activities of commonly prescribed pancreatic enzyme supplements.

- Give **indications for surgery** in persons with chronic pancreatitis.
  - Intractable pain
  - Suspicion of malignancy
    - Common bile duct (CBD duct)
    - Pancreatic duct (PD)[a]
    - Duodenum
    - Blood vessels[b]
  - Symptomatic pseudocysts[b]

[a]If present with other complications

[b]Both surgical and endoscopic drainage procedures are possible

Printed with permission: Mihaljevic AL, et al. *Best Practice & Research Clinical Gastroenterology* 2008; 22(1): 170.

- Give post-operative complications from **pancreatic resection**.

  - Pancreas      – Pancreatitis
    - Fistula

  - Bile duct      – Leak
    - Cholangitis

  - Stomach      – Gastroparesis
  - Surgical site      – Skin wounded infection
    - Intra-abdominal abscess

  - Pancreatic pseudocyst
    - Prevalence in chronic pancreatitis, 25%
    - Communication with pancreatic duct, 70%
    - Complications of pseudocysts, 20% to 40%
    - Diagnostic ERCP-associated risk of infection, 15%
    - Surgical decompression of cyst
      - Long-term success rate, 90%
      - Recurrence of
        - Pseudocyst, 10%
        - Pain, 5%
      - Operative mortality, 3%

**Autoimmune Pancreatitis** (AIP)

➢ Definition

  - Autoimmune pancreatitis (AIP) is a distinct process of chronic periductal inflammation, whirling interstitial, fibrosis, sclerosis, and obliterative phlebitis and atrophy of acinar cells of the pancreas, associated with IgG4-associated systemic disease (ISD) affecting pancreas, bile ducts, salivary glands, kidneys, retroperitoneum, and lymph nodes

  - Focal, but usually diffuse involvement of pancreas with irregular narrowing of pancreatic duct, swelling of parenchyma, from periductive lymphoplasmacytic, infiltration, storiform fibrosis, obliterative phlebitis (infiltrative surrounds venules but not arterioles), and IgG4 positive immunostaining of ≥ IgG4 positice cells per HPF

  - Type I, lymphoplasmacytic sclerosing pancreatitis, and type II idiopathic duct centric pancreatitis

➢ Demography

  - More frequently males (80%), over 50 years (80%)

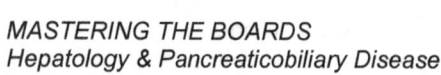

- Clinical
  - Pain is not a prominent feature

- Laboratory
  - ↑ IgG4 antibody
  - The IgG4 antibody also reacts to the PBP (plasminogen-binding protein) of H. pylori.
  - Other organs may have similar inflammatory infiltration
  - Elevated serum IgG4 is 75% sensitive and 93% specific for AIP; IgG4 > 2x ULN are highly specific, but ↑ IgG4 may also be seen in 1.5% of pancreatic cancers

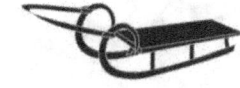

*MASTERING THE BOARDS*
*Hepatology & Pancreaticobiliary Disease*

A.B.R. Thomson

- ➢ Diagnosis

- Give the **Mayo Clinic HISOR diagnostic criteria** for the diagnosis of autoimmune pancreatitis (AIP), and the features characteristic for the diagnostic groups.
  - Histology
    - Periductal lymphoplasmacytic infiltrate with
      - Obliterative phlebitis and storiform fibrosis
      - Storiform fibrosis with abundant IgG4 cells (>10 IgG4 cells/HPF)
  - Imaging
    - Typical
      - Diffusely enlarged pancreas
      - Delayed 'rim' enhancement
      - Diffusely irregular
      - Attenuated main pancreatic duct
    - Other
      - Focal pancreatic mass/enlargement
      - Focal pancreatic ductal stricture
      - Pancreatic atrophy
      - Calcification
      - Pancreatitis
  - Serology
    - ↑ serum IgG4 level (normal 8-140 mg/dL)
  - Other organ involvement
    - Biliary strictures
      - Hilar/intrahepatic
      - Persistent distal
    - Gland involvement
      - Parotid/lacrimal gland
      - Mediastinal lymphadenopathy
      - Retroperitoneal fibrosis
  - Response to steroid therapy
    - Resolution or marked improvement of pancreatic /extrapancreatic manifestation with corticosteroid therapy

Abbreviations: HPF, high power field; IgG4, immunoglobulin G4

503

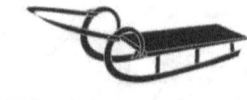

**Japan Pancreas Society** criteria for the diagnosis of AIP

➢ Diagnostic criteria: criterion I must be present together with criterion II and/or III

I.  Imaging criterion
   o Diffuse narrowing of the main pancreatic duct with
      - Irregular wall (more than one third the length of the entire pancreas)
      - Enlargement of the pancreas

II. Laboratory criterion
   o ↑ serum gammaglobulin and/or IgG or autoantibodies

III. Histopathologic criterion
   o ↑ lymphoplasmacytic infiltrate and
   o Dense fibrosis

Abbreviations: AIP, autoimmune pancreatitis; IgG, immunoglobulin G

Printed with permission: Gardner, et al. *AM J Gastroenterol* 2009; 104: 1620-1623.


**Diagnostic Groups**

   o Group A: diagnostic pancreatic histology
      - Presence of one or more of the following criteria:
         ▪ Specimen demonstrating the full spectrum of LPSP
         ▪ >10 IgG4 cells/HPF on immunostatin of pancreatic lymphoplasmacytic infiltrate

   o Group B: typical imaging and serology
      - Presence of all the following criteria:
         ▪ CT or MRI scan showing diffusely enlarged pancreas with delayed and 'rim' enhancement
         ▪ Pancreatogram showing diffusely irregular pancreatic duct
         ▪ ↑ serum IgG4 levels

   o Group C: response to corticosteroids
      - Presence of all the following criteria:
         ▪ Unexplained pancreatic disease after negative workup for other etiologies
         ▪ ↑ serum IgG4 and/or other organ involvement confirmed by presence of abundant IgG4 positive cells
         ▪ Resolution or marked improvement of pancreatic and/or extrapancreatic manifestations with corticosteroid therapy

504

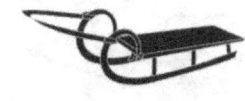

Abbreviations: AIP, autoimmune pancreatitis; CT, computed tomography; HPF, high power field; IgG, immunoglobulin G; LPSP, lymphoplasmacytic sclerosing pancreatitis; MRI, magnetic resonance imaging

Printed with permission: Gardner, el. *AM J Gastroenterol* 2009; 104: 1620-1623.

➢ Diagnostic imaging

- o CT/MRI shows "sausage-shaped" enlargement of pancreas, peripheral (RIM) enhancement, and delayed enhancement; ERCP shows characteristic diffusely irregular and narrowed pancreatic duct

• Give diagnostic imaging manifestations of autoimmune pancreatitis.

- o Abdominal ultrasound, EUS
    - – Pancreas
        - ▪ Hypoechoic
        - ▪ Diffusely enlarged
- o CT
    - – Pancreas
        - ▪ Enlarged
        - ▪ "Sausage-shaped"
        - ▪ IV contract
            - – Delayed/prolonged
    - – Rim around the pancreas (delayed images)
    - – Mass effect from focal swelling
    - – Pancreatic duct
        - ▪ Diffuse or segmental narrowing (strictures)
        - ▪ Atypical imaging features:
            - – Pancreatitis
            - – Focal pancreatic mass
            - – Focal pancreatic duct stricture
            - – Pancreatic atrophy
            - – Persistent distal biliary stricture
- o MRI, MRCP
    - – Pancreas
        - ▪ Diffusely enlarged ($\downarrow T_1$ – and $\uparrow T_2$ – weighted intensity)
        - ▪ Atrophy
        - ▪ Calcifications
    - – Pancreatic duct
        - ▪ Attenuated main duct
        - ▪ Biliary strictures
- o ERCP
    - – Pancreatic duct
        - ▪ Diffuse or segmental narrowing from strictures

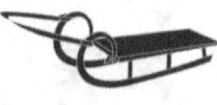

See Sleisenger and Fordtran's Gastrointestinal and Liver Disease. 10<sup>th</sup> Edition. *Saunders/Elsevier*, Philadelphia, 2016, Table 59.1, page 1002.

- Give a comparison of the diagnostic imaging of autoimmune chronic pancreatitis (AIP) versus alcoholic chronic pancreatitis (ACP).

| Site | ACP | AIP |
|------|-----|-----|
| o Duct | – Duct dilation | ▪ Duct narrowing |
| o Pseudocyst | – Common | ▪ Rare |
| o Calcification or stone | – Common | ▪ Rare |
| o Pancreatic parenchyma | – Atrophy | ▪ Enlargement |

Printed with permission: Dite P, et al. *Best Practice & Research Clinical Gastroenterology* 2008; 22(1): pg. 136.

---

SO YOU WANT TO BE A GASTROENTEROLOGIST!

- Within the context of chronic pancreatitis, distinguish the histological features of Autoimmune chronic pancreatitis (ACP) from Idiopathic duct centric chronic pancreatitis (IDCCP)

| | ACP | IDCCP |
|---|-----|-------|
| o Cells | – ↑ lymphocytes<br>– ↑ plasma cells<br>– IgG4 positive | ▪ Neutrophils, as well as lymphocytes and plasma cells |
| o Veins | – Obstructive phlebitis | |
| o Fibrosis | – "Wharled" (aka LPSP [lymphoplastic sclerosing pancreatitis] | |

---

➢ Histopathology

  o Two forms

   – Lymphoplasmacytic sclerosing pancreatitis (LPSP)

   – Idiopathic duct centric chronic pancreatitis (IDCP)

    ▪ Less common than LPSP

  o Dense infiltration of pancreas with T lymphocytes and plasma cells which express IgG4 on their surface, possibly directed towards UBR$_2$ (ubiquitin-protein ligase E3 component N- recognin).

➢ Treatment

  o Consistent response to 30-40 mg prednisone, tapering with improvement in serum IgG4 and imaging

506

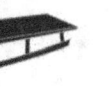

- Give the expected response to steroid therapy in AIP.

| Category | Criteria |
|---|---|
| ○ Pathological features | – ↓ periductal lymphoplasmacytic infiltrate with obliterative phlebitis (LPSP)<br>– IgG4 positive cells<br>– ↓ lymphoplasmacytic infiltrate with fibrosis |
| ○ Serology | – ↓ elevated serum IgG4 level |
| ○ Other organ involvement | – ↓ parotid/lacrimal gland involvement<br>– ↓ mediastinal lymphadenopathy<br>– ↓ retroperitoneal fibrosis |
| ○ Steroid therapy | – Resolution of pancreatic/extrapancreatic manifestations with steroid therapy |

Abbreviation: LPSP, lymphoplasmacytic sclerosing pancreatitis

Printed with permission: Dite, Petr., et al. *Best Practice & Research Clinical Gastroenterology* 2008; 22(1): pg. 138.

"Everyone wants to live on top of the mountain, but all the happiness and growth occurs while you're climbing it."

Andy Rooney Og Mandino

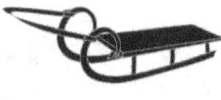

# PANCREATIC CYSTS AND TUMOURS

➤ Causes/associations

- Give types of of cystic and cystic-appearing lesions of the pancreas.
  - ○ Congenital true cysts
    - – Polycystic disease
    - – Von Hippel-Lindau disease
    - – Cystic fibrosis
    - – Dermoid cysts
  - ○ Inflammatory
    - – Pseudocysts
    - – Abscess
    - – Hydati cyst
  - ○ Angiomatous cysts
  - ○ Cystic neoplasms
    - – *Mucinous tumours*
      - ▪ Mucinous cystadenoma (aka macrocystic adenoma) and cystadenocarcinoma
      - ▪ Intraductal mucin hypersecreting neoplasm (aka mucinous ductal ectasia)
    - – *Non-mucinous tumours*
    - – Serous cystadenoma (aka microcystic adenoma)
      - ▪ Papillary cystic tumour
      - ▪ Cystic cavitation of pancreatic adenocarcinoma or lymphoma
  - ○ Acquired cysts
    - – Central cavitary necrosis
    - – Pseudocyst
    - – Parasitic cyst
  - ○ Misdiagnosed nonpancreatic lesions
    - – Splenic artery aneurysm
    - – Choledochal cyst
    - – Mesenteric cyst
    - – Duodenal duplication cyst or diverticulum
    - – Lesser sac biloma
    - – Lymphangioma
    - – Hypoechoic solid tumour
  - ○ Metastases, with cystic component

Printed with permission: Degen L, et al. *Best Practice & Research Clinical Gastroenterology* 2008; 22(1): 92.

508

> Diagnosis

- Give the diagnostic features of types of pancreatic cysts.

| Cyst Type | EUS Features | Fluid Appearance | Cytology | CEA | Amylase |
|---|---|---|---|---|---|
| o SCA | - Microcystic, honeycombed, 20% macrocystic | • Thin, clear, some- times bloody | • Cuboidal cells clear glycogen- positive cytoplasm | Low | Low |
| o MCN* | - Macrocystic | • Viscous, clear | • Mucin-rich fluid, columnar mucin-positive cells, with variable atypia | High | Low |
| o IPMN* | - Duct dilation<br>• Main duct (MD – IPMN)<br>• Branch duct (BD – IPMN)<br>• Malignant potential MD >> BD – IPMN | • Viscous, clear | • Mucin-rich fluid, columnar mucin-positive cells, with variable atypia | High | High |
| o PP | - Macrocystic, thick wall<br>- Unilocular, internal debris | • Thin, dark, non- mucinous | • Inflammatory cells without evidence of mucin or epithelial cells | Variable | High |
| o PET (cystic) | - Variable | • Variable, typically non- mucinous | • Small cells, scant cytoplasm, monomorphic nuclei | Un- known | Low |
| o SPT | - Mixed solid and cystic | • Bloody | • Papillary structures, macrophages, myxoid stroma, monomorphic neoplastic cells | Low | Low |
| o LEC | - Solid, hetero- geneous<br>- Subtle posterior enhancement | • Thick and milky, gray or frothy | • Anucleated squamous cells, lymphocytes | Variable | Low |

509

Abbreviations: EUS: Endoscopic ultrasound; IPMN, intraductal papillary mucinous neoplasm; LEC, lymphoepithelial cysts; MCN, mucinous cystic neoplasms; PD: Pancreatic duct; PET, pancreatic endocrine tumour; PP, pancreatic pseudocysts; SCA, serous cystadenoma; SPT, solid pseudopapillary tumours

Printed with permission: Fasanella KE, and McGrath K. *Best Practise and Research Clinical Gastroenterology* 2009; 23:35-48; Brugge WR. *2009 ACG Annual Postgraduate Course*:231-234.

- Give a comparison of the viscosity, amylase, concentration, CEA and CA2-4 levels, and cytological findings in pancreatic serous cystadenoma, benign and malignant mucinous cystic neoplasm (MCN), intraductal papillary mucinous tumour (IPMT) and pseudocyst (PC).

| Parameter Analyzed | Serous Cystadenoma | MCN-Benign | MCN-Malignant | IPMT | PC |
|---|---|---|---|---|---|
| o Viscosity | ↓ | ↑ | ↑ | ↑ | ↓ |
| o Amylase | ↓ | ↓ | ↓ | ↑ | ↑ |
| o CEA | ↓ | ↑ | ↑ | ↑ | ↑ |
| o CA 19-9 | ↓ | ↓/↑ | ↑ | ? | ↓ |
| o Cytologic findings | Usually negative, rarely cuboidal cells | Occasionally mucinous epithelial cells | Benign – occasional mucinous epithelial cells | Papillary cluster of mucinous cells | Histiocytes |

Note:

- o CEA, CA19-9, amylase
  - – Suggestive of pseudocyst vs neoplasm
  - – Size itself not an indicator of need to drain pseudocyst for symptoms

Adapted from: Sleisenger and Fordtran's Gastrointestinal and Liver Disease. 10th Edition. Saunders/Elsevier, Philadelphia, 2016, Table 60-7, page 1039.

510

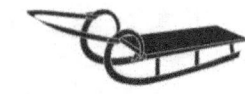

- Give a comparison of pancreatic serous versus mucinous cystadenoma.

|  | Serous Cystadenoma (SCA) | Mucinous Cystadenoma (MCA) |
|---|---|---|
| o Sex | - Female (2-3:1) | • Female (~100%) |
| o Age | - 60s | • 60s |
| o Ethanol abuse | - No association | • No association |
| o Pancreatic history | - Yes (uncommon) | • Yes (uncommon) |
| o Malignant potential | - No (rare) | • Yes |
| o Location | - Evenly distributed body/tail | • Body/tail |
| o Locularity | - Multiple small | • Multilocular |
| o Calcifications | - Central sunburst or stellate | • Peripheral, curvilinear |

- Give a comparison of IPMT versus pancreatis pseudocyst.

|  | IPMT | Pseudocyst (PC) |
|---|---|---|
| o Sex | -Male (3-4:1) | • Male |
| o Age | -60s | • Variable |
| o Ethanol abuse | -No association | • Yes |
| o Pancreatic history | -Yes uncommon | • Yes uncommon |
| o Malignant potential | -Yes | • No |
| o Location | -Head | • Head |
| o Locularity | -Multilocular | • Unilocular |
| o Calcifications | -No | • No, unless associated with chronic pancreatitis |

Adapted from: Scheiman JM. *AGA Institute Postgraduate Course* 2006: pg. 586.

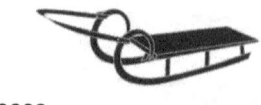

511

- o The three major types of pancreatic cysts (SCA, MCP, IPMN, PC) are seen in patients in their 60s.
- o The age of presentation of PC is variable.
- o SCA and MPA are more common in women, IPMT and PC are more common in men.
- o Malignant potential is
  - High in MCA and IPMT
  - Low in SCA and PC
- o A history of pancreatitis is uncommon in SCA, MCA, and IPMN.

- Give a comparison of SCA, MCA, IPMTand PC in terms of location, locularity and calcifications.

| | | SCA | MCA | IPMT | PC |
|---|---|---|---|---|---|
| o | Location | B/T | B/T | H | H |
| o | Multilocular | - | + | 60% | - |
| o | Calcification | Central sunburst or stellate | Peripheral, curvilinear | - | + (unles associated with chronic alcoholic pancreatitis) |

> Treatment

- Give the traditional therapeutic approach to the therapy of cystic lesions.

| | | Pseudocyst | Serous | Mucinous | Malignant |
|---|---|---|---|---|---|
| o | Head | Drain | Monitor | Monitor | Resect |
| o | Body | Drain | Monitor | Resect | Resect |
| o | Tail | Resect | Resect* | Resect* | Resect |

- o Cyst fluid CGA < 3.1 mg/ml suggests serious cystadenomas, whereas CEA > 480 mg/ml suggest mucinous fluid

*Approach varies with risk of surgery

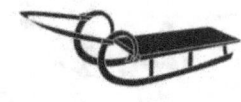

**Pseudocysts** (PC)

➤ Definitions

- Pseudocyst
  - Non-epithelized fluid collection > 4 wk old as a consequence
  - Caused by
    - Trauma from disruption of pancreatic duct (PD)
    - Acute pancreatitis (AP)
    - Chronic pancreatitis (CP)
  - The acute pseudocyst may become chronic "..... as a sequelae of chronic pancreatitis and downstream pancreatic ductal obstruction with fibrotic strictures or stones" (Sleisenger and Fordtran's Gastrointestinal and Liver Disease. 9th Edition. *Saunders/Elsevier*, Philadelphia, 2010, page 1039).

- Localized necrosis
  - Pancreatic tissue → Cause a leak in → Cystic space filled
  - Pancreatic plus peripancreatic fat necrosis     the pancreatic duct     with amylase-rich fluid

- "...a fluid collection that persists for 4 to weeks and becomes encapsulated by a wall of fibrous or granulation tissue (Sleisenger and Fordtran's Gastrointestinal and Liver Disease. 9th Edition. Saunders/Elsevier, Philadelphia, 2010, page 941).

- Usually or adjacent to the pancreas, but occasionally seen in pelvis or chest

- Conceptually, fluid filled sacs, sometimes with necrotic pancreatic debris

- Pseudocyst plus liquefied necrotic debris after 5 to 6 weeks may be termed WOPN (walled off pancreatic necrosis)

- Walled-off pancreatic necrosis (WOPN)
  - Internal debris in WOPN, rather than fluid in pseudocyst
    - Predictor of poor outcome
  - Nasocystic or PEG-cystic cavity drain
  - Necrosectomy, 90% success rate within 4 mon

513

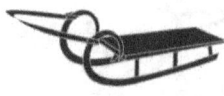

- Give clinical, diagnostic imaging and laboratory features that distinguish pseudocysts from cystic neoplasms of the pancreas.

| Feature | Pseudocyst | Cystic neoplasm |
|---|---|---|
| ❖ Clinical | | |
|   o Gender | - More commonly male | ▪ Usually female |
|   o Age | - 30-40 years | ▪ 60-70 years |
|   o Alcohol abuse | - Common | ▪ Uncommon |
|   o History of acute or chronic pancreatitis | - Common | ▪ Uncommon |
|   o Diagnostic imaging* | | |
|     - Septae | - | + |
|     - Unilocular | + | + |
|     - Multi-locular | - | + |
|     - Solid component | - | + |
|     - Calcification | + | + |
|     - Mural nodules of wall | | |
|   o Communication between cyst and pancreatic duct on ERCP | - 70% | ▪ Rare (except for IPMN) |
| ❖ Cyst fluid | | |
|   o Amylase | - High | ▪ Low |
|   o CEA, CA19-9 | - Low | ▪ High |
|   o Cytology | - Inflammatory cells | ▪ Glycogen<br>▪ Mucin-containing cells<br>▪ Malignant cells |

Abbreviations: CEA, Carcinoembryonic antigen; CT, computed tomography; EUS, endoscopic ultrasound; US, ultrasonography

Adapted from: Sleisenger and Fordtran's Gastrointestinal and Liver Disease. 10th Edition. Saunders/Elsevier, Philadelphia, 2016, Table 60-6, page 1039.

514

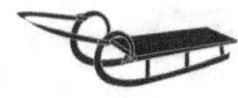

*MASTERING THE BOARDS*
*Hepatology & Pancreaticobiliary Disease*

A.B.R. Thomson

➢ Treatment

- Give indications for treatment of a person with a pancreatic pseudocyst.
  - o Pseudoaneurysm formation
  - o Fistula formation into adjacent viscera
  - o Expansion of the pseudocyst producing abdominal pain
  - o Expansion of the pseudocyst producing duodenal or biliary obstruction
  - o Abscess formation.
  - o Pancreatic ascites (tracking of pancreatic juice into the peritoneal cavity or pleural space)
  - o Pleural effusion
  - o Rupture
  - o >6 cm, 6 weeks after episode of pancreatitis
  - o Concern for malignant cystic lesion

Adapted from: Kim HC, et al. *Acta Radiol*. 2008;49(7):727-34; and Christensen NM, et al. *Am J Surg*. 1975;130(2):199-205.

Drainage
  - o EUS drainage better if necrotic cyst not infected (i.e., abscess)
  - o PCD (percutaneous drainage)
    - – More prolonged drainage if connection with pancreatic duct
  - o Do a dynamic high resolution CT after drainage to rule out pseudoaneurysm

## Serous Cystadenoma

➢ Laboratory
  - o Cyst filed with clear, watery fluid (no mucin)
  - o Cytology of fluid may show cuboidal cells with glycogen-rich cytoplasm.

➢ Diagnostic imaging
  - o Body or tail of pancreas
  - o Many tiny cysts
  - o Fibrous septa
  - o Honeycomb appearance

515

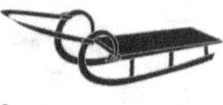

- o Scar with stellate appearance
- o Stellate scar may be calcified
- o Central. "sunburst" calcification (on CT scan)
- o No communication with pancreatic duct

➢ Prognosis
- o Rarely malignant (3%)

## Mucinous Cystic Neoplasm (MCN)

➢ Laboratory
- o Thick mucus material (or blood)
- o Fluid in cyst
  - – ↑ CEA
  - – In benign MCN
- o Cytology shows
  - – Adenocarcinoma cells
  - – Columnar

➢ Diagnostic imaging
- o May be benign, but in individual patient assume to be malignant
- o Body or tail of pancreas
- o Thick wall
- o Occasional septa
- o Stroma (ovarium-like)
- o Mucinous epithelial cells with atypia
- o No communication with pancreatic duct on ERCP/MRCP larger cysts with nodules in wall are more likely to be malignant than benign MCN.
- o Lesions are never mutifocal, so once the single lesion is removed, surveillance is not necessary.

➢ Prognosis
- o 5-year survival rate after resection of tumour, 30% to 63%

516

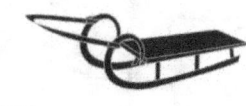

## Intraductal Papillary Mucinous Neoplasms (IPMN)

> SO YOU WANT TO BE A GASTROENTEROLOGIST!
>
> In the context of a pancreatic tumour and
> - Patient — no pain or weight loss
> - Tumour — large, but no obstruction of biliary tree
> - Blood test — ↑ LDH (lactate dehydrogenase)
>
> - Give the most likely pathological diagnosis.
>
>   o Only 1% of pancreatic tumours are lymphomas or extranodal non-Hodgkin lymphomas, and the typical patient-, tumour- and its characteristics are given above.

➤ Definition

  o "…. Papillary neoplasms within the main pancreatic duct showing mucin hypersecretion that often leads to duct dilation and chronic obstructive pancreatitis.

  o Thick (viscous) mucous with ↑ CEA, ↑ amylase

➤ Demography

  o Male: female ratio: 1-2.4

  o Mean age of diagnosis
    - 65 years

➤ Genetics

  o As compared with pancreatic adenocarcinoma
    - In IPMN there are more frequent molecular changes in SKT 11/LKB1 inactivation and PIK3CA mutation
    - Less frequent mutations in K-Ras and P53 tumour suppressor genes, P16 and DPC4

  o In IPMN, there is ↑ expression of
    - Fascin (an actin-bundling protein), methylated PPENK
    - Human telomerase reverse transcriptase

517

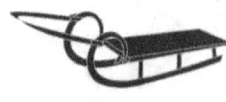

- ➢ Types
  - o Main, branched or main plus branched (mixed) pancreatic ducts
  - o Main duct IPMNs are more likely to become malignant and to grow faster: 63% develop HGD/cancer in 5 years, vs 15% for branched chain IPMNs

- ➢ Clinical
  - o Symptoms arise from mucin distending involved pancreatic duct; (may see mucus extruding from ampulla on ERCP)
  - o 5-year survival rate after resection, > 75%
  - o Main duct IPMN or branching chain IPMN > 3 cm are more likely to be malignant.

- ➢ Laboratory
  - o Increased serum bilirubin predicts the presence of malignancy
  - o ↑ CEA in 80-95% of IPMNs

- • Give the significance of ↑ amylase concentration in the fluid aspirated from a pancreatic cyst.
  - o Amylase in a gut aspirate only signifies that the cyst which contained the fluid was in commutation with a pancreatic branch duct or main duct.

- ➢ Diagnostic imaging
  - o MRI
  - o CT
    - – CT using pancreatic protocol (detects IPMN in 97% of cases)
  - o MRCP
    - – Breath-hold MRCP
    - – MRCP with secretin (S-MRCP),
    - – MRCP is superior to CT to demonstrate communication between ducts, and cyst morphology
  - o EUS
  - o ERCP
  - o PET scanning sensitivity, 57-90%; specificity, 85-97%
  - o Exclude pancreas divisium (MRCP, 100% accurate; CT, sensitivity 90%, specificity, 97%)

518

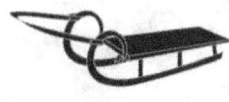

➢ Histopathology
  - Cytology
    - Columnar mucinous epithelial cells with variable atypia
  - Grape-like cluster of cysts, localized or diffuse dilation of main pancreatic duct, patulous ampulla of Vater
  - Lesions of main or bronchial pancreatic ducts, with proliferation of the mucinous epithelium leading to ductal and cystic dilation
  - 20-30% of IPMNs are multifocal, arising from a field defect in the entire pancreas that can cause multiple primary neoplasms.
  - Range histologically from benign, low grade (LGD), or high grade dysplasia to invasive cancer, with various grades of histology, probably being present with the same specimen

➢ Treatment
  - Chemotherapy
  - Cyst ablation with ethanol or paclitaxel (a chemotherapeutic agent which inhibits the disassembly of microtubules and induces apoptosis with complete resolution of cysts in 79%, may be reasonable for IPMNs with low risk of malignancy:
    - No symptoms
    - < 3 cm size
    - Main duct < 6 mm
    - No mural nodules, thickness or septations
  - Endoscopy
    - NG (nasogastric) drain
    - Stent

519

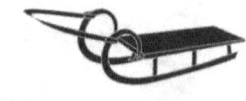

- Give the pros and cons of nasogastric drains versus pancreatic stents.

| Nasogastric Drain | Stent |
|---|---|
| o Pros | |
|    – Flushing and fluoroscopy at any time | • Easy, quick, dislocation rare<br>• Not disabling, patients stay mobile, feel better |
| o Cons | |
|    – Discomfort; easily dislocated; leads to immobilization of patients, nose-pain; flushing often futile and tedious, no direct control during flushing | • No flushing<br>• Control needs endoscopic session |

Printed with permission: Giovanni M. *Best Practice & Research Clinical Gastroenterology* 2004; 18(1): pg.192.

- o Surgery
    - – Sendai guidelines for resection
    - – After surgical resection, invasive > 40%, non-invasive > 70%; resections recur in a median of 20 months, and 58% of these recurrences involve distal sites.

- Give the **Sendai Guidelines** for resection of IPMNs.

| | | |
|---|---|---|
| o Symptomatic | – All IPMN (MD- and BD – IPMN) with symptoms | |
| o Asymptomatic | – All MD-IPMNs<br>– BP-IPMNs > 3 cm | |
| o EUS | – All IPMN with<br>   • Nodules<br>   • Thickening | |
| o CEA | – > 192 | |
| o Surveillance EUS, ERCP, MRCP (CT scan) | – Enlargement on surveillance every 6-12 mon | |

An ↑ CEA > 192 in IPMN predicts future or present malignant degeneration.

520

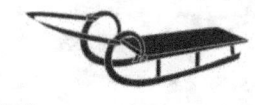

# Pancreatic Duct Adenomatous Cancer (PDCa)

➤ Demography

- o Incidence $10/10^5$

- o Prevalence
  - Because the mortality rate is so high, prevalence figures are meaningless

- o 10% are metastatic
  - Pancreas supplied by splanchnic artery
  - Renal cell , especially late

- o 1% endocrine

---

A curiosity!

Persons with annular pancreas have an ↑ risk of developing hepatopancreatic adenocarcinoma.

---

➤ Pathology

- o Most pancreatic carcinomas are from duct cells (PDCa), and may secrete mucin.

- o Site
  - Pancreas
    - 70% H (head of pancreas)
    - 150% B (body)
    - 15% T (tail)
  - Wall of duodenum
  - Ampullary of Vater
  - Distal bile duct (aka common bile duct)

➤ Causes/associations

- Give genetic and non-genetic causes/associations of pancreatic cancer.
  - o Familial

| Number of First Degree Relatives Affected | ↑ Relative Risk |
|---|---|
| 1 | 2.3x |
| 2 | 6x |
| 3 | 32x |

521

- o Hereditary pancreatitis
  - Cationic trypsinogen (CT)
  - CFTR
  - SPINK
- o Genetic abnormalities
  - Familial atypical mole and multiple melanoma (FAMMM)
    - Germline p16 mutation
  - Hereditary breast cancer
    - Germline BRCA2 mutation
  - Oncogenes
    - K-Ras mutations (90%) and p53 (70%) mutations (occur early and indicate tumour induction by exogenous carcinogens)
  - TP53, APC4 (aka SMAD4) mutations (occur late)
  - EGF (epidermal growth factor) receptors
  - SONIC hedgehog product
  - Inactive tumour suppression gene (p59, p16 [DKN2A])
  - Familial pancreatic cancer
  - Familial ovarian and breast cancer
- o Polyp syndromes
  - Familial adenomatous polyposis (FAP)
  - HNPCC (Lynch) mismatch MLH1, MSH2, BRCH2
  - Peutz-Jeghers syndrome (PJS)
  - Cowden syndrome (CS)
- o Lifestyle
  - Smoking
    - ↑ risk 1.5 x
    - Interacts to further increase risk in
      - Alcoholism
      - $GSTT_1$
  - Alcohol
  - High-saturated fat (red meat) low vegetable/low vitamin diet
- o Diet
  - Low intake of
    - Fresh fruits
    - Vegetables
    - Selenium

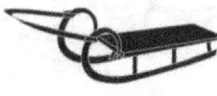

522

- o Drugs
  - – 7-fold increased risk after exposition to dichlorodiphenyltrichloroethane or deviates (e.g., ethylene)
- o Metabolic
  - – Chronic pancreatitis, especially when the pancreatitis is due to
    - ▪ Alcohol
    - ▪ Cystic fibrosis
    - ▪ Other forms of hereditary pancreatitis
    - ▪ Tropical pancreatitis
  - – Diabetes mellitus
  - – Partial gastrectomy
- o Miscellaneous
  - – Cystic fibrosis
  - – Fanconi anemia
  - – Familial adenomatous polyposis (FAP)
  - – Ataxia telangiectasia
  - – Neuroendocrine tumours (NET)

Adapted from: Keller J, et al. *Best Practice & Research Clinical Gastroenterology* 2007; 21(3): pg. 522.

- • Give precursor lesions for PDCa.

Because the mortality rate for pancreatic ductal cancer (PDCa) is so high, it is important to recognize precursor lesions so that early diagnosis and possibly better survival will occur.

- o PIN    – Pancreatic intraepithelial neoplasia
- o MCN    – Mucinous cystic neoplasms
- o IPMN   – Intraductal papillary mucinous neoplasms
- o SPT    – Solid pseudopapillary tumour
  - ▪ 20% risk of solid-pseudopapillary carcinoma
  - ▪ Abnormal expression of β-catenin and p120
  - ▪ ↓ expression of E-cadherin protein, or E-cadherin protein localized to cell nucleus
- o Cystic islet cell tumour
- o Serous cystadenomas may rarely (3%) be malignant (serous cystadenocarcinoma)

Note: Early events include K-Ras mutation and p16 loss, whereas late events include TP53 and APC4/SMAD4 loss.

523

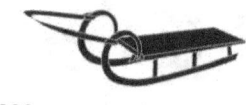

➤ Laboratory

  ○ ↑ **CA19-9** (tumour marker) occurs in
    – 70% to 80% of persons with pancreatic adenocarcinoma
    – Some persons with biliary obstruction and cholangitis

  ○ The tumour marker CA 19-9 has a sensitivity of 86% and a specificity of 87% to diagnose pancreatic ductal cancer (PDCa).

  ○ CA19-9 may be falsely positive in the presence of jaundice or cholangitis (-a-b).

  ○ Because CA 19-9 is not suitable for screening, the diagnosis of PDCa is usually made by diagnostic imaging of the abdomen.

Sleisenger and Fordtran's Gastrointestinal and Liver Disease. 9th Edition. Philadelphia, 2010, page 1014.

➤ Diagnostic imaging

  ○ Cystic neoplasms may mimic a pseudocyst, especially when there are nodules or internal septations.

• Give diagnostic imaging tests of PDCa.

  ○ Abdominal ultrasound

  ○ Helical CT pancreatic protocol
    – Dual-phase scanning after Po/Iv contrast, with pancreatic arterial phase at 40 sec and portal venous phase at 70 sec after IV contrast agent is given.
    – Oral contrast, to distinguish between pancreas and duodenum
    – Hypoattenuating –adenocarcinoma
    – Hyperattenuating – neuroendocrine tumour
    – 10% are isoattenuating, so use indirect signs
    – Indirect signs
      ▪ Dilated PD, CBD, double duct (PD+CBD)
      ▪ Mass effects
      ▪ Pancreatic atrophy
      ▪ Abnormal pancreatic contour
      ▪ 97% correct diagnosis of PDCa
      ▪ 100% accurate in predicting unresectable disease
      ▪ 85% of persons predicted to have resectable disease by CT turn out to actually have unresectable disease

524

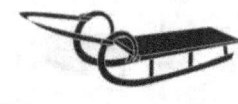

o MRI, MRA, MRV, MRCP
  – Magnetic resonance imaging
  – Gadolinium contrast used for MRA, MRV, MRCP
  – Image weighting
    ▪ $T_1$ – MRI (solid)
    ▪ $T_2$ – MRCP (fluid)
  – Use MRI to directly biopsy pancreatic mass
  – Staging sensitivity for PCa
    ▪ MRI      84%
    ▪ CT              91%

o PET (positron emission tomography using radioactive fluorodeoxyglucose [FDG} F18)
  – Shows focal area of ↑ uptake of FDG in pancreas, and "hot spots" (↑ FDG uptake) of metastases in liver.
  – Does not show details of anatomy of pancreas, s do CT or MRI.
  – Performance characteristics: sensitivity of 95% to detect malignant pancreatic tumours.

See Feldman M., et al. Sleisenger and Fordtran's Gastrointestinal and Liver Disease. 9th Edition. *Saunders/Elsevier*, Philadelphia, 2010, Table 60.8, page 1027; Epidemiologic and Biological Characteristics of Pancreatic Cystic Neoplasms)

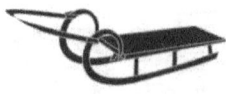

➢ Endoscopy

  o ERCP (endoscopic retrograde cholangiopancreatography)
    - Evaluation of recurrent pancreatitis (avoid in chronic pain syndromes)
    - Pancreatic duct disruptions or leaks
    - Symptomatic pancreatic pseudocysts
    - Drainage of pancreatic necrosis
    - Palliative stenting

  o EUS (endoscopic ultrasound)
    - Diagnostic procedure in acute and chronic pancreatitis
    - Consider before transmural drainage of pancreatic fluid collection/necrosis/pseudocyst
    - Pancreatic mass < 2 cm
      • Sensitivity
        - EUS 98%
        - CT    91%

526

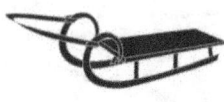

- Usually used to complement CT for staging
- More sensitivity than CT to determine if there is vascular invasion
- Suitable to obtain biopsy (FNA, fine needle aspiration), as also is CT
- Useful for celiac plexus block
- Types of EUS
  - Radial (Olympus) 360° perspective
  - Linear (for sampling or injection) (Pentax)
- "EUS is superior to CT for detection of co-existent [pancreatic] malignancy [in a pseudocyst] particularly when the lesion is small" *Saunders/Elsevier,*
- EUS also has the substantial advantage of FNA.

- o Contrast-enhanced harmonic EUS (CH-EUS)
  - Visualizes pancreatic parenchymal perfusion and the microvasculature
  - Determined hypo-enhancement pattern diagnosed ductal carcinoma with high sensitivity and specificity.
  - Superior to multi-detector-row computed tomography (MDCT) in distinguishing small ductal carcinomas from other tumours.
  - Combining CH-EUS with EUS-FNA improves the sensitivity with which EUS-FNA identifies ductal carcinomas.

Source: Kitano M et al. Am J Gastroenterol 2012; 107: 303-310.

➢ Histopathology

- Give the names of immunohistochemical markers which may be used to confirm that a tumour in the pancreas is mucus secreting, and is not derived from acinar or neuroendocrine cells of the pancreas.
  - o Markers for mucin
    - $MUC_1$, $MUC_2$, $MUC_4$
    - CEA (carcinoembryonic antigen)
    - CA 19-9, Ca 125
    - $DuPan_2$
  - o Markers for cytokeratins
    - 7, 8, 18, 19 (cytokeratin 7 is usually absent from pancreatic tumours arising from acinar or neuroendocrine cells).

527

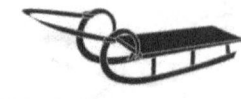

> Treatment

❖ Surgery (for resectable lesion)

- Give factors which usually preclude surgery for pancreatic cancer (i.e., patient is not a surgical candidate).
  - o Metastases
  - o Ascites
  - o Mental caking
  - o Large celiac axis node
  - o Vascular involvement
  - o Degree of involvement of circumference of vessel reflects likelihood of vessel invasion

- Give a description and draw a picture of the **Whipple Procedure**.

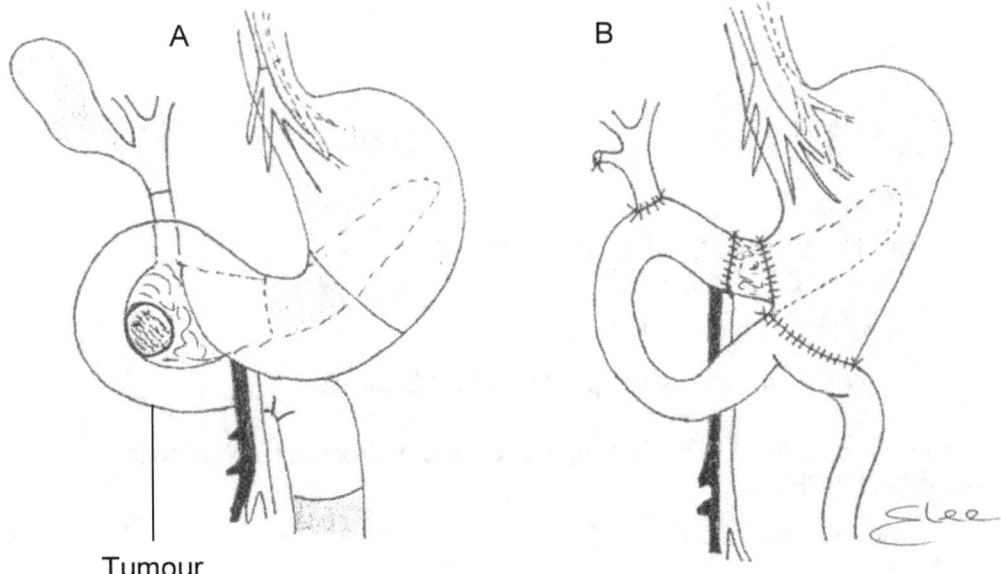

Tumour

A.  o An en bloc resection of the distal stomach, duodenum, common duct, and head of the pancreas containing the pancreatic neoplasm is performed (areas removed are not shaded).
    o A cholecystectomy and truncal vagotomy are also performed.

B.  o Gastrointestinal continuity is restored by performing a pancreaticojejunostomy, a choledochojejunostomy, and a gastrojejunostomy.

Adapted from: Reber, H.A and Way, L.W: The pancreas. In Dunphy, J.E, and Way, L.,W [eds.]. *Current Surgical Diagnosis and Treatment*, 3rd Ed. Los Altos, Calif. Lange Medical Publications, 1977.

528

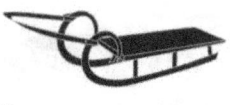

- Non-resectable
  - Endoscopic stenting
  - Laparoscopy
  - Laparotomy
    - Chemoradiation
  - Pain control

- ❖ Chemoradiation Therapy
  - Chemotherapy agents
    - Gemcitabine / 5-FU
      - 2 months longer survival
      - Palliation for fit patients (pain control)
    - Taxol
      - Inject directly into PCa mass
  - Radiation
    - Palliation
    - Focal radiation

- ❖ Pain control
  - Celiac plexus neurolysis (CPN) (CP bock)
    - EUS or CT directed
  - Local anesthesia given before CPN
  - 50 mcg/hr – fentanyl patch post CPN for 2 weeks

- Give complications of CPN/CPB (celiac plexus neurolysis (CPN) / celiac plexus block (CPB).
  - Postural hypotension
  - 2 wk worsening of pain, before pain / quality of life improve
  - Diarrhea (2%) 48 hours post CPN (celiac plexus neurolysis) / CPB (celiac plexus block)

529

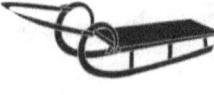

## Non-Adenomatous Cancers of the Pancreas

➢ Types

- Give types of non-adenomatous acinar or ductal tumours of the pancreas.
  - o Lymphoma
    - – High index of suspicion
    - – Flow cytometry needed
    - – Round
    - – Discrete
    - – More hypoattenuating
  - o NET (neuroendocrine tumour)
    - – Functioning
    - – Non-functioning
      - ▪ Gastrinoma
      - ▪ Insulinoma
      - ▪ Glucagonoma
      - ▪ VIPomas
      - ▪ Somatostatinoma
  - o AIP (autoimmune pancreatitis)
  - o TB (tuberculosis)

## Pancreatic Neuroendocrine Tumours (NET)

- Non-functioning
  - o > 50% are malignant
  - o Usually in pancreatic head
  - o Often large
  - o Have worse survival compared to functioning pancreatic neuroendocrine tumours
  - o Resect all sporadic tumours, or if > 2 cm in MEN I

530

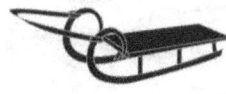

- Functioning

## *Gastrinoma*

- o 1 per year/$10^6$ population
- o Malignant ~ 66%
- o 20% associated with MEN I
- o > 50% of sporadic and > 70% of hereditary gastrinomas are in the duodenum
- o Resection of all sporadic gastrinomas and in MEN I if > 2.5 cm

## *Insulinoma*

- o 1 per year/$10^6$ population
- o Benign in ~90%
- o Solitary in 95%
- o <2 cm in 85-90%
- o 4% are MEN I
- o In MEN I patients insulinomas are multiple in 90%
- o Enucleation if solitary; pancreatic
- o tomy if multiple
- o Clinical features
  - Neuroglycopenia (90%)
    - Amnesia or coma (47%)
    - Confusion (80%)
    - Visual changes (59%)
    - Convulsions (17%)
    - Altered consciousness (38%)
  - Sympathetic overdrive (60-70%)
    - Weakness (56%)
    - Sweating (69%)
    - Tremors (24%)
    - Palpitations (12%)
    - Hyperphagia (14%)
  - Obesity (<50%)

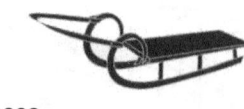

## Glucagonoma

➤ Demography

- o Occur in 10-15% of patients
- o Frequently multiple (>30%)
- o Tumours >3 cm are aggressive (metastases)
- o

➤ Clinical

- o Migratory necrolytic erythema (70-90%)
- o Weight loss (80%)
- o Diarrhea (25%)
- o Thromboembolism (15%-25%)
- o Glossitis, chelitis (15%-40%)
- o Psychiatric symptoms (0%-17%)

➤ Laboratory

- o Glucose intolerance (40%-90%)
- o Normochromic, normocytic anemia (35%-90%)
- o Hypoaminoacidemia (80%)

Adapted from: Metz, D.C., and Jensen, R.T. *Gastroenterology* 2008; 135: 1469-1492.

➤ Treatment

- o Resect lesion if > 3 cm in the body/tail and if > 2 cm in the pancreas head
- o Tumours < 1 cm require yearly follow-up by CT or MRI from an early age

## VIPoma

➤ Definition

- o Neuroendocrine tumour, usually (> 80%) of the pancreatic tail, secreting ↑ PNM-27 (vasoactive intestinal peptide)

532

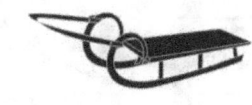

- Pathophysiology
  - ↑ PHM-27 in VIPoma NET tumour
  - PHM-27 shares a common precursor with VIP2
  - When ↑ PHM-27 → VIP-like actions → ↑ activity of adenylate cyclase → ↑ cAMP
    - → ↑ Cl⁻ secretion (diarrhea)
    - → Secondary hyperaldosteronism

---

**SO YOU WANT TO BE A GASTROENTEROLOGIST!**

- Give the pathophysiology of the flushing, bones disease and hyperglycemia which occur in VIPoma.
  - Flushing          - Vasodilation
  - Bone disease       - ↑ osteolysis of bone
  - Hyperglycemia      - Glycogenolytic effect of VIP

---

- Clinical
  - ↑ VIP → WDHH syndrome
    - Watery diarrhea
    - Hypokalemia → renal and heart failure
    - Achlorhydra

- Laboratory

Serum VIP levels are increased with VIPoma, especially when the patient is having diarrhea (levels may fluctuate).

- Give other causes of chronic diarrhea which may also be associated with ↑ VIP, but without an associated secreting pancreatic endocrine tumour.
  - Laxative abuse
  - Short bowel syndrome (surgical resection of a portion of the small bowel)
  - Radiation enteritis

533

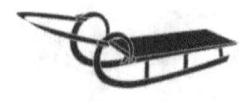

- ➤ Pathology
  - o Single tumour
  - o Large
  - o ~ 75% in tail of pancreas
  - o High rate of metastases

- ➤ Treatment
  - o Octreotide (benefit does not always reflect changes in blood levels of VIP)
  - o Surgical resection
  - o Caution alert: do not use in pregnancy (risk of uterine ischemia)

## Somatostatinoma

- ➤ Clinical

| | Somatostatinoma | |
| --- | Pancreatic | Intestinal |
| o Diabetes mellitus | 95 | 20 |
| o Gallbladder disease | 94 | 40 |
| o Steatorrhea | 85 | 10 |
| o Hypochlorhydria | 85 | 15 |
| o Diarrhea | 75 | 25 |
| o Weight loss | 50 | 35 |

- ➤ Treatment
  - o Local
    - – Liver resection
    - – Chemoembolization
    - – Radiofrequency ablation
  - o Systemic
    - – Somatostatin analogues
    - – Somatostatin receptor radionuclide therapy
    - – MIBG radionuclide therapy
    - – Chemotherapy, especially for poorly differentiated tumours

Printed with permission: Alexakis N, and Neoptolemos JP. *Best Practice & Research Clinical Gastroenterology* 2008; 22(1): 199.

534

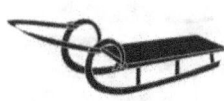

# CONGENITAL ABNORMALITIES

## Annular Pancreas

➢ Incidence

  o Annular pancreas (AP) – 100/10$^5$

  o **Embryonic development** of the pancreas
    - At about 4 weeks of gestation (A), dorsal and ventral buds are formed from the duodenum.
    - At 6 weeks (B), the ventral pancreas extends toward the larger dorsal pancreas.
    - By about 7 weeks (C), fusion of dorsal and ventral pancreas has occurred and ductular anastomosis is beginning.
    - At birth (D), the pancreas is a single organ, and ductular anastomosis is complete.

Printed with permission: Sleisenger and Fordtran's Gastrointestinal and Liver Disease. 9th Edition. Saunders/Elsevier, Philadelphia, 2010, Figure 55-10, page 915

➢ Embryology

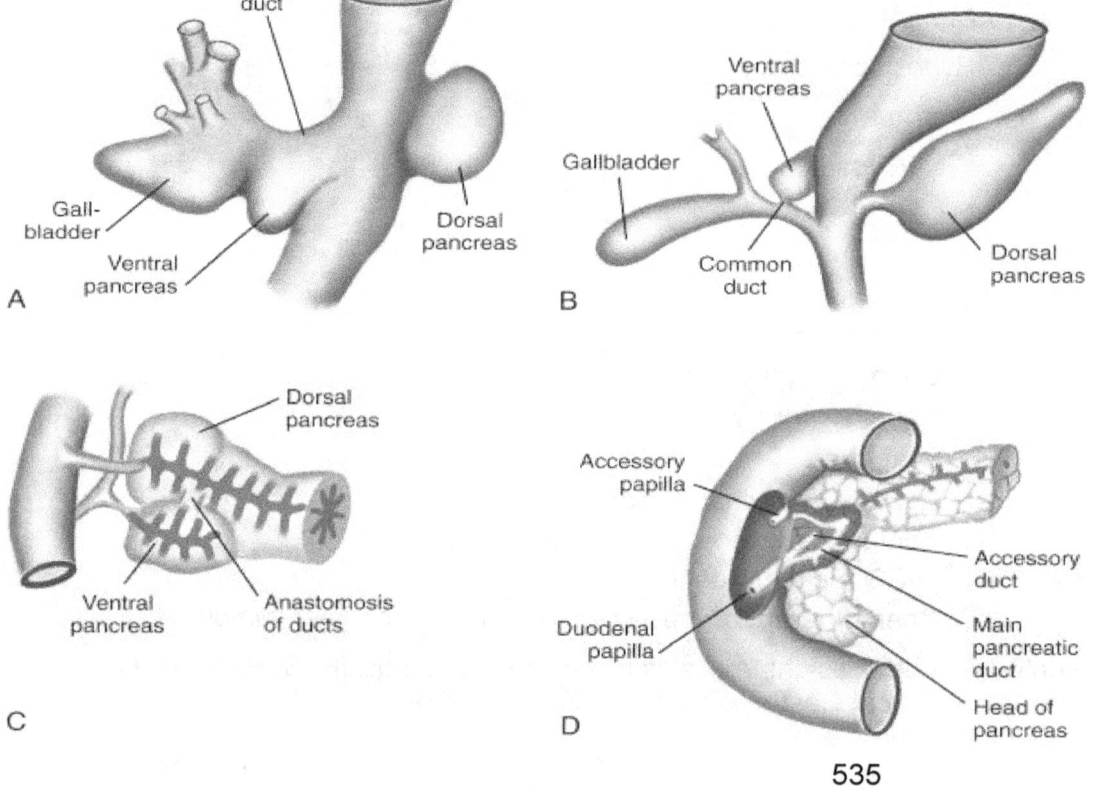

535

- ➤ Clinical (in adults)
    - ○ Pancreatitis
    - ○ Biliary obstruction

- ➤ Diagnostic imaging
    - ○ Abdominal film
        - – "double bubble" sign (from foregut obstruction)
    - ○ CT scan
        - – Enlarged head of pancreas
        - – No focal mass
    - ○ MRCP
    - ○ ERCP
        - – "ring like" pancreatic duct surrounding the duodenum plus normal pancreatic duct (failure of the normal left ventral bud of the pancreas of fully rotate during normal embryological development)
    - ○ Laparotomy

- ➤ Treatment
    - ○ Surgical duodenostomy

## Cystic Fibrosis (CF) Involving the Pancreas

- ➤ Genetics
    - ○ CFTR (Cystic Fibrosis Transmembrane Conductance Regulator)
        - – A peptide which functions as an anion channel
        - – $Cl^-$ and $HCO_3^-$ pass through this channel, causing alkaline pancreatic fluid secretion.
        - – In the pancreas, CFTR is in the apical membrane of the pancreatic duct cell.
    - ○ Regulator domains
        - – CFTR is regulated by way of three regulatory domains
            - ▪ NBD (nucleoside binding domain) 1 and 2
            - ▪ R (regulatory) domain
                - – R domain binds to cytoplasmic glutamine to stimulate $Cl^-$ secretion.
                - – $NBD_{1/2}$ binds to cytoplasmic ATP to stimulate $HCO_3^-$ secretion.
                - – The conformation of the CFTR protein changes depending upon whether it is bound to $NBD_{1/2}$.

536

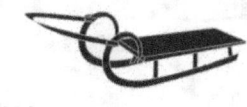

- o Second messengers
  - – Regulates $NBD_1$, $NBD_2$ and the R domain of CFTR.
  - – For CFTR, second messenger system includes
    - • ATP
    - • PKA
    - • $Ca^{2+}$
    - • Glutamate (intra-acinar cell)
  - – The second messenger system in turn is stimulated by secretin and VIP as well as Ach.
    - • Secretin/VIP → receptors →↑ cAMP → ↑ PKA (protein kinase A)-mediated phosphorylation of R domains of CFTR.
    - • Ach → ↑ $Ca_i^{2+}$ (intracellular $Ca^{2+}$)
- o Mutations
  - – Numerous genetic mutations of CFTR have been described.
  - – The commonest genetic mutation in CFTR is ΔF508, a three-base pair deletion of the phenylalanine-coding codon 508.
  - – When there are major mutations in CFTR alleles, the function of CFTR is lost.
  - – When CFTR no longer functions normally as a regulated anion channel in the apical membrane of the pancreatic duct cell, mucus is not hydrated, ducts are blocked and tissue atrophies.
- o Modifiers
  - – There may be modifier genes, or environmental factors which influence the clinical features of CF (gastric fibrosis).
  - – A modifier gene interacts with a susceptibility gene to "increase the risk of developing a pathological outcome" (Sleisenger and Fordtran's Gastrointestinal and Liver Disease. 10th Edition. Saunders/Elsevier, Philadelphia, 2010, Table 57.1, page 949).

➤ Clinical

- o Many organs are affected in CF, and vary with the nature of the genetic changes e.g., alter the impact and environmental factor on causing pancreatitis, such as alcohol damage leading to pancreatitis.
- o The clinical impact of CFR, a susceptibility gene, may also be affected by an unidentified modifier gene.

537

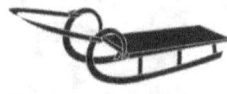

- Give GI/hepatobiliary manifestations of cystic fibrosis.
  - Esophagus
    - Gastroesophageal reflux
  - Stomach
    - Peptic ulcer disease
  - Small bowel
    - Fat malabsorption
    - Mecomium ileus
    - Ileal atresia
    - Intussusception
  - Colon
    - Volvulus
    - Distal intestinal obstruction syndrome (meconium equivalent)
    - Fecal masses
    - Constipation
    - Impaction
    - Rectal prolapse
    - Hemorrhoids
  - Peritoneum
    - Peritonitis
  - Pancreas
    - Nutritional failure caused by pancreatic insufficiency
    - Diabetes
    - Calcification
    - Maldigestion
    - Fat soluble vitamin deficiencies
    - Steatorrhea and azotorrhea
  - Gallbladder
    - Gallstones
    - Atrophic gallbladder
  - Liver
    - Hepatomegaly
    - Focal biliary cirrhosis (FBC)
    - Cirrhosis
    - Portal hypertension
    - Non-alcoholic fatty liver disease (NAFLD)
    - Premature death

538

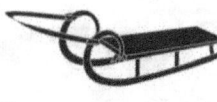

Adapted from: Sleisenger and Fordtran's Gastrointestinal and Liver Disease. 10th Edition. Saunders/Elsevier, Philadelphia, 2016, Box 57.2, page 953.

- Give **non-GI/Hepatobiliary manifestations** of cystic fibrosis in the adult.
  - Eyes
    - Venous engorgement
    - Retinal hemorrhage
  - Lungs
    - Sinusitis
    - Nasal polyposis (secondary to mucous membrane hypertrophy)
    - Lower respiratory infections
    - Bronchiectasis
    - Chronic infection with Pseudomonas aeruginosa
  - Endocrine
    - Glucose intolerance
    - Diabetes mellitus
  - GU
    - Male infertility (sterility; congenital bilateral absence of vas deferens [CBAVD]), epididymis, and seminal vessels)
    - Female infertility (increased viscosity of vaginal mucous)
  - Nutrition
    - Clubbing
    - Short stature
  - Skeletal
    - Retardation of bone age
    - Demineralization
    - Hypertrophic pulmonary osteoarthropathy
  - Other
    - Salt depletion through excessive loss of salt via the skin
    - Heat stroke
    - Hypertrophy of apocrine glands
  - Premature death

Adapted from: Sleisenger and Fordtran's Gastrointestinal and Liver Disease. 10th Edition. Saunders/Elsevier, Philadelphia, 2016, Box 57.2, page 953.

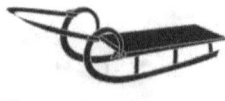

- ➢ Laboratory
  - o CF - diagnosis
    - – Sweat chloride testing
    - – Nasal bioelectrical response
    - – Rectal potential difference
    - – Genetic testing
  - o CF – complications (steatorrhea)
    - – ↓ fat soluble vitamins
- •
- ➢ Diagnostic imaging

---

## SO YOU WANT TO BE A GASTROENTEROLOGIST!

- • Give radiological features of meconium ileus / DIOS (distal intestinal obstruction syndrome).
  - o Proximal ileum
    - – Hypertrophy of wall
  - o Distal ileum
    - – Dilation, or
    - – Narrowing from inspissated meconium
  - o Bead-like appearance from pellets of meconium
  - o Air/gas
    - – Little air or air-fluid levels
    - – Bubbles of gas in meconium
  - o Colon
    - – Empty
    - – Microcolon
  - o Associated
    - – Volvulus
    - – Atresia
    - – Ascites
    - – Calcification
    - – Intussusception
    - – Rectal prolapse
    - – Cancer
      - ▪ Stomach
      - ▪ Small intestines
      - ▪ Pancreas
      - ▪ Biliary tree

540

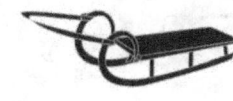

- ➢ Pathology
- • Give pathological features of the pancreas in cystic fibrosis.
  - o Inspissated secretions in ducts
  - o Blockage extends to acinar cells
  - o Epithelial flattening and atrophy
  - o Dilation of acini with calcium-rich eosinophilic concretions
  - o Pseudocysts
  - o Hyperplasia and necrosis of ductular and acinar cells
  - o Inflammation (mild, chronic)
  - o Fibrosis
  - o Calcification
  - o Late loss of islet of Langerhans (glucose intolerance is common, but CFRD [cystic fibrosis-related disease] is uncommon).

- ➢ Treatment
  - o Pancreatic enzyme supplements
    - – Enteric-coated minimicrospheres with/without gastric acid inhibition (H2RAs, PPIs)
  - o Nutritional support begins with 2 tablets with meals and adjust the dose to maintain normal growth, and correct symptoms such as steatorrhea.
    - – Calories
    - – Protein
    - – FSV (fat soluble vitamins) A, D, E, K
  - o Anti-oxidants e.g., vitamin E
  - o Manage complications
  - o Genetic consultation re family testing

- • Give the **adverse effects** of long-term use of high dose pancreatic enzyme supplements.
  - o Mouth, Anus
    - – Irritation
  - o Kidney
    - – ↑ uric acid (high purine conent of supplements) → hyperuricouria → renal calculo
  - o Colon
    - – Strictures (fibrosing colopathy)

541

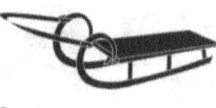

**Pancreas Divisum** (PD)

- ➢ Definition
    - o A congenital abnormality caused by: "failure of the dorsal and ventral pancreatic ducts to fuse".
    - o Most of the pancreatic secretions then drain ".......through the relatively small dorsal duct of Santorini and minor [accessory] papilla rather than the ventral duct of Wirsung and the major papilla" (Sleisenger and Fordtran's Gastrointestinal and Liver Disease. 10th Edition. Saunders/Elsevier, Philadelphia, 2016, page 931).

- ➢ Genetics
    - o CFTR gene (and at a lower level, SPINK1 and PRSS1) mutations and pancreas divisum might be cofactors associated with the occurrence of acute recurrent or chronic pancreatitis.
    - o In patients with CFTR gene mutations, pancreas divisum is found in 47%
    - o The frequency of pancreas divisum is the same in patients with idiopathic pancreatitis, chronic alcoholic pancreatitis, and in controls without any pancreatic diseases (5-7%).

- ➢ Treatment
    - o Sphincterotomy of minor papilla or placement of stent in minor (accessory) papilla may be helpful for symptoms of pancreatitis (acute or chronic), especially with pain characteristic of acute recurrent pancreatitis.
    - o Pancreas divisum controversial cause of pancreatitis ().

Source: Bertin C, et al. Am J Gastroenterol 2012; 107: 311-317.

"Setting goals is the first step in turning the invisible into the visible."

Tony Robbins

542

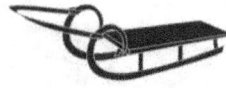

# ABBREVIATIONS

| | |
|---|---|
| AIP | Autoimmune pancreatitis |
| CCK | Cholecystokinin |
| CT | Computed tomography |
| CT | Cationic trypsinogen |
| EUS | Endoscopic ultrasound |
| FNA | Fine needle aspiration |
| HGD | High grade dysplasia |
| HPF | High power field |
| IAP | Ideopathic acute pancreatitis |
| IgG | Immunoglobulin G |
| IgG4 | Immunoglobulin G4 |
| IPMN | Intraductal pancreatic mucinous neoplasia |
| ISD | IgG4-associated systemic disease |
| LEC | Lymphoepithelial cysts |
| LGD | Low grade dysplasia |
| LPSP | Lymphoplasmacytic sclerosing pancreatitis |
| MCN | Mucinous cystic neoplasms |
| MDCT | Multidetectable CT |
| MRCP | Magnetic resonance cholangiopancreatography |
| MRI | Magnetic resonance imaging |
| NG/NJ | Nasogastric/nasojejunal |
| PD | Pancreatic duct |
| PET | Pancreatic endocrine tumour |
| PP | Pseudopapillary tumours |
| S-MRCP | MRCP with secretin |
| SOD | Sphincter of Oddi dysfunction |
| ULN | Upper limit of normal |
| US | Ultrasonography |

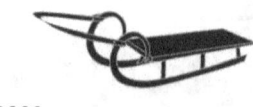

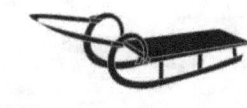

# TABLE OF CONTENTS

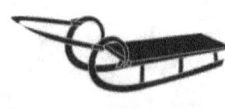

*MASTERING THE BOARDS*
*Hepatology & Pancreaticobiliary Disease*

A.B.R. Thomson

# APPETITE AND FOOD INTAKE

## Satiety Signals (Anorectic Peptides)

- Give the satiety signals arising from the GI tract.

    - Stomach, adipocytes
        - Ghrelin
        - GRP (gastrin-releasing peptide)
        - Leptin

    - Pancreas
        - Insulin
        - NPY (neuropeptide Y)
        - PP (pancreatic polypeptide)

    - Small intestine
        - APO A-IV
        - CCK (cholecystokinin)
        - GLP-1 (glucagon-like peptide 1)
        - Oxyntomodulin
        - PYY (peptide YY)

---

**SO YOU WANT TO BE A GASTROENTEROLOGIST!**

- Give an explanation of the mechanism of the effect of Apo– A IV on producing satiety.

    Apo – A IV

    - Produced in
        - Enterocytes, in response to dietary fat release PYY and NPY → ↑ enterocyte production of Apo – A IV
        - Arcuate nucleus of hypothalamus
    - Anorectic effect of Apo – A IV acts centrally

- Give GI signals which increase appetite.

    Trick question! There is only one GI peptide which stimulates appetite, ghrelin (leplin, lowers appetite; ghrelin, gain in appetite).

---

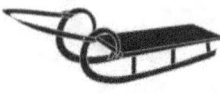

- Give the CNS networks implicated in the control of food intake.
  - Arcuate nucleus – NPY, AGRP, POMC, CART
  - Paraventricular nucleus (PVN) – CRF, TRH, GLP-I
  - Lateral hypothalamic nucleus (LVN) – MSH, Orexin A, B
  - Cortex – Anorexigenic and orexigenic pathway

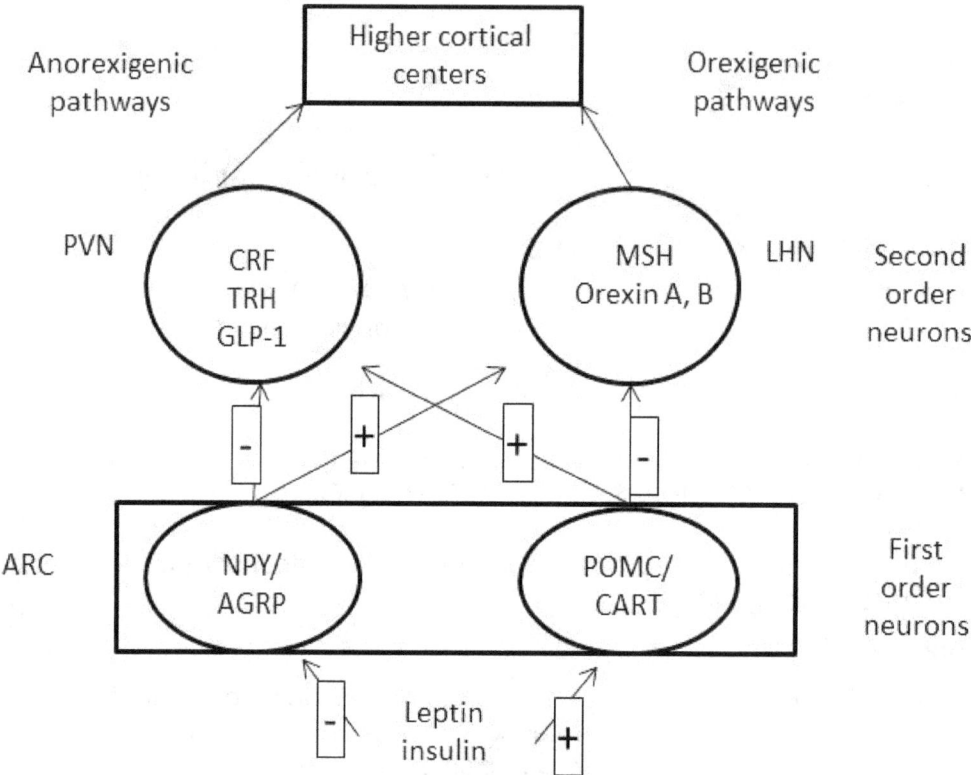

Abbreviations: AGRP, agouti-related protein; ARC, arcuate nucleus; CART, cocaine and amphetamine regulated transcript; CCK, cholecystokinin; CRF, corticotrophin releasing factor; GLP-1, glucagon-like peptide; LHN, lateral hypothalamic nucleus; MSH, melanocyte-stimulating hormone; NPY, neuropeptide Y; NS, nervous system; NTS, solitary nucleus; POMC, proopiomelanocaortin; PVN, paraventricular nucleus; PYY, peptide YY3-36; TRH, thyrotrophin-releasing hormone.

Printed with permission: Foxx-Orenstein AE. *2008 ACG Annual Postgraduate Course Book:* pg. 148.

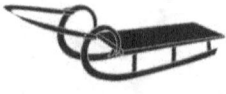

## SO YOU WANT TO BE A NUTRITIONIST!

- Give the steps in the gut-brain-liver axis which helps to maintain even levels of **blood glucose** concentration during fasting.

- ❖ Fasting
  - o ↑ TG breakdown
    - – ↑ FFA
  - o ↑ FFA
    - – ↓ insulin sensitivity
    - – ↑ insulin resistance
    - – ↓ uptake of glucose by muscle
    - – ↑ PPAR α
      - ▪ induced ER proteins
    - – FIT
      - ▪ ½ (fat inducing transcripts)
      - ▪ ½ lead to formation of hepatic lipid droplets
    - – ↑ oxidation of FFA
      - ▪ ↑ acetyl CoA
      - ▪ ↑ ketone bodies
  - o ↑ glycerol
    - – ↑ synthesis of glucose

- ❖ Feeding lipids
  - o ↑ acyl-CoA synthase mediated production of long-chain fatty acyl-coenzyme A
  - o ↑ long-chain fatty acyl-coenzyme A – signals vagal afferents to the nucleus of the solitary tract.
  - o Stimulation of the nucleus of the solitary tract increases glutamatergic neurotransmission through vagal efferents to the liver.

- ❖ Feeding carbohydrates
  - o Rapid absorption of glucose
  - o Increased glutamatergic neurotransmission from the nucleus of the solitary tract decreases hepatic glucose production, even before the ingested carbohydrate is digested and glucose absorbed from the intestine.

548

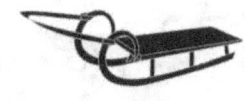

# EATING DISORDERS

- Give the diagnostic criteria for anorexia nervosa.

  o Refusal to maintain minimal normal body weight

  o Intense fear of weight gain

  o Body-image disturbance (e.g., feeling fat when emaciated)

  o Absence of three consecutive menstrual cycles

  o Specific type

    - Restricting type: Person does not regularly engage in binge eating or purging behaviour (e.g., self-induced vomiting, use of laxatives)

    - Binge-eating/purging type: Person regularly engages in eating or purging behaviour (e.g., self-induced vomiting, use of laxatives)

Printed with permission: Williamson DA, et al. *Best Practice & Research Clinical Gastroenterology* 2004; 18(6): pg 1074.

- Give the diagnostic criteria for bulimia nervosa.

  o Episodes of compulsive binge eating

  o Lack of control over eating binges

  o Use of extreme methods for controlling weight (self-induced vomiting, laxative abuse, diuretic abuse, restrictive dieting, or excessive exercise)

  o At least two binge eating episodes per week for at least 3 months

  o Obsessive overconcern with body shape, body weight, and body size

  o Specific type

    - Purging type: Person regularly engages in purging behaviour (e.g., self-induced vomiting, use of laxatives, use of diuretics, or enemas)

    - Non-purging type: Person does not engage in purging behaviour (e.g., self-induced vomiting, use of laxatives, use of diuretics, or enemas)

Note: this table was adapted from the DSM-IV diagnostic criteria for bulimia nervosa

Printed with permission: Williamson DA., et al. *Best Practice & Research Clinical Gastroenterology* 2004; 18(6): pg 1080.

The psychiatric eating disorder bulimia nervosa may be associated with the misuse of laxatives.

- Give clinical features that could confirm your suspicions of a patient's laxative abuse.

  o Vital signs

    - Hypothermia

    - Bradycardia

    - Arrhythmia

549

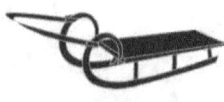

- o Hair
  - Hair loss
- o Teeth
  - Loss of dental enamel
- o Parotids
  - Large parotid glands
- o Skin
  - Dry skin
  - Languor
  - Scars or calluses on the dorsum of hand
- o Ankle
  - Pedal edema

- Give indications for the use of enteral tube feeding (ETF) in the adult patient.
  - o Protein-energy malnutrition (greater than 10% weight loss) with little or no oral intake for 5 days
  - o Less than 50% of the required oral nutrient intake for previous 7-10 days
  - o Severe dysphagia or swallowing-related difficulties, e.g., head injury, strokes, motor neuron disease
  - o Major, full-thickness burns
  - o Massive small bowel resection (in patients with 50-90% small bowel resection, ETF is given to hasten gut regeneration and return to oral intake, often in combination with parenteral nutrition)
  - o Low-output enterocutaneous fistulae* (<500 mL/day)
  - o Conditions where tube feeding would normally be helpful
    - Major trauma
    - Radiation therapy
    - Mild chemotherapy
  - o Conditions where tube feeding is of limited or undetermined value
    - Immediate postoperative period or post-stress period if an adequate oral intake will be resumed within 5-7 days
    - Acute enteritis
    - Less than 10% of the small intestine remaining (parenteral nutrition is usually indicated)
  - o Conditions/situations in which tube feeding should not be used
    - Complete mechanical intestinal obstruction
    - Ileus or intestinal hypomotility
    - Severe uncontrollable diarrhea

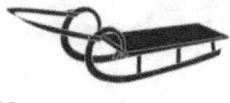

- High-output fistulae
- Severe acute pancreatitis
- Shock
- Aggressive nutritional support not desired by the patient or legal guardian, in accordance with hospital policy and existing law
- Prognosis not warranting aggressive nutritional support

*If the fistula is proximal, the feeding should be distal. If the fistula is distal, sufficient proximal length must be present to allow sufficient absorption. Fistuale due to malignancy, radiation and distal obstruction are unlikely to close spontaneously

Printed with permission: Stratton RJ, and Smith TR. *Best Practice & Research Clinical Gastroenterology* 2006; 20(3): pg. 457.

➢ Complications

- Give **complications** of enteral tube feeding (ETF).
    - o Mechanical
        - – Tube blockage by feed or tube kinking
        - – Tube malposition (e.g., into trachea)
        - – Insertion trauma
        - – *Nasogastric* damage to nasal septum, esophagus, stomach, perforation (rare)
        - – *Gastrostomy/enterostomy* damage to stomach, small bowel, bleeding, peritonitis, leakage, irritation and infection around site
        - – Loss of tube into GI tract
    - o Feed/flow related
        - – Diarrhea or constipation, bloating, cramps
        - – Aspiration pneumonia/regurgitation
    - o Metabolic
        - – Fluid and electrolyte disturbances
        - – Hypo- and hyper-natremia, kalemia, phosphatemia, glycemia
    - o Infections
        - – Infection around ostomy site
        - – Infection of feed or administration set (very rare if commercial feed and set used according to guidelines)
    - o Organ dysfunction
        - – Aspiration pneumonia may precipitate respiratory distress
    - o Psychological
        - – Effects on self-image
        - – Anxiety and depression
        - – Social isolation (if unable to eat, if confined to bed/home)

Printed with permission: Stratton RJ, and Smith TR. *Best Practice & Research Clinical Gastroenterology* 2006; 20(3): pg. 459.

551

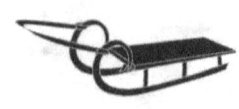

# MALNUTRITION

- o Normal values
    - – Basal energy expenditure approximately 0.8 kcal/min, or 1150 kcal/day
    - – Recommended daily energy intake, ~ 22 to 25 kcal/kg.
- ➢ Assessment
- • Give methods of nutritional assessment.
    - o Subjective global assessment
        - – History
            - ▪ Changes in weight (< 90% IBW [ideal body weight])
            - ▪ Changes in dietary intake
            - ▪ Gastrointestinal symptoms
            - ▪ Functional capacity
            - ▪ Stress of disease
        - – Physical examination
            - ▪ Loss of subcutaneous fat
            - ▪ Muscle wasting: deltoids, quadriceps, biceps, supra/subscapular muscles
            - ▪ Edema: ankles, sacrum, ascites
            - ▪ Skin rashes
            - ▪ Eye changes
            - ▪ Neurological changes
        - – Indirect calorimetry

- ➢ Classification
    - o Well nourished
        - – No history or physical findings of malnutrition
    - o Moderately malnourished
        - – Weight loss 5-10% of usual body weight (UBW)
        - – Mild signs of malnutrition
    - o Severely malnourished
        - – Weight loss 10% of UBW
        - – Severe signs of malnutrition

- ➢ Laboratory
    - o Albumin, pre-albumin, transferrin, retinol-binding protein, lymphocyte count, WBC
        - – 24-hour urinary urea nitrogen, nitrogen balance
        - – Creatinine-height index
        - – Delayed cutaneous hypersensitivity
        - – Muscle function

552

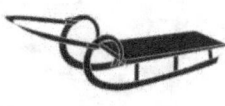

- o Anthropometric measurements
  - – Height, weight, ideal body weight, usual body weight, BMI
  - – Weight as percent IBW or UBW; % weight loss
  - – Triceps skinfold thickness, mid-arm circumference, and others
- o Techniques to assess body composition
- o Bio-impedance
- o Imaging: DEXA scan (bone density) and CT scan
- o Dilution radioisotope methods, whole body counting (total body $K^+$)

Abbreviations: BMI, body mass index ($kg/m^2$); IBW, ideal body weight; UBW, usual body weight

Adapted from: Sleisenger and Fordtran's Gastrointestinal and Liver Disease. 10th Edition. Saunders/Elsevier, Philadelphia, 2016, page 76-80.

➤ Causes/associations

• Give a classification of the causes of malnutrition, and indicate how these can be suspected from a directed history.

| Etiologies | History |
| --- | --- |
| o Decreased diet intake and decreased assimilation | – Unintentional weight loss >10% body wt<br>– Decreased food intake<br>  ▪ Socioeconomic<br>  ▪ Anorexia<br>  ▪ Self-restricted diets e.g., alcoholism |
| o Increased metabolism<br>  – Critical acute illness<br>  – Chronic inflammation | ▪ Critical illness<br>▪ Gastrointestinal symptoms<br>  – Dysphagia<br>  – Nausea/vomiting<br>  – Chronic diarrhea<br>  – Abdominal pain (sitophobia [fear of eating]) |
| o Increased losses | – Chronic diarrhea, vomiting |
| o Mixed metabolic abnormality | – HIV/AIDS<br>– Cancer<br>– Chronic liver disease<br>– Heart failure<br>– COPD<br>– Chronic infection(e.g., TB) |

Printed with permission: Alberda C, et al. *Best Practice & Research Clinical Gastroenterology* 2006; 20(3): pg.427.

# INCREASED BODY MASS INDEX/OBESITY

➤ Definition

- Give a definition of adult obesity, and state the effect on the risk of comorbidities.

| Classification | BMI (kg/m$^2$) | Risk of Comorbidities |
|---|---|---|
| o Normal range | 18.5-24.9 | Average |
| o Overweight | $\geq$ 25.0 | |
| o Preobesity | 25.0-29.9 | Increased |
| o Obesity class I | 30.00-34.9 | Moderate |
| o Obesity class II | 35.00-39.9 | Severe |
| o Obesity class III | $\geq$ 40.0 | Very severe |

Abbreviations: BMI, body mass index

Printed with permission: Formiguera X, and Canton A. *Best Practice & Research Clinical Gastroenterology* 2004; 18(6): pg 1126.

- o Optimal waist circumference
  - – Women   < 35 inches / 88 cm
  - – Men   < 40 inches / 102 cm
- o BMI (wt (kg) / height (m$^2$))

| Definition | BMI, kg/m$^2$ |
|---|---|
| – Normal | < 25 |
| – Overweight | 25 – 29.9 |
| – Obese | $\geq$ 30 |
| – Severe obesity | $\geq$ 40 (or > 35 plus comorbidities) |

➤ Demography

- o Increased body mass index (BMI) above 25 kg/m$^2$ is seen in about two thirds of Americans, and of these one third have a BMI > 30 kg/m$^2$.

- o Obesity is associated with many morbidities such as diabetes mellitus, systemic hypertension, musculoskeletal problems, and fatty liver disease (simple steatosis, non-alcoholic steatohepatitis).

554

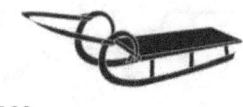

> Diagnosis

- Give the diagnostic criteria for the "**Metabolic Syndrome**".

| Risk Factor | | Abnormal Level |
|---|---|---|
| o Waist circumference | – Men<br>– Women | >102 cm<br>>88 cm |
| o Fasting blood glucose | | ≥100 mg/dl |
| o Serum triglyceride | | ≥ 150 mg/dl, or under treatment with fibrates |
| o Serum HDL cholesterol | - Men<br>- Women | <40 mg/dl<br><50 mg/dl |
| o Arterial blood pressure | | ≥ 130/ ≥85 mmHg, or under pharmacologic treatment |

Abbreviations: DBP, diastolic blood pressure; SBP, systolic blood pressure

Printed with permission: Cortez-Pinto H, and Camilo ME. *Best Practice & Research Clinical Gastroenterology* 2004;18(6): pg 1092.

> Complications

- Give GI/liver complications of obesity.
    - o Esophagus - GERD, Barrett esophagus, adenocarcinoma
    - o Stomach – Retention, adenoma carcinoma, gastric cardia cancer
    - o Colon – Hemorrhoids, diverticulosis, colorectal cancer (CRC), non-specific abdominal pain
    - o Liver (NAFLD, SS/NASH), cirrhosis, hepatocellular cancer (HCC)
    - o Pancreas – Pancreatitis, cancer
    - o Gallbladder – Stones, cancer

Abbreviations: NAFLD, non-alcoholic fatty liver disease; NASH, non-alcoholic steatohepatitis; SS, simple steatosis

Printed with permission: Freeman HJ. *Best Practice & Research Clinical Gastroenterology* 2004; 18(6): 1169.

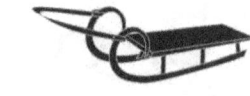

- Give **complications** of obesity.

Obesity and triglyceride-derived toxic lipid metabolites accumulate in ectopic tissues and lead to multiorgan dysfunction, T2DM and CVD.

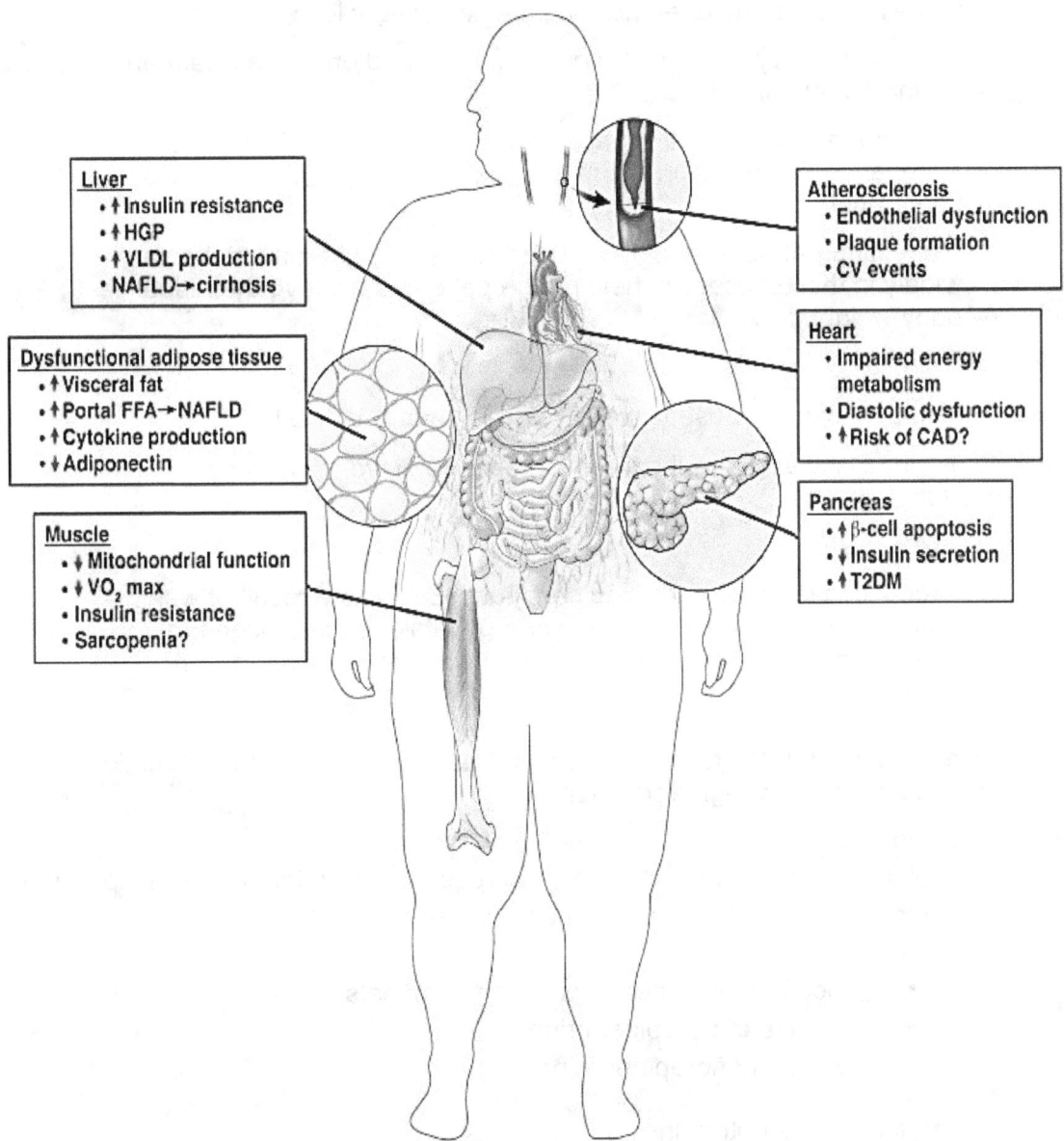

**Liver**
- ↑ Insulin resistance
- ↑ HGP
- ↑ VLDL production
- NAFLD→cirrhosis

**Dysfunctional adipose tissue**
- ↑ Visceral fat
- ↑ Portal FFA→NAFLD
- ↑ Cytokine production
- ↓ Adiponectin

**Muscle**
- ↓ Mitochondrial function
- ↓ VO$_2$ max
- Insulin resistance
- Sarcopenia?

**Atherosclerosis**
- Endothelial dysfunction
- Plaque formation
- CV events

**Heart**
- Impaired energy metabolism
- Diastolic dysfunction
- ↑ Risk of CAD?

**Pancreas**
- ↑ β-cell apoptosis
- ↓ Insulin secretion
- ↑ T2DM

  - Morbidity (BMI > 40 kg/m$^2$) reduces life expectancy.

Printed with permission: Cusi K. Gastroenterology. 2012;142(4):711-725.

> Treatment

- o The only effective treatment is long-term reduced calorie intake, in conjunction, in selected patients, with bariatric surgery

- o Drug used to reduce appetite or to produce a mild malabsorption lead to very modest and often non-maintained weight loss.

- o Bariatric surgery remains the only effective and enduring treatment for morbid obesity.

- o Because physicians will increasingly be caring for patients who experience complications from their bariatric surgery, this topic is important to consider.

- o Many different approaches are used to lose weight, and these vary widely in their success in helping the patient to achieve their ideal body weight.

Maintaining achieved purposeful weight loss is usually difficult.

- Give processes which make the maintenance of weight loss so challenging.

  - o Recidivism

  - o Reduction in basal energy expenditure (BEE) as a result of weight loss, requiring an even further ↓energy intake even though the ideal body weight has been achieved with the initial short-term dieting.

- Give classes of drugs to treat obesity in addition to behavior modification (diet, exercise) for weight reduction.

  - o Sympathomimetric
    - Noradrenergic sympathomimetic drugs, phentermine and diethylpropion
    - Only approach for short-term use (no more than 3 months)
    - ↑ satiety
      - ▪ ↓ food intake by acting on nerve terminals
      - ▪ ↑ release of norepinephrine
      - ▪ ↓ uptake of norepinephrine

  - o Serotonergic (sibutramine)
    - Blocks orexigenic and stimulates anorexigenic systems
    - Serotonin agonist (lorcaserin)
    - Selective agonist of serotonin 2C receptor → ↓ food intake

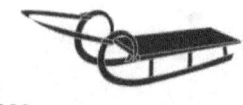

- 10 mg po bid provided
  - % of persons losing ≥ 5% of baseline weight in 1 year:
    - Lor  47.5
    - PL  20.3%
    - TG  ~20%
  - % of persons maintaining weight loss in second year:
    - Lor  67.9%
    - PL  50.3%
    - TG  ~18%
- TG in terms of weight loss ~ 3 kg to 4 kg/year
  - ↓ SBP/DBP, HR, total/LDL cholesterol, CRP, fibrinogen, fasting glucose and insulin concentrations in blood
- Because lorcaserin is a selective agonist of the serotonin 2 C receptor, rather than the 2B serotonin receptor, there should be no lorcaserin-associated cardiac valvular disease (such as was seen with fenfluramine).

o Pancreatic lipase inhibition
  - Orlistat (Xenical®)

Abbreviations: CRP, C-reactive protein; DB, diastolic blood pressure; Lor, lorcaserin; PL, placebo; SBP, systolic blood pressure; TG, therapeutic gain


➢ Pharmacology

o Inhibits activity of pancreatic lipase

o 120 mg po tid, continued loss of weight at one year, as % of initial body weight

| | |
|---|---|
| – "placebo" (lifestyle changes) | 5.5 to 6.6 |
| – Orlistat plus lifestyle changes | 8.5 to 10.2 |
| – Therapeutic gain | 1.9 to 4.7 |

➢ Adverse effects

o GI
  - Nausea
  - Fatty/oily stools/spotting 12-48 hours after a high fat meal
  - Increased defecation frequency
  - Liquid stools
  - Fecal urgency
  - Flatulence
  - Flatus with fecal discharge
  - Fecal incontinence

558

- o  Nutrition  –  ↓ absorption of fat soluble vitamins A, D, E
  –  ↓ weight
- o  Liver  –  Uncertain association of liver injury
  –  $3 / 10^5$ orlistat users
- o  Kidney  –  Oxalate-induced acute renal injury

- Give the mechanisms of the development of acute oxalate-induced renal injury in persons taking orlistat.
  - o  Orlistat → ↓ digestion of TG → ↑ TG in stool → ↑ binding of $Ca^{2+}$ - less $Ca^{2+}$ -oxalate and ↑ luminal oxalate - ↑ absorption of oxalate → ↑ oxalate excretion by kidney, with ↑ deposition of oxalate in renal parenchyma
  - o  Note: $Ca^{2+}$ - oxalate in the lumen of the intestine requires the fatty acids (Fas) removed from dietary TG (triglyceride), in order for the luminal $Ca^{2+}$ to become bound to FAs ($Ca^{2+}$ - FA), then for the oxalate to be absorbed by the intestine, and excreted into the urine.

- Endocannaboids: CB-1 antagonists
  - o  Clinically meaningful weight loss is off-set by psychiatric AEs
  - o  Not approved for use

- Anti-depressants
  - o  Bupropion
    - –  SR 300-400 mg/day
    - –  Especially useful for prevention of weight gain when smokers stop smoking
    - –  Alters the metabolism of norepinephrine
  - o  Fluoxetine
    - –  60 mg po per day
    - –  SSRI (selective serotonin reuptake inhibitor)

- Diabetes – Treating drugs
  - o  Metformin
    - –  ↓ hepatic glucose production
    - –  ↑ insulin sensitization in peripheral tissue
    - –  ↑ anorexic effect

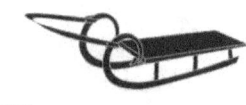

- o Metformin very modest weight loss when used or prevention of diabetes (~2.5% of initial body weight)
- o Other oral diabetic drugs give only minimum weight loss

- **GLP-1 mimetic**
  - o ↑ glucose-dependent insulin secretion
  - o ↓ appetite
  - o Slows gastric emptying

- **Others (not established)**
  - o Anti-epileptics
  - o NPY antagonists
  - o Anti-ghrelin agents
  - o GH (growth hormone) fragment
  - o Dietary supplements

Adapted from: Palamara KL, et al. *Cardiol Rev* 2006;14(5):238-58.


## MICRONUTRIENTS DEFICIENCIES

- Give the principle causes of micronutrient deficiencies.

| | | |
|---|---|---|
| o Reduced intake | – | Sitophobia |
| | – | Complicated meals |
| | – | Underlying disease (tumour) |
| o Impaired absorption | – | Rapid emptying |
| | – | Poor mixing of food and duodenal juice |
| | – | Pancreaticocibal asynchrony |
| | – | Bacterial overgrowth |
| | – | Rapid transit |
| o Disturbed distribution/metabolism | – | Enterohepatic circulation ↓ |
| | – | Enteropancreatic circulation ↓ |
| | – | Micronutrient interactions |
| o Increased loss | – | Occult bleeding |
| | – | Disturbed protein binding |
| | – | Increased renal elimination |

Printed with permission: Schölmerich J. *Best Practice & Research Clinical Gastroenterology* 2004; 18(5): pg.917-933.

Clinical Pearl / Gem:

- o In patients with diarrhea and skin rash (vesicular pustular plagues, red, scaling) on face and leg, think of Zn (zinc) deficiency.

---

Clinical caution:

- o Vitamin E deficiency is common in patients with cirrhosis (cholestasis → ↓ absorption of fat soluble vitamins → vitamin E deficiency
- o The neurological signs of vitamin E deficiency are similar to those of HE (hepatic encephalopathy).
- o Don't confuse the two; when in doubt, give vitamin E (tocopherol 1000 IU per day) to the patient with HE.

- Give the neurological signs which suggests vitamin E deficiency.
  - o Ataxia
  - o Gait abnormalities
  - o Hyporeflexia
  - o Peripheral neuropathy

- Give the ocular signs of vitamin A (retinol) deficiency.
  - o Eyes
    - Night blindness
    - Dry eyes (xerophthalmia)
    - Corneal xerosis
    - Conjunctival xerosis

"Success isn't something that just happens – success is learned, success is practiced and then it is shared."

Sparky Anderson

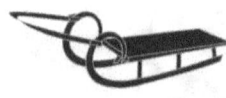

# REACTIONS TO FOOD

- ❖ Immunological
  - o Skin
    - – Immediate gastrointestinal hypersensitivity
    - – Oral allergy syndrome
    - – Acute urticaria
    - – Atopic dermatitis
    - – Acute angioedema
  - o Lung
    - – Acute bronchospasm
    - – Asthma
  - o Gut
    - - Esophagus
      - ▪ Eosinophillic esophagitis
    - - Small bowel
      - ▪ Celiac disease
      - ▪ Dermatitis herpetiformis (DH)
      - ▪ Cow's milk enteropathy
      - ▪ Food protein-induced enterocolitis
    - - Food protein-induced proctocolitis or proctitis
    - - Eosinophilic gastroenteritis

- ❖ Non-immmunological
- • Give non-immunological adverse reactions to food or food additives.
  - o Allergic eosinophilic gastroenteritis
  - o Eosinophilic esophagitis
  - o Food intolerance (non-immune mechanisms)
  - o Food protein-induced enterocolitis syndromes
  - o Food toxicity or food poisoning
  - o Idiosyncratic reactions
  - o Metabolic reactions
  - o Pharmacological reactions
  - o Physiological reactions
  - o Psychological reactions

Adapted from: Sleisenger and Fordtran's Gastrointestinal and Liver Disease. 10th Edition. Saunders/Elsevier, Philadelphia, 2016, Box 10.2, page 151; Box 10.3, page 152; Table 10.2, page 157.

➢ Treatment

- Give a management approach to the patient with suspected food allergies as a cause of GI symptoms.
  - o Establish foods and food additives that reproducibly cause symptoms
    - Careful history, including diet history
    - Elimination diet
    - Skin testing and/or RAST
    - Consider IgG testing
    - Food antigen challenge
  - o Exclude and manage other disorders that may mimic GI food allergy
  - o Initiate treatment for food allergies
    - Elimination diet
    - Avoidance of specific foods
    - Medications for after accidental exposure (antihistamines, epinephrine, corticosteroids)
    - Preventive measures (oral cromoglycate, avoid co-precipitating factors, e.g., medications)
    - Education about hidden sources of antigens and cross-reacting foods

Adapted from: Ferreira CT, and Seidman E. *J Pediatr* (Rio J) 2007;83(1):7-20.

"Attitude is a little thing that makes a big difference."

Winston Churchill

563

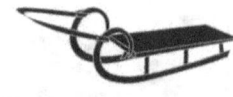

# ABBREVIATIONS

| | |
|---|---|
| AGRP | Agouti-related protein |
| ARC | Arcuate nucleus |
| BMI | Body mass index |
| CART | Cocaine and amphetamine regulated transcript |
| CCK | Cholecystokinin |
| CNS | Central nervous system |
| COPD | Chronic obstructive pulmonary disease |
| CRF | Corticotrophin releasing factor |
| GLP-1 | Glucagon-like peptide |
| IBW | Ideal bodyweight |
| LHA | Lateral hypothalamic area |
| LHN | Lateral hypothalamic nucleus |
| MSH | Melanocyte-stimulating hormone |
| NPY | Neuropeptide Y |
| NAFLD | Non-alcoholic fatty liver disease |
| NASH | Non-alcoholic steatohepatitis |
| NPY | Neuropeptide Y |
| NS | Nervous system |
| NTS | Solitary nucleus |
| POMC | Proopiomelanocortin |
| PVN | Paraventricular nucleus |
| PYY | Peptide YY3-36 |
| SS | Simple steatosis |
| TRH | Thyrotrophin-releasing hormone |
| UBW | Usual body weight |

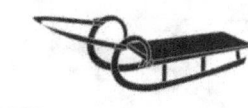

# MISCELLANEOUS

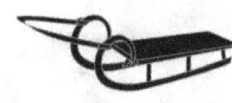

# TABLE OF CONTENTS

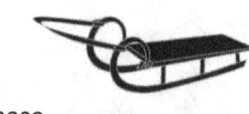

*MASTERING THE BOARDS*
*Hepatology & Pancreaticobiliary Disease*

A.B.R. Thomson

# GI THERAPY AND PREGNANCY

- For the following GI conditions, give the medications for a pregnant women to avoid during attempts to become pregnant.
  - Nausea/vomiting
    - Cisapride
  - Dyspepsia, GERD
    - Sodium bicarbonate
    - Omeprazole
    - Bismuth subsalicyclate (for *H. pylori* eradication)
    - Misoprostol ($PGE_2$)
  - EGD/colonoscopy
    - Avoid EGD in first trimester (T1) (because you can't monitor the fetus)
    - Full colonoscopy rarely indicated
    - Avoid diazepam, propofol in T1 (for sedation)
  - Liver disease
    - Interferon
    - Ribavirin
    - B blockers
    - Penicillamine
  - Liver transplant
    - Mycophenolate
    - Sirolimus
  - Constipation
    - Castor oil
    - Mineral oil
    - Tegaserod
  - Diarrhea
    - Kaopectate
    - Alosetron
  - IBD
    - Methotrexate
    - Ciprofloxacin
  - IBS
    - Amitriptyline
    - Nortriptyline
    - Imipramine
    - SSRIs
    - Bismuth

Adapted from: Kane S. *AGA Institute 2007 Spring Post Graduate Course Syllabus* pg. 511-513.

568

## MICROBIOLOGY

- Give the advantages and disadvantages of common microbiological techniques.

| Technique | Method | Advantage | Disadvantage |
|---|---|---|---|
| ○ Culture | - Bacteria grown on selective mediums | ▪ Cheap, widely available, and easy to use | - Grossly underestimates fecal populations |
| ○ PCR-T/DGGE denaturing/temperature gradient gel electrophoresis | - Using either temperature or a denaturing agent to separate DNA strands, which are then run on a gel | ▪ Very useful in detecting difference in bacterial populations | - Does not identify bacteria unless bands on the gel are cut and sequenced |
| ○ FISH (fluorescent *in situ* hybridization) | - Oligonucleotide probes designed to hybridize with specific species | ▪ Allows spatial organization of microbiota to be studied | - Slow, will only detect the bacteria probed for |
| ○ Quantitative PCR | - Specific primers detect either individual species or genus | ▪ Can detect small number of bacteria and quantify them | - Laborious |
| ○ 16S rDNA sequencing | - Bacterial DNA isolated and ribosomal DNA cloned and then sequenced | ▪ Enormous quantities of data at individual species level | - Very costly, available in only a few specialist centres |

Printed with permission: Parkes GC, et al. *AJG* 2008;103: pg. 1561.

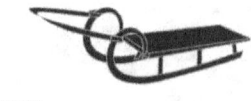

569

# HIV/AIDS

- Pathophysiology: Mechanisms of HIV transmission into the gastrointestinal tract.
  - Once released from the basal surface of the epithelial cell, HIV-1 infects CCR5+ lymphocytes in the lamina propria.
  - Virus efficienctly replicates in activated CD4+ T cells of the lamina propria.
  - The distribution of HIV coreceptors within the mucosa may also permit infection of cells central to antigen presentation such as macrophages and dendritic cells.
  - Dendritic cells of the lamina propria express C type lectin that traps the virus and assists in the dissemination of HIV-1 from the gastrointestinal tract to secondary lymphoid organs.
  - After 2 weeks of infection T cell death occur by cell lysis apoptosis and by cytotoxic lymphocytes, resulting in rapid depletion of lamina propria CD4+ T cells.

Abbreviation: CCR, CC-chemokine receptors

Source: Siew C. Ng & Brian Gazzard. *Nat Rev Gastroenterol. Hepato* 2009;6:592-607, page 594.

- Clinical
- Give liver diseases/conditions which occur even in  in HIV-infected persons.
  - HCV (coinfection in 25%) - faster development of fibrosis, poorer response to HCV treatment
  - HBV, HBV-associated ↑ mortality
  - Alcohol liver disease (associated lifestyle)
  - NAFLD (fat redistribution from HAART [ lipodystrophy]))
  - Cholangiopathy (intra- and extra-hepatic)
  - Asymptomatic ↑ in transaminases, alkaline phosphatase
  - Kaposi sarcoma
  - Opportunistic infection
    - Cholangiopathy: mycobacterium
    - Fungal: cryptological, histological, coccidiomycosis, extra pulmonary pneumacystitis carcinoma
  - Nodular regenerative hyperplasia (vasculopathy)

Adapted from: Sleisenger and Fordtran's Gastrointestinal and Liver Disease. 10th Edition. Saunders/Elsevier, Philadelphia, 2016, Box 34.6, page 551.

570

- Give non-hepatic gastrointestinal manifestations of HIV infected persons.
  - Upper gastrointestinal tract
    - Esophagitis
    - Esophageal ulcers (eg caused by cytomegalovirus or candida spp.
  - Small intestine and colon
    - HIV associated enteropathy
    - HIV associated diarrhea
  - Anorectal
    - Non-specific proctitis
    - Anal fistula and/or abscess and/or fissure
    - Rectal ulcers
    - Weight loss and wasting

Printed with permission: Siew C. Ng & Brian Gazzard. *Nat Rev Gastroenterol Hepato* 2009;6:592-607: page 595

- Give causes of **abdominal pain** in patients with HIV/AIDS, not including non-AIDS specific conditions.

| Organ | Causes |
|-------|--------|
| ○ Stomach | |
|    – Gastritis | ▪ CMV<br>▪ Cryptosporidia |
|    – Focal ulcer | ▪ Proteinuria<br>▪ CMV<br>▪ PUD |
|    – Outlet obstruction | ▪ Cryptosporidia<br>▪ CMV<br>▪ Lymphoma<br>▪ PUD |
|    – Mass | ▪ Lymphoma<br>▪ KS<br>▪ CMV |
| ○ Small bowel | |
|    – Enteritis | ▪ Proteinuria<br>▪ Cryptosporidia<br>▪ CMV<br>▪ MAC |
|    – Obstruction | ▪ Lymphoma<br>▪ KS |
|    – Perforation | ▪ CMV<br>▪ Lymphoma |

571

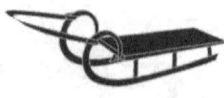

| Organ | Causes |
|---|---|
| o Colon | |
| – Colitis | ▪ Proteinuria |
| | ▪ CMV |
| | ▪ Enteric bacteria |
| | ▪ HSV |
| – Obstruction | ▪ Proteinuria |
| | ▪ Lymphoma |
| | ▪ KS |
| | ▪ Intussusception |
| – Perforation | ▪ CMV |
| | ▪ Lymphoma |
| | ▪ HSV |
| – Appendicitis | ▪ KS |
| | ▪ Cryptosporidia |
| | ▪ CMV |
| o Liver, spleen | |
| – Infiltration | ▪ Proteinuria |
| | ▪ Lymphoma |
| | ▪ CMV |
| | ▪ MAC |
| o Biliary tract | |
| – Cholecystitis | ▪ Proteinuria |
| | ▪ CMV |
| | ▪ Cryptosporidia |
| | ▪ Microsporidia |
| – Papillary stenosis | ▪ CMV |
| | ▪ Cryptosporidia |
| | ▪ KS |
| – Cholangitis | ▪ CMV |
| o Pancreas | |
| – Pancreatitis | ▪ CMV |
| | ▪ KS |
| | ▪ Pentamidine |
| | ▪ Ddl |
| – Tumour | ▪ Lymphoma |
| | ▪ KS |

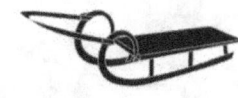

| Organ | Causes |
|---|---|

- o Mesentery, peritoneum
  - – Infiltration
    - MAC
    - Cryptococcus spp.
    - Istoplasmosis
    - Tuberculosis
    - Coccidioidomycosis
    - Toxoplasmosis
    - KS
    - Lymphoma

Abbreviations: AIDS, acquired immunodeficiency syndrome; CMV, cytomegalovirus; ddl, didanosine; HSV, herpes simplex virus; KS, Kaposi sarcoma; MAC, Mycobacterium avium complex; PUD, peptic ulcer disease

## ABDOMINAL PAIN

- Give unusual causes of abdominal pain.
  - o Epiploic appendicitis
    - – Inflamed fat tags on anti-mesenteric border of colon
    - – CT scan changes
      - Focal, oval of fat on anti-mesenteric side of colon (often on left side)
      - Inflammatory stranding
      - Penetrating vein → thrombosed → linear central attenuating line
  - o FMF (familial Mediterranean fever)
    - – Defect in FMF gene on chromosome 16 → abnormal pyrin → ↑ IL-1β → inflammation
    - – Inflammation of
      - Peritoneum
      - Pleura
      - Arthritis
      - Skin (cellulitis-mimicking)
    - – Family history
    - – May be triggered by exercise

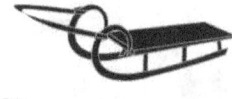

- Give the feature which raise suspicion for familial Mediteranean fever (FMF).
  - "Mediterranean origin" (Italy, Greece, Turkey, Middle East)
  - Family history
    - Acute abdomen
    - Pleurisy
    - Arthritis
    - Skin rash
    - Amyloidosis
  - Laboratory
    - ↑ ESR
  - Treatment
    - Colchicine prophylaxis
    - Avoid surgery

- Give causes of **RUQ pain**.
  - Peptic ulcer disease (gastric or duodenal ulcer)
  - Pancreatitis
  - Hepatitis
  - Cholecystitis
  - Renal colic
  - Pneumonia/pleurisy
  - Empyema/pericarditis
  - Coronary artery disease

- Give four '**red flag**' situations that indicate that surgery is necessary in the patient with an **acute abdomen**.
  - Progressive abdominal distension
  - Tender abdominal mass with fever and hypotension (abscess)
  - Septicemia plus abdominal findings
  - Suspected bowel ischemia (acidosis, fever, tachycardia)
  - Deterioration of patient while on conservative treatment

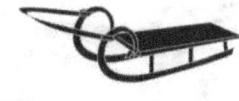

## GUM HYPERTROPHY

- Give causes of gum hypertrophy.

  - Gingivitis (e.g., from smoking, calculus, plaque, Vincent's angina (fusobacterial membranous tonsillitis)

  - Drugs

  - Phenytoin

  - Pregnancy

  - Scurvy (vitamin C deficiency: the gums become spongy, red, bleed easily and are swollen and irregular)

  - Leukemia (usually monocytic)

Adapted from: Talley NJ and O'Connor S. 4th ed. Oxford. *Blackwell Science* 2001 .

## HALITOSIS

- Give non-dental causes of halitosis.

  - Infection
    - Poor oral hygiene
    - Putrid (due to anaerobic chest infections with large amounts of sputum)

  - Metabolic
    - Fetor hepaticus (a sweet smell)
    - Ketosis (diabetic ketoacidosis results in excretion of ketones in exhaled air, causing a sickly sweet smell)
    - Uremia (fish breath: an ammoniacal odour)

  - Drugs
    - Alcohol (distinctive)
    - Paraldehyde
    - Cigarettes, tobacco

Adapted from: Talley NJ and O'Connor S. 4th ed. Oxford. *Blackwell Science* 2001.

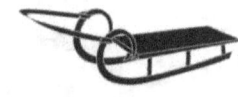

# MULTISYSTEM DISORDERS

- Give conditions which may affect every organ system, including the GI tract.

    o Infection
    - AIDS/HIV
    - Coccidiomycosis
    - Syphilis
    - Tuberculosis
    - Whipple disease

    o MSK
    - Amyloidosis
    - Lupus
    - Sarcoidosis

- Give when to suspect secondary amyloidosis of GI tract / liver.

    o Secondary (reactive, such as GI/liver) AA amyloid fibrils (Primary AL amyloid)
    - CVS
        - Restrictive cardiomyopathy
        - Heart failure (HF)
    - CNS/PNS
        - Peripheral neuropathy
    - Kidney
        - Proteinuria
        - Nephrotic syndrome
    - GI
        - Gastroparesis
        - Diarrhea
        - Bleeding (vascular friability → mucosal erosions)
    - Liver (diffuse process)
        - Hepatomegaly
        - Ascites
        - AP >> ALP

    o MSK
    - Adult Still disease
    - Ankylosing spondylitis
    - Juvenile idiopathic arthritis
    - Psoriatic arthropathy
    - Rheumatoid arthritis

576

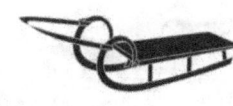

- o Chronic infections
  - − Bronchiectasis
  - − Osteomyelitis
  - − Tuberculosis
  - − Skin abscesses (usually from injected drug abuse)
- o Immunodeficiency states
  - − Common variable immunodeficiency
  - − HIV or AIDS
- o Hereditary periodic fevers
  - − Familial Mediterranean fever (FNF)
  - − Hyperimmunoglobulin D syndrome
  - − Muckle Wells syndrome
  - − TNF receptor-associated periodic syndrome
- o IBD
  - − Crohn disease
  - − Ulcerative colitis
- o Neoplasia
  - − Castleman disease
  - − Renal cell carcinoma
  - − Adenocarcinoma of the lung, gut, and urogenital tract
- o Systemic vasculitis
  - − Behcet disease
  - − Systemic lupus erythematosus

Printed with permission: Prayman T. et al. *Nature Reviews, Gastroenterology and Hepatology* 2009;6:608-617, Box 1:page 611.

---

MCQ Alert: Congo red deposits in submucosal blood vessels, staning green with polarized light
- − Think reactive (AA) amyloidosis

---

577

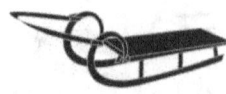

> Treatment

| Disease | Aim of Treatment | Example of Treatment |
|---------|------------------|----------------------|
| ○ AA amyloidosis | - ↓ acute phase response<br>- ↓ production of serum amyloid A protein | ▪ Anti-inflammatory and immunosuppressive therapy in patients with rheumatoid arthritis and Crohn disease (e.g., anti TNF antibodies) Colchicine for patients with Familial Mediterranean fever<br>▪ Surgery for patients with osteomyelitis and rare cytokine producing tumours |
| ○ AL amyloidosis | - Suppress production of monoclonal immunoglobulin light chains | ▪ Ascites |
| ○ Hereditary amylodosis | - Eliminate source of genetically variant protein | ▪ Orthotopic liver transplantation for patients with familial amyloid polyneuropathy |
| ○ B2 microglobulin amyloidosis | - Reduce plasma concentration of B2 microglobulin | ▪ Renal transplantation |

Printed with permission: Macmillan Publishers Ltd: Prayman T. et al. *Nature Reviews, Gastroenterology and Hepatology* 2009;6:608-617, Table 2: page 614

"Courage is what it takes to stand up and speak; courage is also what it takes to sit down and listen."

Winston Churchill

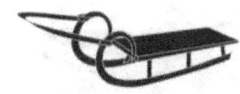

*MASTERING THE BOARDS*
*Hepatology & Pancreaticobiliary Disease*

A.B.R. Thomson

## NAILS

- Give conditions of causing alteration in the normal appearance of the nails of the hands.
  - Terry nails
    - Whitening of the proximal 80% of the nail, leaving a small rim of peripheral reddening.
    - Seen in
      - Older people
      - Heart failure
      - Cirrhosis
      - Non-insulin dependant diabetes.
  - Red half moons in nail beds (variety of Terry nails, also described by Terry)
    - Lunula that is red and also called the nails of cardiac failure
  - Azure half moons in nail beds
    - The nails of Wilson disease
    - The lunulae are light blue.
  - Muehrcke lines
    - Two arcuate white lines parallel to the lunula and separated by normal nail.
    - Because they are located in the nail bed (not the nailplate). Muehrcke's lines do not progress with the growth of the nail.
    - They are seen in patients with hypoalbuminemia (< 2 gm/100 ml), and disappear with its resolution.
  - Beau lines
    - Transverse grooves on the fingernails of patients recovering from a serious illness
  - Meese lines (aka Reynolds or Aldrich lines)
    - Transverse white lines distal to the cuticle.
    - Seen in
      - Arsenical or thallium poisoning
      - Cancer chemotherapy
      - Hodgkin lymphoma
      - Other systemic disorders (such as severe cardiac or renal disease).

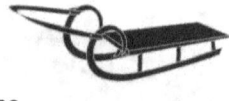

- Nail pitting
  - Early but non-specific sign of psoriasis
- Yellow nail syndrome
  - A yellowish colour of the nail plates due to abnormal lymphatic circulation.
- Brittle nails
  - Seen in various dysmetabolic states such as
    - Hyperthyroidism
    - Malnutrition
    - Iron or calcium deficiency
  - They are characterized by
    - Irregular, frayed, and torn nail borders
- Splinter hemorrhages
  - Linear red hemorrhages
  - Extending from the free margin of the nail bed toward the proximal margin.
  - Seen with
    - Subacute bacterial endocarditis
    - Trichinosis
    - Trauma
- Leukonychia-white nails, beginning at the lunula-may be normal; seen in cirrhosis, leprosy, arsenic poisoning, vasomotor disturbance of fingers

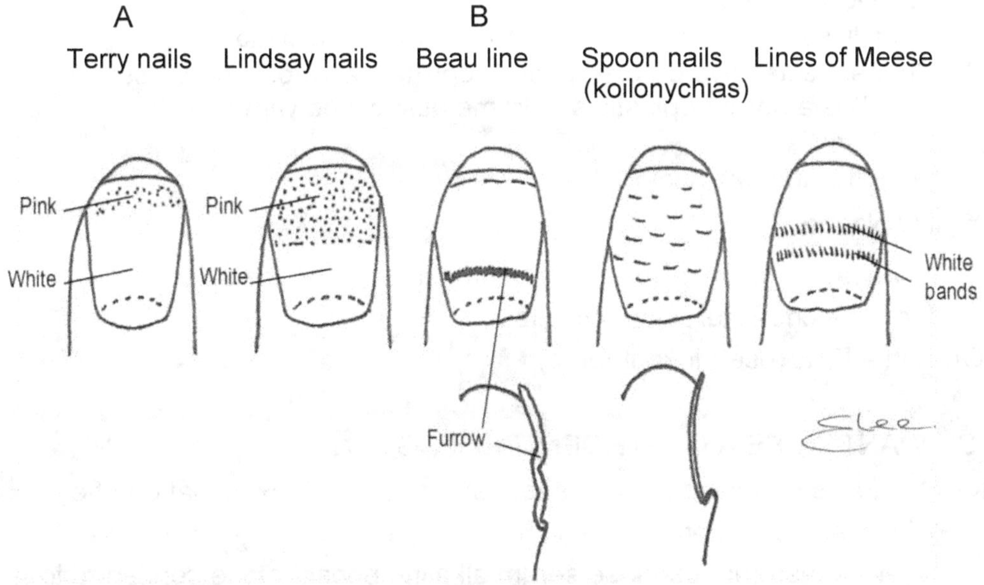

A                       B

Terry nails   Lindsay nails   Beau line   Spoon nails   Lines of Meese
                                   (koilonychias)

Adapted from: Mangione S. Physical Diagnosis Secrets. *Hanley & Belfus*, Philadelphia, 2000, page 412.

580

**SKIN**

- o Acanthosis nigrans
  - – Black velvety rash, typically in/on
    - ▪ Axillar
    - ▪ Nape of neck
    - ▪ Hands
  - – Associated with
    - ▪ Cancer (paraneoplastic syndrome)
      - – Stomach
      - – HCC
      - – Lung
    - ▪ Metabolic syndrome
- o Acrodermatitis enteropathica (zinc deficiency)
  - – Associations
    - ▪ Alcoholism
    - ▪ TPN (total parenteral nutrition)
    - ▪ Chronic diarrhea
      - – Crohn disease
      - – Celiac disease
  - – Caution: the patient suspected to having refractory celiac disease, and have red scaling, vesiculopustular plaque and legs, think of zinc deficiency, the correction of which may allow the gluten enteropathy to respond to a gluten-free diet.
- o Seborrheic keratosis
  - – Usually small areas, of no common morbid association
  - – Sudden, extensive outbreaks of Seborrheic keratosis (aka Leser-Trelat) is a paraneoplastic syndrome associated with cancer
    - ▪ Lung
    - ▪ GI (Stomach, Colon, Liver, Pancreas)
- o Yellow plaque
- • Give GI causes of yellow plagues, the GI mucosa, or on the skin.
  - o In mucosa – cholesterol embolization
  - o On skin – PXE (pseudoxanthoma)

---

**SO YOU WANT TO BE A GASTROENTEROLOGY!**
- • Give GI causes of angiod streaks seen on fundoscopic examination of eyes.
  - o PXE (pseudoxanthoma elasticum)
  - o Paget disease (but because serum alkaline phosphatase concentration is increased, your reflex might be to think of cholestatic liver disease)

---

581

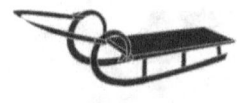

*MASTERING THE BOARDS*
*Hepatology & Pancreaticobiliary Disease*

A.B.R. Thomson

# ABBREVIATIONS

| | |
|---|---|
| ACTH | Adrenocorticotropic hormone |
| AIDS | Acquired immunodeficiency syndrome |
| ALP | Alkaline phosphatase |
| BMT | Bone marrow transplantation |
| CMV | Cytomegalovirus |
| CSS | Churg-Strauss syndrome |
| dDI | didanosine |
| EBV | Epstein-Barr virus |
| EGFR | Epidermal growth factor receptor |
| GH | Growth hormone |
| GI | Gastrointestinal |
| HSV | Herpes simplex virus |
| KS | Kaposis sarcoma |
| LES | Lower esophageal sphincter |
| LGV | Lymphogranuloma venereum |
| MAC | Mycobacterium avium complex |
| MCT | Medullary carcinoma of the thyroid |
| MCTD | Mixed connective tissue disease |
| MEN | Multiple endocrine neoplasia |
| NAAT | Nucleic acid amplification testing |
| PAN | Polyarteritis nodosa |
| PO | Orally |
| RPR | Rapid plasma regain test |
| SBP | Spontaneous bacterial peritonitis |
| SLE | Systemic lupus erythematous |
| SOS | Sinusoidal obstruction syndrome |
| STI | Sexually transmitted infection |
| TMP- SMX | Trimethoprim sulfamethoxazole |
| TPHA | Treponema pallidum hemagglutination assay |
| TPPA | Treponema pallidum particle agglutination |
| VEGF | Vascular endothelial growth factor |
| VIP | Vasoactive intestinal polypeptide |

582

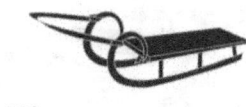

*MASTERING THE BOARDS*
*Hepatology & Pancreaticobiliary Disease*

A.B.R. Thomson

## REFERENCES

Available online at www.giandhepatology.com

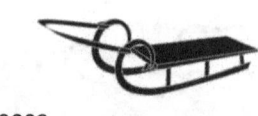

*MASTERING THE BOARDS*
*Hepatology & Pancreaticobiliary Disease*

A.B.R. Thomson

# INDEX

Note: Page number followed by f and t indicates figure and table respectively.

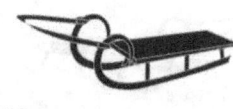

585

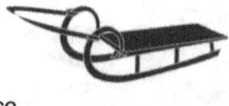

586

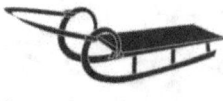

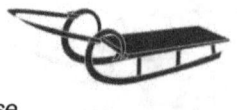

590

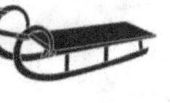

clinical, 214–216, 214t
Dress syndrome and, 221
histopathology, 217
methods and metabolism, 212
methotrexate and, 218t–219t
mushroom poisoning and, 220
oral contraceptive agents, 220
pathophysiology, 213–214

**E**

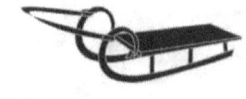

**F**

Familial mediterranean fever (FMF), 573–574
Familial pancreatitis, 462
Fatty liver disease
    biopsy in, 32t
    causes/associations, 28
    clinical, 29–30
    diagnostic imaging for, 31–32
    FFL, 33–37
    histopathology, 32–33, 32t
    laboratory findings for, 30–31
    NAFLD and, 29–30
    pathogenesis, 23–28
FFA. *See* Free fatty acids
FFL. *See* Focal fatty liver
Fibrolamellar hepatocellular cancer (FLHCC), 381
    *vs.* focal nodular hyperplasia, 362t
FibroSpect II, 38
FibroSure. *See* Fibro test
Fibro test, 38
Fitz☐Hugh☐Curtis (FHC) syndrome, 96, 179
"Flares" of acute hepatitis, 135t–136t, 136–138
FLHCC. *See* Fibrolamellar hepatocellular cancer
FMF. *See* Familial mediterranean fever
FNH. *See* Focal nodular hyperplasia
Focal fatty liver (FFL), 33–37, 363
    macrovesicular steatosis, causes of, 34
    Mallory bodies, 36–37
    microvesicular steatosis, causes of, 34
    NASH, biopsy lesions of, 35
Focal nodular hyperplasia (FNH)
    case self test studies, 408, 408f
    causes/associations, 360
    definition, 359
    demography, 359
    diagnostic imaging, 360–361
    *vs.* fibrolamellar hepatocellular cancer, 362t
    *vs.* hepatic adenoma, 361t
    histopathology, 359
    treatment, 362
Food/food additives, reactions to
    immunological, 562
    non-immunological, 562
    treatment, 563
Free fatty acids (FFA), 27

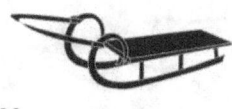

# G

Gallbladder
anatomical overview, 416
cancer, 453
Hartmann pouch and, 416
polyps, 92
tumours, 92
Gallstone pancreatitis, 486
Gamma glutamyl transpeptidase (GGT), 17, 17t
Gastric antral vascular ectasia (GAVE)
*vs.* portal hypertensive gastropathy, 258t
Gastrinoma, 531
GAVE. *See* Gastric antral vascular ectasia
GGT. *See* Gamma glutamyl transpeptidase
GI therapy, 568
GI tract, 23
Glucagonoma, 532
Ground-glass hepatocytes, 112
Gum hypertrophy, 575

# H

HA. *See* Hepatic adenoma
HAA. *See* Hepatic artery aneurysm
Halitosis, 575
Hartmann pouch, 416
HAV. *See* Hepatitis A virus
HBcAb-IgM, 107
HBeAg, 107
HBsAb, 107
HBsAg, 107
HBV. *See* Hepatitis B virus
HCC. *See* Hepatocellular cancer
HCV. *See* Hepatitis C virus
H63D heterozygote, 184
H63D homozygote, 184
HDV. *See* Hepatitis D virus
HE. *See* Hepatic encephalopathy
HELLP syndrome
clinical, 331
definition, 329
demography, 329
diagnosis, 332
histopathology, 333
laboratory abnormalities, 332–333
pathophysiology, 329–331

*MASTERING THE BOARDS*
*Hepatology & Pancreaticobiliary Disease*

A.B.R. Thomson

594

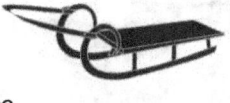

595

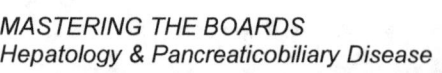

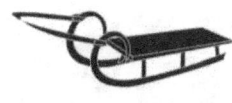

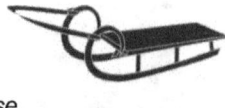

Barcelona Clinic Liver Cancer classification, 374, 374f
hypervascularity on ultrasound, 375
Okuda staging system, 373t

surveillance for, 376–377, 376t
treatment, 378–380, 379t, 380t
Hepatocytes
canalicular membrane of, 5
CMA and, 6
desmosomes and, 6
endoplasmic reticulum and, 5
nuclei of, 5
sinusoidal membrane of, 5
ubiquitin/proteasome pathway and, 6
"Hepatofugal" blood flow, 254–255
Hepatoportal sclerosis (HPS), 268
Hepatopulmonary syndrome (HPS)
clinical, 309–310
definition, 308
diagnostic imaging, 310
laboratory findings, 310
pathophysiology, 309
pulmonary function testing for, 310
treatment, 311
Hepatorenal syndrome (HRS)
definitions, 289
demography, 290
diagnosis, 292, 292t–293t
pathophysiology, 291–292
prevention, 294
treatment, 293–294
types, 290t
Hereditary hemochromatosis (HH)
with celiac disease, 194
diagnostic algorithm, 187f
diagnostic imaging for, 188
differential diagnosis, 189–192
genetics

C282Y/H63D compound heterozygote, 184
C282Y heterozygote, 184
C282Y homozygote, 183–184
H63D heterozygote, 184
H63D homozygote, 184
no HFE mutations, 184

histopathology, 188–189
indications for, 188
interventions for, 194t
laboratory findings in, 186

598

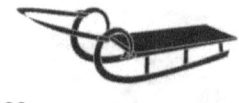

Immunoprophylaxis, for HBV infection, 113, 114t
INF. *See* Interferon
Inflammasomes, 24–25
Inherited metabolic disorders of liver, 182t, 211, 211t
INR. *See* International normalized ratio
Insulinoma, 531
Interferon (INF), 317t
     adverse effects of, 128
     contraindications, 129
     for HBV infection, 123, 128t
     for HCV infection, 160t, 161–162, 161t–165t, 166–167
     Lamivudine *vs.,* 130t
Intermediate filaments, 8
International normalized ratio (INR), 18
Intraductal papillary mucinous neoplasms (IPMN)
     clinical, 518
     definition, 517
     demography, 517
     diagnostic imaging, 518–519
     genetics, 517
     histopathology, 519
     laboratory, 518
     nasogastric drains *vs.* pancreatic stents, 520t
     Sendai Guidelines for resection, 520
     treatment, 519–520
     types, 518
Intrahepatic cholestasis of pregnancy (ICP), 327t–328t
     clinical, 323–324
     demography, 322
     histopathology, 324
     laboratory, 324
     pathophysiology, 322
     prognosis, 324t
     risk factors, 323
     treatment, 325–326, 325t
IPH. *See* Idiopathic portal hypertension
IPMN. *See* Intraductal papillary mucinous neoplasms
Ischemic hepatitis, 238–239
Ito cells. *See* Hepatic stellate cells (HSC)


**J**
Jaundice
     causes/associations, 339
     differential diagnosis, 340
     with lymphoma, 344
     in neonate, 340

600

pathophysiology, 338

# K
Kala-azar, 178

Kasabach☐Merritt syndrome, 356

King's College Criteria (KCC) risk stratification criteria for liver
transplantation, 250

Kupffer cells, 6, 214

# L
Lamivudine, 129t, 130, 130t

Lamuvidine, 317t

Laparoscopic cholecystectomy, 444

Laxative abuse, 549–550

Leptospirosis, 177

Lipolysis/lipogenesis, balance of, 27

Liver

biopsy, 36

disease (*See also specific disease*)

ALD, 42–52

Child-Pugh (CP) classification of, 21t, 22t

fatty, 23–41

MELD score and, 22

monogenic causes of, 28

peri-operative mortality rates, 22

pre- and post-operative care, 19–20

on predicting post-operative mortality, 20–21

in pregnancy, 321, 321t

PSC, 85–94

pulmonary complications of, 307–315

echinococcal ("hydratid") cyst, 180–181

enzymes tests, 12

function tests, 12

inherited metabolic disorders of, 182t

pathogenesis, 24

pregnancy and, 316–337

pseudotumour of, 178

pyogenic abscess, 178

vascular diseases of, 225–240

Liver transplantation (LT), 52

assessment

of liver donors, 390

UNOS listing criteria, 388–389

clinical, 385

601

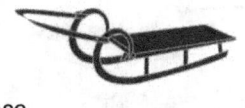

603

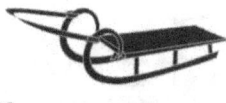

*MASTERING THE BOARDS*
*Hepatology & Pancreaticobiliary Disease*

A.B.R. Thomson

in Wilson disease, 196
Non-alcoholic steatohepatitis (NASH), 23, 29
    biopsy criteria for diagnosis of, 33
    biopsy lesions of

                                            grades, 35
                                          stages, 35

    case self test studies, 400, 400f
    to NAFLD, 29–30
    treatment, 39–41, 41t
Non-cirrhotic portal hypertension, 208
Non-skin solid organ tumours, 396
Non-viral infectious causes of hepatitis, 96
NRH. *See* Nodular regenerative hyperplasia
Nucleosides, for HBV infection, 123, 129t, 130–131
Nucleotides, for HBV infection, 123, 129t, 130–131


**O**
Obesity
    on acute pancreatitis, 482
    adverse effects, 558–560
    complications of, 555–556, 556f
    definition, 554, 554t
    demography, 554
    diagnosis, 555t
    GI/liver complications of, 555
    metabolic syndrome, criteria for, 555t
    pharmacology, 558
    treatment, 557–558
Obstructive chronic pancreatitis, 498
OCA. *See* Oral contraceptive agents
Octreotide, 317t, 318
OHS. *See* Ovarian hyperstimulation syndrome
Okuda staging system of HCC, 373t
OP. *See* Osteoporosis
Oral contraceptive agents (OCA), 220
Orthodeoxia, 310
Osler☐Weber☐Rendu disease (OWRD), 268–269
Osteomalacia, 95
Osteoporosis (OP), 95
Ovarian hyperstimulation syndrome (OHS), 273
OWRD. *See* Osler☐Weber☐Rendu disease


**P**
Paget disease, 581

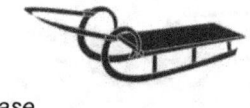

605

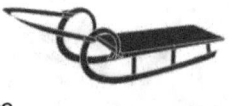

606

609

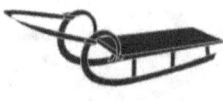

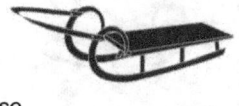

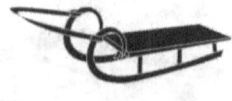

*MASTERING THE BOARDS*
*Hepatology & Pancreaticobiliary Disease*

A.B.R. Thomson

## V

Vaccination
- for HAV infection, 98
- for HBV infection, 98, 111–114
- for HCV infection, 98

Vascular diseases of liver, 225–240
- Budd□Chiari syndrome, 226–230
- hepatic artery aneurysm, 239–240
- hepatic artery thrombosis/stenosis, 236, 236t–237t
- ischemic hepatitis, 238–239
- portal colopathy, 225
- portal vein stenosis, 236
- portal vein thrombosis, 234–235
- sinusoidal obstruction syndrome, 230–231
- splenic vein thrombosis, 237–238

Veno-occlusive Disease. *See* Sinusoidal obstruction syndrome (SOS)

VHLD. *See* Von Hippel□Lindau disease

VIPoma, 532–534
- clinical, 533
- definition, 532
- laboratory, 533
- pathology, 534
- pathophysiology, 533
- treatment, 534

Viral hepatitis, 46t
- comparison of, 97t
- HAV, 97, 98, 99–100
- HBV, 97, 98, 101–139
- HCV, 97, 98, 140–172
- of liver, 97–99
- mortality during pregnancy, 98
- *vs.* symptomatic gallstones, 320t
- treatment, 99

Virologic breakthrough, HBV, 133

Vitamin A deficiency, 561

Vitamin E deficiency, 561

Von Hippel□Lindau disease (vHLD), 225

## W

Wall-echo shadow sign, 435

Walled-off pancreatic necrosis (WOPN), 485

Weil syndrome. *See* Leptospirosis

Whipple procedure, 528, 528f

Wilson disease (WD)
- ceruloplasmin levels in, 201

clinical features, 197–199
definition, 195, 195f
histopathology, 199
iron deficiency in, 201
laboratory features, 200
liver copper, measurement of, 201
NAFLD in, 196
pathophysiology, 196–197
in pregnancy, 337
scoring system, 203t
screening, 205
tests for diagnosis, 200–204, 200t–201t, 202f, 203t
treatment, 204–205

ammonium tetrathiomolybdate, 205
chelating therapy, 205
D-penicillamine, 204–205
Trientine, 205

Window period, HBV infection, 109
WOPN. *See* Walled-off pancreatic necrosis

## Y
Yellow plaque, 581

## Z
Zinc deficiency. *See* Acrodermatitis enteropathica

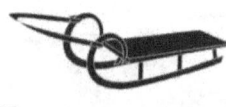

www.ingramcontent.com/pod-product-compliance
Lightning Source LLC
Chambersburg PA
CBHW081713220526
45468CB00008B/1824

* 9 7 8 1 9 8 1 9 4 3 5 0 0 *